Atypical Antipsychotics

Medical Psychiatry

ADDITIONAL VOLUMES IN PREPARATION

Atypical Antipsychotics
From Bench to Bedside

edited by
John G. Csernansky
Washington University School of Medicine
St. Louis, Missouri, U.S.A.

John Lauriello
University of New Mexico
Albuquerque, New Mexico, U.S.A.

MARCEL DEKKER, INC.   NEW YORK · BASEL

Library of Congress Cataloging-in-Publication Data
A catalog record for this book is available from the Library of Congress.

ISBN: 0-8247-5412-3

This book is printed on acid-free paper.

Headquarters
Marcel Dekker, Inc., 270 Madison Avenue, New York, NY 10016, U.S.A.
tel: 212-696-9000; fax: 212-685-4540

Distribution and Customer Service
Marcel Dekker, Inc., Cimarron Road, Monticello, New York 12701, U.S.A.
tel: 800-228-1160; fax: 845-796-1772

Eastern Hemisphere Distribution
Marcel Dekker AG, Hutgasse 4, Postfach 812, CH-4001 Basel, Switzerland
tel: 41-61-260-6300; fax: 41-61-260-6333

World Wide Web
http://www.dekker.com

The publisher offers discounts on this book when ordered in bulk quantities. For more information, write to Special Sales/Professional Marketing at the headquarters address above.

Preface

The past decade has seen a tremendous advance in the treatment of psychotic disorders; one could almost say a second golden age of antipsychotic discovery. As chlorpromazine (Thorazine®) ushered in an era of unprecedented antipsychotic medications and their successful, but not curative, impact on psychiatric practice, so too clozapine (Clozaril®) launched an aggressive introduction of a growing number of "atypical antipsychotics."

The term atypical antipsychotic implies different things to different people. For some, atypical connotes that these compounds are not the typical ones used. This was certainly true a decade ago, but not now. There are currently more prescriptions for these newer medications than for drugs developed prior to clozapine's approval in the United States.

Atypicality also may denote a potentially different clinical outcome. For nearly 30 years, pharmaceutical development focused on producing drugs with more specific dopamine-receptor blockade so that the dose needed for effect became smaller and smaller. This line of development was based on an animal and human model of induced parkinsonism. If a rat became stiff or cataleptic, then the compound was seen as a promising antipsychotic. Unfortunately, none of these antipsychotics could reliably produce an antipsychotic effect without extrapyramidal side effects (EPS). Clozapine was the first approved antipsychotic that showed antipsychotic effect at doses below those that cause EPS. In fact, clozapine has little or no EPS. The development of other atypical antipsychotics continues to follow the same rule as clozapine: effect without stiffness. One extremely important outcome of reduced EPS would be a reduction in the incidence of the potentially irreversible, hyperkinetic movement disorder tardive dyskinesia.

On a receptor level, all the atypicals share a relatively complicated multi-receptor-blockade picture, in sharp contrast to typical antipsychotics such as haloperidol (Haldol®) that are mainly D2-receptor blockers.

However, the older typical drugs also share some of these qualities and therefore do not conclusively distinguish the two groups.

Finally, atypicals are reported to have broader effects, aside from treating psychosis, than typical antipsychotics. This has been an area of great research and parallels the wider use of antidepressants beyond the treatment of depression. However, one should be aware that typical antipsychotics have been also used for nonpsychotic patients, although with some trepidation due to the fears of irreversible tardive dyskinesia.

In this book the authors present up-to-date, cutting-edge information on the basic and clinical science of the atypical antipsychotics. The book is geared toward the nonresearcher but assumes that the reader desires the background basic science as well as the clinical science and practice. The book is divided in two parts, which can be read independently. The first part enlists psychiatric researchers to explain the basic science of antipsychotic treatment. The second utilizes the expertise of clinical researchers on the various applications of atypical antipsychotics in a variety of populations. The two sections are complementary; for example, the basic science of brain imaging, especially positron emission tomography, is covered in the first part while the clinical use of brain imaging is covered in the second.

The first part, on the basic science, includes chapters on the underlying pathophysiology of schizophrenia and the mechanism of atypical antipsychotics and effects of atypical antipsychotics on gene expression. The section also covers the neurophysiogical effects of these medications, animal models that explain the action of atypicals, and, finally, the use of neuroimaging in humans to elucidate the mechanism of action of atypicals. The chapters in the clinical science section include a brief descriptive survey of psychotic disorders as well as discussions on the acute and long-term efficacy of atypical antipsychotics and the effects of atypicals on the CNS as measured by neuroimaging modalities. Finally, chapters on the use of atypicals in children, affective disorders, and a review of new approaches to drug development are presented.

This is an exciting time to be treating severe mental illness, and the advent of the atypical antipsychotics is truly a watershed event. We hope this book can share both the ideas and the excitement of these potential developments.

John Csernansky
John Lauriello

Contents

Contributors

Mark E. Bardgett, Ph.D. Department of Psychology, Northern Kentucky University, Highland Heights, Kentucky, U.S.A.

Peter F. Buckley, M.D. Professor and Chair, Department of Psychiatry and Health Behavior, Medical College of Georgia, Augusta, Georgia, U.S.A.

Juan R. Bustillo, M.D. Department of Psychiatry, University of New Mexico, Albuquerque, New Mexico, U.S.A.

Pierre Chue, FRCPC Associate Clinical Professor, Department of Psychiatry, University of Alberta, Edmonton, Alberta, Canada

Robert R. Conley, M.D. Professor and Chief, Inpatient Research Program, Maryland Psychiatric Research Center, University of Maryland, Baltimore, Maryland, U.S.A.

John G. Csernansky, M.D. Gregory B. Couch Professor of Psychiatry, Washington University School of Medicine, St. Louis, Missouri, U.S.A.

Jennifer Dallas Department of Psychiatry and Health Behavior, Medical College of Georgia, Augusta, Georgia, U.S.A.

Scott Filippino Washington University School of Medicine, St. Louis, Missouri, U.S.A.

Oliver Freudenreich, M.D. Director, MGH First-Episode and Early Psychosis Program, Department of Psychiatry, Massachusetts General Hospital and Harvard Medical School, Boston, Massachusetts, U.S.A.

Donald C. Goff, M.D. Director, MGH Schizophrenia Program, Department of Psychiatry, Massachusetts General Hospital and Harvard Medical School, Boston, Massachusetts, U.S.A.

Deanna L. Kelly, Pharm.D., BCPP Assistant Professor, Maryland Psychiatric Research Center, University of Maryland, Baltimore, Maryland, U.S.A.

John Lauriello Associate Professor and Vice Chairman, Department of Psychiatry; Executive Medical Director of the UNM Psychiatric Center; Psychiatry Chief, Clinical Operations; and Director of the Schizophrenia Research Group, University of New Mexico, Albuquerque, New Mexico, U.S.A.

Rhoshel Lenroot Fellow, Child and Adolescent Psychiatry, Department of Psychiatry, University of New Mexico, Albuquerque, New Mexico, U.S.A.

Donna L. Londino, M.D. Assistant Professor, Department of Psychiatry and Health Behavior, Medical College of Georgia, Augusta, Georgia, U.S.A.

Stephen R. Marder, M.D. Professor and Vice Chair, Department of Psychiatry and Biobehavioral Sciences, David Geffen School of Medicine at UCLA, and Chair, Department of Psychiatry, and Director, Mental Illness Research, Educational, & Clinical Center (MIRECC), VA Greater Los Angeles Healthcare System, Los Angeles, California, U.S.A.

Patricio O'Donnell, M.D., Ph.D. Professor, Center for Neuropharmacology & Neuroscience, Albany Medical College, Albany, New York, U.S.A.

Joseph M. Pierre, M.D. Assistant Clinical Professor, Department of Psychiatry and Biobehavioral Sciences, David Geffen School of Medicine at UCLA, and VA Greater Los Angeles Healthcare System, Los Angeles, California, U.S.A.

Bryan L. Roth, M.D., Ph.D. Professor, Departments of Biochemistry, Psychiatry, and Neurosciences and National Institute of Mental Health Psychoactive Drug Screening Program, Case Western Reserve University Medical School, Cleveland, Ohio, U.S.A.

Laura M. Rowland, Ph.D. Department of Psychiatry, University of New Mexico, Albuquerque, New Mexico, U.S.A.

Martha Sajatovic, M.D. Associate Professor, Department of Psychiatry, Case Western Reserve University School of Medicine, Cleveland, Ohio, U.S.A.

Melvin Shelton, M.D., Ph.D. Assistant Professor, Department of Psychiatry, Case Western Reserve University School of Medicine, Cleveland, Ohio, U.S.A.

Edna Stirewalt Department of Psychiatry and Health Behavior, Medical College of Georgia, Augusta, Georgia, U.S.A.

Lisa Wiggins, M.S. Department of Psychiatry and Health Behavior, Medical College of Georgia, Augusta, Georgia, U.S.A.

1

Atypical Antipsychotic Drugs: Theories of Mechanism of Action

Scott Filippino and John G. Csernansky

*Washington University School of Medicine,
St. Louis, Missouri, U.S.A.*

I. INTRODUCTION

The advent of antipsychotic drugs occurred via a process that is both colorful and serendipitous. Ironically, war was the force that initially propelled the development of this group of drugs that has helped bring peace to so many patients with schizophrenia. The phenothiazines and their derivatives, including methylene blue, were well known to 19th-century industrial chemists, but largely as dyes. Then, when methylene blue was discovered to possess antimalarial properties, numerous additional derivatives of methylene blue were synthesized by the Germans in World War I and by the Allies in World War II for this purpose. At the time, quinine, a derivative of a tropical tree bark, was the only treatment for malaria, and access to the trees that produced quinine was very tenuous. Thus, the development of a synthetic antimalarial became strategically essential for modern armies who conducted global campaigns.

While the Germans succeeded in synthesizing quinacrine, the Allies chanced upon the aminoalkyl phenothiazines. Although such compounds lacked antimalarial properties, painstaking work by French researchers demonstrated that these drugs had antihistamine properties superior to other compounds available at the time. The development of this new class of antihistamines led to the synthesis of promethazine.

Soon after World War II, Henri Laborit, a surgeon of the French navy, began experimenting with novel forms of anesthesia that blended narcotics, sedatives, and hypnotics (1). He noted that promethazine was useful in combination with anesthetic agents for reducing perioperative stress, and suggested the development of a new antihistamine that would be more sedating than promethazine. The compound developed by the Rhône-Poulenc Laboratories in 1951 to satisfy this need was chlorpromazine. Laborit and his colleagues then observed that while chlorpromazine produced the desired sedation, it also produced a type of disinterest in their surgical patients that they felt might be useful in psychiatric patients with agitation.

By 1952, several French psychiatrists, including Delay, Deniker, Harl, Hamon, Paraire, and Velluz, had begun to test chlorpromazine in patients with schizophrenia and other psychotic disorders, and while there remains some debate about who should be given credit for the first use of this drug, there is certainly no debate about its profound effects on the treatment of psychiatric patients.

Under the trade name Largactil (and later Thorazine), chlorpromazine was soon made available to psychiatrists throughout the world, and a number of studies confirmed its value in treating schizophrenia. Perhaps the most important of these studies was that of the U.S. Veterans Administration Collaborative Study Group, led by Leo Hollister. This study not only definitively demonstrated chlorpromazine's efficacy using a controlled clinical trial design, but did so at a time in American history when most clinicians were focused on psychoanalysis and resistant to the idea that schizophrenia had a biological basis and could be chemically treatable.

Soon after the availability of antipsychotic drugs became widespread, clues to their mechanism of action began to appear. In a paper in 1963 (2), Arvid Carlsson and Margit Lindqvist noted that haloperidol and chlorpromazine "exerted a characteristic effect on the metabolism of brain catecholamines" and suggested that the most likely mechanism of doing so was to "block monoaminergic receptors in the brain." It took only a few more years to isolate the particular monoamine affected by antipsychotics. In 1964, Anden, Roos, and Werdnius noted elevated metabolites of dopamine in rabbit striatum after chlorpromazine or haloperidol (3), and in 1970 Anden and colleagues examined the ability of numerous antipsychotics to block monoamine receptors in rats (4), and concluded that "the most potent and specific neuroleptics seemed to influence mainly the brain [dopamine] receptors." Later, several subtypes of dopamine receptors were discovered, and the relationship between antipsychotic activity and dopamine receptor blockade became narrowed to the D_2 subtype.

Perhaps ironically, the first atypical antipsychotic drug, clozapine, was synthesized by Wander Pharmaceuticals in 1959; yet, it would take almost three decades before this drug would trigger a second pharmacological revolution in psychiatry. In another irony of antipsychotic drug development, the potential of clozapine as an antipsychotic drug was initially overlooked because its pharmacologic profile suggested it would not produce effects on the brain's motor pathways. Thus, in the context of beliefs that antipsychotic efficacy and extrapyramidal effects were always linked, clozapine was considered to be "defective" (5). Nonetheless, despite this label, psychiatrists in Germany, Switzerland, and Austria worked with clozapine throughout the 1960s and were impressed with its success in the treatment of patients with schizophrenia, especially those that had been resistant to other drugs (6). After several patients in Finland developed lethal agranulocytosis (7), clozapine was withdrawn from further use. Fortunately, clozapine's superiority in treating otherwise resistant patients was not forgotten, and in 1988, the results of a double blind study were reported comparing clozapine with chlorpromazine in treatment resistant patients (8). The results of this study gave the first indisputable evidence of clozapine's superiority over the typical antipsychotic, chlorpromazine, and rapidly led to clozapine's introduction into clinical use in the United States under FDA guidelines designed to reduce the risk of undetected agranulocytosis.

II. MECHANISMS OF ACTION: WHAT MAKES A DRUG ATYPICAL?

Soon after clozapine's introduction as an antipsychotic in the United States, it soon became the pharmacological prototype for a new generation of antipsychotic drugs. The fact that clozapine was effective as an anti-psychotic drug but only rarely produced acute adverse effects on the motor system that had been previously linked to the blockade of dopamine D_2 receptors suggested that there might be new pharmacological avenues to achieving an effective antipsychotic drug. Moreover, clozapine was found not to elevate plasma levels of prolactin (i.e., a neurohormone whose release is under dopaminergic control), which further challenged the notion that efficacy and side-effects of antipsychotic drugs were inseparably linked by the common mechanism of dopamine D_2 receptor blockade. Thus, the search began for other drugs that might be able to capture the "atypical" properties of clozapine without its limiting propensity to cause agranulocytosis.

Receptor binding studies revealed that clozapine bound to a number of neurotransmitter receptors other than the dopamine D_2 receptor, often with greater affinity than its affinity at the dopamine D_2 receptor. Because of these many other actions of clozapine, a variety of competing theories were brought forward to explain clozapine's atypical profile. In the past decade, one has clearly emerged as dominant – that is, the hypothesis that clozapine's atypical profile is due to its combined antagonist actions at serotonin 5-HT_{2A} and dopamine D_2 receptors (i.e., the 5-HT_{2A}/D_2 hypothesis). As reviewed below, the 5-HT_{2A}/D_2 hypothesis may be credited with inspiring the development of several new atypical drugs. However, other theories have also been brought forward, and two of these (i.e., the fast dissociation hypothesis and the partial D_2 agonist hypothesis) have also been linked to the specific atypical antipsychotic drugs. All three of these popular theories will be reviewed in detail below.

III.   THE 5-HT_{2A}/D_2 HYPOTHESIS

The 5-HT_{2A}/D_2 hypothesis has influenced the development of several of the atypical antipsychotic drugs in use today, including risperidone, olanzapine, and ziprasidone, as well as other agents (e.g., iloperidone) under consideration (9). The origin of this theory lies, in part, in the observation that clozapine is a potent antagonist of 5-HT_{2A} receptors and that blockade of these receptors mitigates antipsychotic drug-induced movement disorders (i.e., catalepsy) in rodents. In an early experiment by Sulpizio and colleagues, clozapine, but not typical antipsychotic drugs, antagonized the effects of fenfluramine, which promotes the release of serotonin from presynaptic stores, on temperature regulation in rodents (10). On the basis of this result, the investigators conjectured that clozapine may "[preserve] a dopamine-serotonin balance" and suggested that clozapine's anti-serotonergic properties deserved further scrutiny. Later experiments then more directly demonstrated the binding of clozapine to serotonin receptors and suggested a similar explanation for the relationship between the blockade of 5HT receptors and clozapine's atypical profile (11).

In regard to these findings and their interpretation, it is important to remember that a relationship between serotonin and the motor pathways of the brain had been established some time before the appreciation of clozapine's atypical profile. In 1975, Costall and associates explored the role of the serotonergic pathways in the production of antipsychotic drug-induced motor abnormalities (12), and showed that lesions of the dorsal or medial raphé nuclei (from which serotonergic neurons arise) in mice reduced haloperidol-induced catalepsy. Similarly, it was also demonstrated that direct injections of serotonin into the nucleus accumbens of rats decreased hyperactivity induced by dopamine injection, and conversely that the ability of typical antipsychotic drugs to reduce dopamine-induced hyperactivity in rats was antagonized by methysergide and cyproheptadine (13). Perhaps, then it should not be surprising that patients with schizophrenia who receive $5\text{-}HT_2$ antagonists demonstrated improvement in antipsychotic drug-induced extrapyramidal side-effects (14,15).

Surprisingly, however, the connection between clozapine's effect on serotonin receptors and the effects of serotonin on the motor pathways of the brain did not draw substantial attention throughout the early 1980s. Rather, clozapine's mechanism of action and its atypical profile were at first hypothesized to occur through its action at special populations of dopamine receptors (16); that is, it blocked mesolimbic dopamine receptors but not mesostriatal neurons where it would produce the extrapyramidal side-effects so typical of other antipsychotic drugs (17). Finally, in 1989, Meltzer brought the action of clozapine on serotonin systems into the foreground, and proposed that clozapine's atypical profile, including its benefits for negative symptoms, were related to its combined blockade of dopamine and serotonin ($5HT_{2A}$) receptors (with a relative preference for serotonin receptors) (18,19). In a seminal article of the $5\text{-}HT_{2A}/D_2$ hypothesis of clozapine's action, Meltzer compared the relative affinity of many atypical and typical antipsychotic drugs on the D_2 and $5HT_{2A}$ receptors to provide convincing support for this hypothesis (20).

In the same year, Meltzer and colleagues also published a metanalysis of receptor binding data to compare the affinities for D_1, D_2, and $5\text{-}HT_{2A}$ receptors in 20 antipsychotic drugs, in conjunction with clinical knowledge of their typicality or atypicality, to generate a discriminant function capable of predicting the properties of an unknown drug (21). Upon testing the discriminant function on the original 20 reference compounds as well as 17 additional drugs, the function correctly predicted the properties of a given drug for 33 of the 37 drugs. Further, the stepwise discriminant function analysis, determined that the pK_i values for D_1 did not significantly contribute to the classification of an antipsychotic drug as typical or atypical. Rather, the atypical and typical antipsychotic drugs were best differentiated by the ratio of their affinities for the $5\text{-}HT_{2A}$ and D_2 receptors alone. Atypical antipsychotic drugs had consistently higher $5\text{-}HT_{2A}/D_2$ ratios than typical drugs.

Given the empirical relationship between drugs with atypical profiles and serotonin receptor blockade, we should now consider the mechanisms that might underlie it. Reviewing the neuroanatomy of the midbrain and basal ganglia (22), it is known that serotonergic fibers from the dorsal raphé project to the cell bodies of dopamine neurons in the substantia nigra, and decrease the firing rate of these dopamine neurons via activation of $5\text{-}HT_2$ receptors (23,24). Similarly, serotonergic fibers from the dorsal raphé also project to the cortex and the striatum (22), where they exert a negative regulatory role on dopamine release. Thus, by blocking 5-HT$_2$ receptors, atypical antipsychotics may decrease the influence of serotonergic neurons that inhibit dopamine activity. Disinhibition of dopamine neurons would then increase the amount of dopamine released into the synaptic cleft, and since the occupancy of dopamine receptors by antipsychotic drugs can be influenced by the concentration of endogenous dopamine, antipsychotic drug-induced dopamine receptor blockade and the extrapyramidal side-effects produced by such a blockade would be mitigated. In addition, some atypical antipsychotic drugs also act as agonists at 5-HT$_{1A}$ autoreceptors located on the 5-HT$_2$ neurons, thereby providing a secondary mechanism by which such drugs could block serotonergic activity in the brain.

It has also been hypothesized that hypodopaminergia in the prefrontal cortex may be the underlying cause of the negative symptoms of schizophrenia (25,26). As noted above, serotonergic neurons synapse on and down-regulate activity of dopaminergic neurons in the prefrontal cortex, and therefore, antagonism of cortical 5-HT$_2$ receptors on dopamine neurons that exert this inhibitory effect would be expected to increase dopamine in the prefrontal cortex and so alleviate the negative symptoms of schizophrenia. This hypothesis is also interesting in that it suggests a basis for the often observed similarity between the negative symptoms of schizophrenia and the extrapyramidal side-effects of antipsychotic drugs.

Given the generally wide acceptance of the 5-HT$_{2A}$/D$_2$ hypothesis, it is notable that the receptor bindings profiles for several of the atypical antipsychotics developed since the reintroduction of clozapine into practice appear to be consistent with it. As previously mentioned, many of the atypical antipsychotic drugs now marketed in the United States were selected for development, at least in part, because of their strong blockade of 5-HT$_{2A}$ receptors relative to D$_2$ receptors. In a recent study comparing the receptor binding profile for risperidone, ziprasidone, olanzapine, and sertindole using cloned human receptors, all of these drugs were found to have substantially higher affinities for 5-HT$_{2A}$ receptors than for D$_2$ receptors – in many cases, the observed difference in affinities was an order of magnitude or more (27). In a different study, a similar binding profile has also been demonstrated in quetiapine (28). Finally, even the newest of the atypical antipsychotic drugs, aripiprazole, has substantial affinity for the 5-HT$_{2A}$ receptor where it also acts as an antagonist, even though much has been attributed to its actions as a partial agonist at D$_2$ receptors (see below).

However, one cannot explain the efficacy of all apparently atypical antipsychotic drugs according to their blockade of 5HT$_{2A}$ receptors. Remoxipride, an effective atypical antipsychotic drug whose use is now limited due to high incidence of aplastic anemia (29), does not block 5-HT$_{2A}$

receptors (30) and its 5-HT$_{2A}$/D$_2$ pK_i ratio may even be smaller than that of haloperidol. Likewise, amisulpride – an atypical drug available outside of North America – has no binding at all to 5-HT$_{2A}$ receptors (31).

IV. THE "FAST DISSOCIATION" HYPOTHESIS

In the late 1900s, another hypothesis to explain the atypical profile of clozapine and at least some of the atypical drugs emerged that focuses on how antipsychotic drugs bind to and then detach from the D$_2$ receptor – that is, the fast dissociation rate hypothesis. To review the pharmacology of drug–receptor interactions briefly, it is important to note that the equilibrium binding constants (i.e., K$_d$ and K$_i$) frequently discussed in reference to the affinity of a drug for a particular receptor actually represent the ratio of the drug's dissociation rate constant (k_d) to its association rate constant (k_a). In other words, drugs with a high affinity for a neurotransmitter receptor (i.e., a low K$_d$) have a relatively slow dissociation rate constant (i.e., a smaller number in the numerator) and a relatively fast association rate constant (i.e., a larger number in the denominator). Conversely, drugs with relatively weak affinity for a given receptor (i.e., a higher K$_d$) may have either a relatively fast dissociation rate constant or a relatively slow association rate constant. Specifically, proponents of the fast dissociation rate hypothesis assert that atypical antipsychotic drugs in general have a fast dissociation rate from D$_2$ receptors as compared to typical antipsychotic drugs. This key feature, especially coupled with relatively low occupancy of D$_2$ receptors at clinical doses, may thus explain the capacity of endogenous dopamine to mitigate blockade of the D$_2$ receptor and so reduce the propensity of such drugs to cause extrapyramidal side-effects (32).

Ironically, some support for this hypothesis can also be gleaned from the results of Meltzer's analysis of atypical and typical antipsychotic drugs. As reviewed above, Meltzer and colleagues differentiated typical and atypical antipsychotic drugs on the basis of the ratio between their affinity for 5-HT$_{2A}$ and D$_2$ receptors using a discriminant function (21). However, they also noted that the affinities of these drugs for the D$_2$ receptor were much more discriminating than their affinities for the 5-HT$_{2A}$ receptor. This finding raises the possibility that atypical antipsychotic drugs might be discriminated only by having a relatively low affinity for the dopamine D$_2$ receptor, perhaps because of a fast dissociation rate constant.

This hypothesis has also gleaned support from earlier studies (33–35), the results of which suggest that there were different thresholds of D$_2$ receptor occupancy for antipsychotic efficacy and for inducing extrapyramidal side-effects. Specifically, Kapur and colleagues systemically assessed the clinical consequences of varying degrees of D_2 receptor occupancy (28–87%) by haloperidol (33), and determined that the antipsychotic effects of this drug coincide with 65% occupancy and that extrapyramidal side-effects coincides with receptor occupancies above 78%. In other experiments, the 65% threshold for antipsychotic efficacy has also been found to apply to other atypical antipsychotic drugs, such as olanzapine (36) and risperidone (37). In the case of ziprasidone, similar studies suggest that clinically effective doses achieve 77% occupancy of the D_2 receptor (38). Even in drugs such as clozapine and quetiapine, where D_2 occupancy at steady state tends to be lower than the proposed threshold, the proponents of this hypothesis point out that these two drugs do produce the required degree of D_2 occupancies for at least several hours after dosing (39–41). Thus, an atypical antipsychotic drug must achieve the required degree of dopamine D_2 receptor occupancy, but avoid a level of occupancy above this that would trigger extrapyramidal side-effects.

Unlike the $5\text{-}HT_{2A}/D_2$ hypothesis, the fast dissociation hypothesis can gain support from the existence of atypical antipsychotic drugs that have little or no affinity for 5-HT receptors, such as remoxipride and amisulpiride. This hypothesis is also consistent with observations that when $5\text{-}HT_{2A}/D_2$ antagonists are administered in excessive doses, the critical threshold of D_2 occupancy can be exceeded and extrapyramidal side-effects will occur, regardless of the drug's action at $5\text{-}HT_2$ receptors (33). Also of interest in regard to this hypothesis is a recent study of an isomer of clozapine with identical affinity for the $5\text{-}HT_2$, D_1, and D_4 receptors, but a tenfold greater affinity for the $5\text{-}HT_{2A}/D_2$ receptor, which appears to lack atypical properties in animal models (42). Finally, this hypothesis suggests caution in comparing the effects of typical and atypical antipsychotic drugs, especially when the typical drug is administered at a dose that is likely to produce D_2 receptor occupancy in excess of the critical threshold (43).

But how would a fast dissociation rate favor the capacity of a drug to achieve the required critical threshold of dopamine D_2 receptor blockade? Kapur, Seeman, and colleagues have outlined a series of arguments in regard to this question (44,45). For example, they assert that having a fast dissociation rate would allow the drug that is interacting with the receptor complex to respond more quickly to rapid changes in the availability of the endogenous transmitter, dopamine. All antipsychotic drugs must compete with endogenous dopamine for occupation of the D_2 receptors, and in regard to this competition, it is notable that the affinity of many typical antipsychotics (e.g., haloperidol, fluphenazine) is high compared to dopamine, while the affinity of many atypicals (e.g., clozapine, quetiapine, ziprasidone) is more similar to dopamine (46). So, in the event of a burst of dopamine into the synaptic space that might be required for normal neuronal function, the endogenous dopamine would be able to displace some of the atypical drug but not the typical drug. In this way, atypical drugs can "attenuate dopamine transmission with lesser distortion of phasic physiologic signaling" (46). However, with regard to the argument that atypical drugs must have an affinity for the dopamine D_2 that is relatively similar to dopamine, it is important to point out that some atypical drugs (e.g., risperidone, aripiprazole) have an affinity for the D_2 receptor that is far greater than dopamine and on par with haloperidol. Thus, not all atypical antipsychotic drugs fit the model proposed by the fast dissociation hypothesis.

V. THE PARTIAL AGONIST HYPOTHESIS

The partial agonist hypothesis is perhaps the newest of the hypotheses put forward to explain the properties of atypical antipsychotic drugs, insofar as there is only one successful drug to which one can point to support it – that is aripiprazole. The partial agonist hypothesis shares one of the basic concepts of the fast dissociation hypothesis in that both hypotheses assert that a drug may become atypical because of the way in which it interacts with the dopamine D_2 receptor. In addition, both the partial agonist hypothesis and fast dissociation hypothesis suggest that there are advantages to drugs that allow the dopamine receptor complex to retain a certain ambient level of activity.

Before discussing the history of the partial agonist hypothesis, it is useful to review the basic pharmacology of a partial agonist drug. Partial agonists can bind to their target receptors with affinities that are high and completely comparable to those of full agonists or antagonists. However, once bound, they activate the receptor only to a partial degree – this level of activation is referred to as the intrinsic activity of the drug. Thus, the behavior of a partial agonist in a neural system is highly dependent on the availability of the endogenous agonist. When tissue concentrations of the endogenous agonist are high (and thus the receptors would be almost completely activated), the addition of a partial agonist would have the effect of inhibiting or antagonizing the system. On the other hand, when tissue concentrations of the endogenous agonist are low, the addition of a partial agonist would have the effect of stimulating the system. Of recent interest in regard to the monoamine systems of the brain, some receptors have been shown to transmit a basal signal in the complete absence of agonist (46), and thus compounds that bind to these receptors and antagonize them might be considered to be "inverse agonists." Recently, it has been suggested that at least some antipsychotic drugs may be inverse agonists at dopamine (47,48) and serotonin receptors (49), rather than simply antagonists.

Despite the very recent introduction of aripiprazole for the treatment of schizophrenia, the use of agonists and partial agonists in the treatment of this disorder is not new. In fact, the observation that the full dopamine agonist, apomorphine, has ameliorative effects on psychosis was made in the late 18th century (50), when the director of the Walter Baker Sanitarium wrote that this drug was useful for sedating patients with "the wildest delirium." Then, in 1972, Arvid Carlsson and coworkers noted that severance of axons in the nigrostriatal pathways produced increases in the activity of tyrosine hydroxylase, a key enzyme in the synthesis of dopamine (51). From this, they theorized that the enzyme responsible for the synthesis of dopamine was controlled by so-called "autoreceptors" on the presynaptic terminal of dopamine neurons. At about the same time, Tamminga and colleagues reported that schizophrenic symptoms improved briefly after the administration of apomorphine (52). Taking these two findings together, the hypothesis emerged that dopamine agonists, especially those that could selectively affect presynaptic dopamine autoreceptors could be used to decrease dopamine synthesis and release, and so treat the psychosis of schizophrenia without directly blocking the postsynaptic D_2 receptor.

Unfortunately, studies involving other full dopamine agonists in the treatment of patients with schizophrenia produced mixed results. Bromocriptine and another ergot derivative failed to show antipsychotic efficacy (53). In other experiments, Tamminga and colleagues used N-propyl-norapomorphine and found that it also reduced the symptoms of schizophrenia, but only for a few days (54). These results were interpreted to suggest that full dopamine agonists could cause a desensitization of dopamine autoreceptors, which then led to a loss of efficacy. Thus, proponents of using dopamine agonists to treat schizophrenia began to search for compounds with "special characteristics" to take advantage of this indirect means of reducing dopamine transmission (55). Ultimately, because the concentrations of dopamine were noted to be low in proximity to the presynaptic autoreceptor, partial dopamine agonists were suggested to fulfill this purpose (56). Additionally, if one accepts the hypothesis that schizophrenia is characterized by states of both hyper- and hypodopaminergia, partial agonists might also be seen as dopaminergic stabilizers, that is, able to reduce the transmission of dopamine in locations or at times when it is excessive and to increase it in locations or at times when it is deficient.

Among the first partial agonists to be tried for the treatment of patients with schizophrenia was preclamol [(−)-3-(3-hydroxyphenyl)-N-n-propylpiperidine] or (−)-3-PPP. As with apomorphine, an initial study examining the short term effects of this drug was promising (56). However, studies of longer duration (i.e., 2–3 weeks) did not support its efficacy (57). Also, preclinical experiments suggested that the intrinsic activity of such drugs was inversely proportional to the duration of their effects (56). So, in the case of 3-PPP, it was hypothesized that its intrinsic activity was too high, and strategies for reducing this critical variable, such as combining 3-PPP with full antagonists such as haloperidol or risperidone were considered. However, the solution to this problem ultimately was found in the synthesis of a drug with a lower level of intrinsic activity.

The most recently marketed atypical antipsychotic drug is now aripiprazole, which has very high affinity for the dopamine D_2 receptor (i.e., a fast association rate and a slow dissociation rate), but an intrinsic activity (30%) below that of 3-PPP. Notably, aripiprazole acts as an agonist at the dopamine autoreceptor, but as an antagonist in some (58,59) but not other (60) postsynaptic receptor preparations (depending on the availability of endogenous dopamine). As mentioned above, aripiprazole is also a moderately strong antagonist at $5-HT_{2A}$ receptors. However, its affinity for this receptor is an order of magnitude less than its affinity for the D_2 receptor. Thus, neither fast dissociation, nor a favorable $5-HT_{2A}/D_2$ ratio, appears to be a sufficient explanation for the atypical properties of aripiprazole. Recalling studies with other antipsychotic drugs that showed that doses associated with D_2 receptor occupancies in excess of 78–80% also produced extrapyramidal side-effects, it is intriguing to note that although aripiprazole produces dopamine D_2 receptor occupancy in excess of 90% at clinically relevant doses, it produces only minimal extrapyramidal side-effects (60).

Considering the new perspective on atypicality produced by aripiprazole, it now becomes interesting to question whether other atypical drugs may also have some level of partial dopamine agonist activity as well. In regard to this question, it is interesting to note that in rats depleted of dopamine by reserpine and alpha-methyl-*p*-tyrosine, clozapine can increase the ability of full dopamine agonists to induce hyperlocomotion and stereotypy (61,62). Thus, it may be possible that clozapine, and perhaps other similar drugs, can achieve their atypical status through multiple mechanisms.

VI. OTHER POSSIBLE CONTRIBUTIONS TO ATYPICALITY

While these three hypotheses are currently the most popular, none of them appears to be sufficient to explain the atypical or typical properties of all antipsychotic drug. Of course, there is no compelling reason to assert that there can only be one route to atypicality; different drug may achieve similar clinical profiles through different pharmacological mechanisms. Likewise, it is possible that there are routes to atypicality other than the three that have been discussed so far. These possibilities will be discussed briefly below.

A. 5-HT$_{1A}$ Agonism

The part played by 5-HT$_{1A}$ receptors in achieving antipsychotic efficacy without extrapyramidal side-effects has recently been scrutinized in the context of the 5-HT$_{2A}$/D$_2$ hypothesis. As previously discussed, 5-HT$_{2A}$ blockade appears to increase dopamine levels in the prefrontal cortex, and the ability of atypical drugs to accomplish this is thought to result in superior efficacy in treating negative and cognitive symptoms. Recently, Meltzer and colleagues have suggested that the increase in the prefrontal cortical dopamine transmission may be dependent on 5-HT$_{1A}$ agonism (63). Of particular note is that this group has demonstrated that 5-HT$_{1A}$ antagonists prevent the increase in dopamine levels in the rat prefrontal cortex observed after administration of clozapine, olanzapine, and risperidone (64).

B. Glutamate

Not only is the glutamate receptor system in an ideal position to regulate dopaminergic function, but theories of AMPA-type glutamate receptor hyperfunction and NMDA-type glutamate receptor hypofunction have been proposed to explain symptom production in schizophrenia (65). Anecdotally, drugs that act on NMDA-type glutamate receptors produce psychotic symptoms; PCP and ketamine are well-known examples, and various interactions between the glutamate and dopamine systems in the brain have been extensively documented in both health and disease (66). For example, some neurons in the monkey and rat ventral midbrain immunostain for glutamate and dopamine, and dopamine neurons in cell culture appeared to form glutamatergic synapses (67). Moreover, abnormal glutamate innervation has been noted in the frontal cortices of schizophrenic patients (68). Proponents of the glutamate hypothesis of schizophrenia have asserted that symptom reduction might be achieved by increasing transmission at NMDA-type glutamate receptors, and while glutamate cannot be practically delivered into the CNS owing to toxicity, glycine and glycine analogs that facilitate glutamate transmission at the NMDA site can be safely administered to patients. In some studies, such drugs have been shown to have mild efficacy as an adjuvant therapy to antipsychotic drugs (69). More recently, other approaches to increasing glutamate transmission via glycine have been explored, including the use of specific glycine transporter inhibitors (70).

C. Antipsychotic Drug Actions at Other Dopamine Receptors

During the fervor to explain clozapine's atypicality, it was noted that clozapine had substantial affinity for several dopamine receptors, especially the D_1 receptor and another member of the D_2-type family of dopamine receptors, the D_4 receptor. Returning briefly to Meltzer's analysis of the receptor binding profile of typical and atypical drugs, the affinity of drugs at the D_1 receptor subtype did not appear to be a reliable predictor of drug type. Moreover, specific antagonists of D_1 receptors do not seem to have antipsychotic efficacy, and many existing atypical drugs do not occupy a substantial proportion of D_1 receptors at therapeutic doses (30). At one time, it was theorized that heritable polymorphisms in the D_4 receptor might determine patients' responses to clozapine, but genetic studies of D_4 alleles in patients with schizophrenia failed to confirm this hypothesis (71). Furthermore, specific D_4 antagonists have produced conflicting clinical results at best, though there may be a role for D_4 in dopamine metabolism in mouse striatum (72).

D. Neurotensin

Finally, the role of the neuropeptide neurotensin in antipsychotic efficacy has been considered (73) for almost 20 years. In a recent review, Kinkead, Binder, and Nemeroff note that antipsychotic drugs change the expression of neurotensin mRNA and that neurotensin receptor agonists can alter the effects of antipsychotic drugs in several models of schizophrenia (74).

Like glutamate, neurotensin has been implicated in the regulation of dopamine transmission. In some studies of patients with schizophrenia, apparently abnormal levels of neurotensin in the cerebrospinal fluid appear to be corrected after the administration of antipsychotic drugs (75). Furthermore, the response of the neurotensin system to antipsychotic drugs appears to be a function of the drug's typical or atypical properties (76). Unfortunately, at present, there are no antipsychotic drugs that directly target neurotensin receptors, and whether such drugs will be developed in the future remains under considerable debate (77).

REFERENCES

1. Laborit H, Huguenard P. L'hibernation artificielle par moyens pharmaco-dynamiques et physiques. Presse Med 1951; 59:1329.
2. Carlsson A, Lindqvist M. Effect of chlorpromazine or haloperidol on formation of 3-methoxytyramine and normetanephrine in mouse brain. Acta Pharmacol Toxicol 1963; 20:140–144.

3. Anden NE, Roos BE, Werdinius B. Effects of chlorpromazine, haloperidol, and reserpine on the levels of phenolic acids in rabbit corpus striatum. Life Sci 1964; 3:149.
4. Anden NE, Butcher SG, Corrodi H, Fuxe K, Ungerstedt U. Receptor activity and turnover of dopamine and noradrenaline after neuroleptics. Eur J Pharmacol 1970; 11:303–314.
5. Hippius H. A historical perspective of clozapine. J Clin Psychiatry 1999; 60(suppl 12):22–23.
6. Shen WW. A history of antipsychotic drug development. Compr Psychiatry 1999; 40:407–414.
7. Idanpaan-Heikkila J, Alhava E, Olkinuora M, Palva IP. Agranulocytosis during treatment with clozapine. Eur J Clin Pharmacol 1977; 11:193–198.
8. Kane J, Honigfeld G, Singer J, Meltzer H. Clozapine for the treatment-resistant schizophrenic. A double-blind comparison with chlorpromazine. Arch Gen Psychiatry 1988; 45:789–796.
9. Meltzer HY. Action of atypical antipsychotics. Am J Psychiatry 2002; 159: 153–154.
10. Sulpizio A, Fowler PJ, Macko E. Antagonism of fenfluramine-induced hyperthermia: a measure of central serotonin inhibition. Life Sci 1978; 22:1439–1446.
11. Altar CA, Wasley AM, Neale RF, Stone GA. Typical and atypical antipsychotic occupancy of D2 and S2 receptors: an autoradiographic analysis in rat brain. Brain Res Bull 1986 16:517–525.
12. Costall B, Fortune DH, Naylor RJ, Mardsen CD, Pycock C. Serotonergic involvement with neuroleptic catalepsy. Neuropharmacology 1975; 14:859–868.
13. Costall B, Naylor RJ. Neuroleptic interaction with the serotoninergic-dopaminergic mechanisms in the nucleus accumbens. J Pharm Pharmacol 1978; 30:257–259.
14. Bersani G, Grispini A, Marini S, Pasini A, Valducci M, Ciani N. 5-HT2 antagonist ritanserin in neuroleptic-induced parkinsonism: a double-blind comparison with orphenadrine and placebo. Clin Neuropharmacol 1990; 13:500–506.
15. Ceulemans DL, Gelders YG, Hoppenbrouwers ML, Reyntjens AJ, Janssen PA. Effect of serotonin antagonism in schizophrenia: a pilot study with setoperone. Psychopharmacology (Berl) 1985; 85:329–332.
16. Meltzer HY. Commentary on "Clinical studies on the mechanism of action of clozapine; the dopamine-serotonin hypothesis of schizophrenia in Psychopharmacology 1989"; 99:S18–S27; Psychopharmacology (Berl) 2002; 163:1–3.
17. Chiodo LA, Bunney BS. Typical and atypical neuroleptics: differential effects of chronic administration on the activity of A9 and A10 midbrain dopaminergic neurons. J Neurosci 1983; 3:1607–1619.
18. Meltzer HY. Clozapine: mechanism of action in relation to its clinical advantages. In: Kales A, Stefanos CN, Talbott JA (eds) Recent advances in Schizophrenia. New York: Springer-Verlag, 1990.

19. Meltzer HY. Clinical studies on the mechanism of action of clozapine: the dopamine-serotonin hypothesis of schizophrenia. Psychopharmacology (Berl) 1989; 99(Suppl):S18–S27.
20. Miczek KA. Landmark publications in Psychopharmacology: the first 40 years. Psychopharmacology (Berl) 2001; 153:399–401.
21. Meltzer HY, Matsubara S, Lee JC. Classification of typical and atypical antipsychotic drugs on the basis of dopamine D-1, D-2 and serotonin2 pKi values. J Pharmacol Exp Ther 1989; 251:238–246.
22. Parent A. Human Neuroanatomy, 9th edn, Baltimore: Williams and Wilkins, 1995.
23. Pazos A, Probst A, Palacios JM. Serotonin receptors in the human brain—IV. Autoradiographic mapping of serotonin-2 receptors. Neuroscience 1987; 21:123–139.
24. Ugedo L, Grenhoff J, Svensson TH. Ritanserin, a 5-HT2 receptor antagonist, activates midbrain dopamine neurons by blocking serotonergic inhibition. Psychopharmacology (Berl) 1989; 98:45–50.
25. Davis KL, Kahn RS, Ko G, Davidson M. Dopamine in schizophrenia: a review and reconceptualization. Am J Psychiatry 1991; 148:1474–1486.
26. Knable MB, Weinberger DR. Dopamine, the prefrontal cortex and schizophrenia. J Psychopharmacol 1997; 11:123–131.
27. Schotte A, Janssen PF, Gommeren W, Luyten WH, Van Gompel P, Lesage AS, De Loore K, Leysen JE. Risperidone compared with new and reference antipsychotic drugs: in vitro and in vivo receptor binding. Psychopharmacology (Berl) 1996; 124:57–73.
28. Saller CF, Salama AI. Seroquel: biochemical profile of a potential atypical antipsychotic. Psychopharmacology (Berl) 1993; 112:285–292.
29. Meltzer HY. Atypical antipsychotics. In: Psychopharmacology, The Fourth Generation of Progress Online Edition. American College of Neuropsychopharmacology 2000. www.acnp.org/g4.
30. Seeman P. Atypical antipsychotics: mechanism of action. Can J Psychiatry 2002; 47:27–38.
31. Trichard C, Paillere-Martinot ML, Attar-Levy D, Recassens C, Monnet F, Martinot JL. Binding of antipsychotic drugs to cortical 5-HT2A receptors: a PET study of chlorpromazine, clozapine, and amisulpride in schizophrenic patients. Am J Psychiatry 1998; 155:505–508.
32. Kapur S, Seeman P. Author reply to Meltzer HY: Action of atypical antipsychotics. Am J Psychiatry 2002; 159:153–155.
33. Kapur S, Zipursky R, Jones C, Remington G, Houle S. Relationship between dopamine D(2) occupancy, clinical response, and side effects: a double-blind PET study of first-episode schizophrenia. Am J Psychiatry 2000; 157:514–520.
34. Farde L, Nordstrom AL, Wiesel FA, Pauli S, Halldin C, Sedvall G. Positron emission tomographic analysis of central D1 and D2 dopamine receptor occupancy in patients treated with classical neuroleptics and

clozapine. Relation to extrapyramidal side effects. Arch Gen Psychiatry 1992; 49:538–544.

35. Nordstrom AL, Farde L, Wiesel FA, Forslund K, Pauli S, Halldin C, Uppfeldt G. Central D2-dopamine receptor occupancy in relation to antipsychotic drug effects: a double-blind PET study of schizophrenic patients. Biol Psychiatry 1993; 33:227–235.

36. Tauscher J, Kufferle B, Asenbaum S, Fischer P, Pezawas L, Barnas C, Tauscher-Wisniewski S, Brucke T, Kasper S. In vivo 123I IBZM SPECT imaging of striatal dopamine-2 receptor occupancy in schizophrenic patients treated with olanzapine in comparison to clozapine and haloperidol. Psychopharmacology (Berl) 1999; 141:175–181.

37. Knable MB, Heinz A, Raedler T, Weinberger DR. Extrapyramidal side effects with risperidone and haloperidol at comparable D2 receptor occupancy levels. Psychiatry Res 1997; 75:91–101.

38. Bench CJ, Lammertsma AA, Dolan RJ, Grasby PM, Warrington SJ, Gunn K, Cuddigan M, Turton DJ, Osman S, Frackowiak RS. Dose dependent occupancy of central dopamine D2 receptors by the novel neuroleptic CP-88,059-01: a study using positron emission tomography and 11C-raclopride. Psychopharmacology (Berl) 1993; 112:308–314.

39. Kapur S, Zipursky R, Jones C, Shammi CS, Remington G, Seeman P. A positron emission tomography study of quetiapine in schizophrenia: a preliminary finding of an antipsychotic effect with only transiently high dopamine D2 receptor occupancy. Arch Gen Psychiatry 2000; 57:553–559.

40. Tauscher-Wisniewski S, Kapur S, Tauscher J, Jones C, Daskalakis ZJ, Papatheodorou G, Epstein I, Christensen BK, Zipursky RB. Quetiapine: an effective antipsychotic in first-episode schizophrenia despite only transiently high dopamine-2 receptor blockade. J Clin Psychiatry 2002; 63:992–997.

41. Suhara T, Okauchi T, Sudo Y, Takano A, Kawabe K, Maeda J, Kapur S. Clozapine can induce high dopamine D(2) receptor occupancy in vivo. Psychopharmacology (Berl) 2002; 160:107–112.

42. Kapur S, McClelland RA, VanderSpek SC, Wadenberg ML, Baker G, Nobrega J, Zipursky RB, Seeman P. Increasing D2 affinity results in the loss of clozapine's atypical antipsychotic action. Neuroreport 2002; 13:831–835.

43. Kapur S, Seeman P. Does fast dissociation from the dopamine d(2) receptor explain the action of atypical antipsychotics?: A new hypothesis. Am J Psychiatry 2001; 158:360–369.

44. Kapur S, Seeman P. Antipsychotic agents differ in how fast they come off the dopamine D2 receptors. Implications for atypical antipsychotic action. J Psychiatry Neurosci 2000; 25:161–166.

45. Kapur S, Remington G. Dopamine D(2) receptors and their role in atypical antipsychotic action: still necessary and may even be sufficient. Biol Psychiatry 2001; 50:873–883.

46. Lefkowitz RJ, Cotecchia S, Samama P, Costa T. Constitutive activity of receptors coupled to guanine nucleotide regulatory proteins. Trends Pharmacol Sci 1993; 14:303–307.

47. Strange PG. Agonism and inverse agonism at dopamine D2-like receptors. Clin Exp Pharmacol Physiol Suppl 1999; 26:S3–S9.
48. Strange PG. Antipsychotic drugs: importance of dopamine receptors for mechanisms of therapeutic actions and side effects. Pharmacol Rev 2001; 53:119–133.
49. Rauser L, Savage JE, Meltzer HY, Roth BL. Inverse agonist actions of typical and atypical antipsychotic drugs at the human 5-hydroxytryptamine(2C) receptor. J Pharmacol Exp Ther 2001; 299:83–89.
50. Douglas CJ. Apomorphine as a hypnotic. NY Med J 1900; 71:376.
51. Kehr W, Carlsson A, Lindqvist M, Magnusson T, Atack C. Evidence for a receptor-mediated feedback control of striatal tyrosine hydroxylase activity. J Pharm Pharmacol 1972; 24:744–747.
52. Tamminga CA, Schaffer MH, Smith RC, Davis JM. Schizophrenic symptoms improve with apomorphine. Science 1978; 200:567–568.
53. Tamminga CA, Chase TN. Bromocriptine and CF 25–397 in the treatment of tardive dyskinesia. Arch Neurol 1980; 37:204–205.
54. Tamminga CA, Gotts MD, Thaker GK, Alphs LD, Foster NL. Dopamine agonist treatment of schizophrenia with N-propylnorapomorphine. Arch Gen Psychiatry 1986; 43:398–402.
55. Tamminga CA. Partial dopamine agonists in the treatment of psychosis. J Neural Transm 2002; 109:411–20.
56. Tamminga CA, Cascella NG, Lahti RA, Lindberg M, Carlsson A. Pharmacologic properties of (−)-3PPP (preclamol) in man. J Neural Transm Gen Sect 1992; 88:165–175.
57. Lahti AC, Weiler MA, Corey PK, Lahti RA, Carlsson A, Tamminga CA. Antipsychotic properties of the partial dopamine agonist (−)-3-(3-hydroxyphenyl)-N-n-propylpiperidine(preclamol) in schizophrenia. Biol Psychiatry 1998; 43:2–11.
58. Kiuchi K, Hirata Y, Minami M, Nagatsu T. Effect of 7-(3-[4-(2,3-dimethylphenyl)piperazinyl]propoxy)-2(1H)-quinolinone (OPC-4392), a newly synthesized agonist for presynaptic dopamine D2 receptor, on tyrosine hydroxylation in rat striatal slices. Life Sci 1988; 42:343–349.
59. Kikuchi T, Tottori K, Uwahodo Y, Hirose T, Miwa T, Oshiro Y, Morita S. 7-(4-[4-(2,3-Dichlorophenyl)-1-piperazinyl]butyloxy)-3,4-dihydro-2(1H)-quinolinone (OPC-14597), a new putative antipsychotic drug with both presynaptic dopamine autoreceptor agonistic activity and postsynaptic D2 receptor antagonistic activity. J Pharmacol Exp Ther 1995; 274:329–336.
60. Yokoi F, Grunder G, Biziere K, Stephane M, Dogan AS, Dannals RF, Ravert H, Suri A, Bramer S, Wong DF. Dopamine D2 and D3 receptor occupancy in normal humans treated with the antipsychotic drug aripiprazole (OPC 14597): a study using positron emission tomography and [11C]raclopride. Neuropsychopharmacology 2002; 27:248–259.
61. Jackson DM, Mohell N, Bengtsson A, Malmberg A. Why does clozapine stimulate the motor activity of reserpine-pretreated rats when combined with a dopamine D1 receptor agonist? Eur J Pharmacol 1995; 282:137–144.

62. Ninan I, Kulkarni SK. Partial agonistic action of clozapine at dopamine D2 receptors in dopamine depleted animals. Psychopharmacology (Berl) 1998; 135:311–317.

63. Ichikawa J, Meltzer HY. The effect of serotonin(1A) receptor agonism on antipsychotic drug-induced dopamine release in rat striatum and nucleus accumbens. Brain Res 2000; 858:252–263.

64. Ichikawa J, Ishii H, Bonaccorso S, Fowler WL, O'Laughlin IA, Meltzer HY. 5-HT(2A) and D(2) receptor blockade increases cortical DA release via 5-HT(1A) receptor activation: a possible mechanism of atypical antipsychotic-induced cortical dopamine release. J Neurochem 2001; 76:1521–1531.

65. Kalkman HO. Antischizophrenic activity independent of dopamine D2 blockade. Expert Opin Ther Targets 2002; 6:571–582.

66. Carfagno ML, Hoskins LA, Pinto ME, Yeh JC, Raffa RB. Indirect modulation of dopamine D2 receptors as potential pharmacotherapy for schizophrenia: II. Glutamate antagonists. Ann Pharmacother 2000; 34:788–797.

67. Sulzer D, Joyce MP, Lin L, Geldwert D, Haber SN, Hattori T, Rayport S. Dopamine neurons make glutamatergic synapses in vitro. J Neurosci 1998 18:4588–4602.

68. Deakin FW, Simpson MD, Slater P, Hellewell JS. Familial and developmental abnormalities of front lobe function and neurochemistry in schizophrenia. J Psychopharmacol 1997; 11:133–142.

69. Javitt DC. Glycine modulators in schizophrenia. Curr Opin Investig Drugs 2002; 3:1067–1072.

70. Vandenberg RJ, Aubrey KR. Glycine transport inhibitors as potential antipsychotic drugs. Expert Opin Ther Targets 2001; 5:507–518.

71. Rao PA, Pickar D, Gejman PV, Ram A, Gershon ES, Gelernter J. Allelic variation in the D4 dopamine receptor (DRD4) gene does not predict response to clozapine. Arch Gen Psychiatry 1994; 51:912–917.

72. Wilson JM, Sanyal S, Van Tol HH. Dopamine D2 and D4 receptor ligands: relation to antipsychotic action. Eur J Pharmacol 1998; 351:273–286.

73. Nemeroff CB. Neurotensin: perchance an endogenous neuroleptic? Biol Psychiatry 1980; 15:283–302.

74. Kinkead B, Binder EB, Nemeroff CB. Does neurotensin mediate the effects of antipsychotic drugs? Biol Psychiatry 1999; 46:340–351.

75. Breslin NA, Suddath RL, Bissette G, Nemeroff CB, Lowrimore P, Weinberger DR. CSF concentrations of neurotensin in schizophrenia: an investigation of clinical and biochemical correlates. Schizophr Res 1994; 12:35–41.

76. Binder EB, Kinkead B, Owens MJ, Nemeroff CB. The role of neurotensin in the pathophysiology of schizophrenia and the mechanism of action of antipsychotic drugs. Biol Psychiatry 2001; 50:856–872.

77. Kinkead B, Nemeroff CB. Neurotensin: an endogenous antipsychotic? Curr Opin Pharmacol 2002; 2:99–103.

2

Probing the "Receptorome" Unveils the Receptor Pharmacology of Atypical Antipsychotic Drugs

Bryan L. Roth

Case Western Reserve University Medical School, Cleveland, Ohio, U.S.A.

I. INTRODUCTION

Over the past 14 years, atypical antipsychotic drugs exemplified by clozapine (1) have revolutionized the treatment of schizophrenia (2–4, 125). Despite the fact that atypical antipsychotic drugs are now prescribed more commonly than typical antipsychotic drugs in many areas of the world, there continues to be debate regarding the cost-effectiveness (5) and the clinical superiority of atypical antipsychotic drugs (6). Atypical antipsychotic drugs are distinguished from typical antipsychotic drugs by the following criteria: 1) atypical antipsychotic drugs lack extrapyramidal side effects (EPS) in humans; 2) atypical antipsychotic drugs do not elevate serum prolactin levels in humans; and 3) atypical antipsychotic drugs do not induce catalepsy in rodents. Other studies suggest that atypical antipsychotic drugs reduce suicidality (7) and improve cognition (8) for instance, though not necessarily without serious side effects such as weight gain (9) and other metabolic and cardiovascular side effects (10,11).

The ideal atypical antipsychotic drug would be one that has no motor side effects, does not induce tardive dyskinesia with chronic use, improves cognition and reduces suicidality—all without metabolic or cardiovascular side effects. At present no one atypical antipsychotic drug fulfills all of these criteria. Indeed, there is a large range in the degree of "atypicality" (12), with some "atypicals" such as risperidone having substantial, dose-related risks of EPS (13) and others, such as clozapine (1) and quetiapine (14) having virtually no dose-related EPS within the range of practical or tolerated doses.

The major problem in developing the "ideal atypical antipsychotic drug" is that there is little consensus regarding the molecular targets responsible for the beneficial or the deleterious effects of atypical antipsychotic drugs. In large measure, this is due to the huge number of molecular targets "hit" by drugs like clozapine (see below), although even "cleaner" drugs such as aripiprazole and ziprasidone still "hit" many molecular targets. An additional problem in discovering the set of targets responsible for atypical antipsychotic drug actions relates to the realization, thanks to the sequencing of the human genome, of the tremendous number of potential molecular targets in existence. Indeed, in the case of G-protein coupled receptors (GPCRs), there are 300–400 potential molecular targets, excluding odorant GPCRs, which could be occupied (at least in theory) by atypical antipsychotic drugs. Ideally, one would like to screen the entire *receptorome* (the entire complement of receptors in the genome) to discover the molecular targets responsible for atypical antipsychotic drug actions, although this is not yet feasible with the current technology. For the purposes of this chapter, we will define receptorome to include non-odorant GPCRs only.

In this chapter I summarize what is now known regarding the interactions of typical and atypical antipsychotic drugs with the human receptorome in vitro. Of course because such an analysis is limited merely to in vitro measurements issues such as in vivo receptor occupancy and the effects of doses on in vivo selectivities cannot be addressed adequately. As we will demonstrate, although antipsychotic drugs interact with a large number of molecular targets, it is possible to divide these interactions into those likely to be beneficial and those likely to be deleterious for treatment of schizophrenia. We will use as the main source of information on the receptor pharmacology of antipsychotic drugs a public domain, on-line, searchable database located at: http://pdsp.cwru.edu/pdsp.asp that has been created by the National Institute of Mental Health (NIMH) Psychoactive Drug Screening Program. It is our contention that a detailed understanding of the receptor pharmacology of atypical antipsychotic drugs will allow for the development of novel antipsychotic drugs with improved efficacies and fewer side effects.

II. BIOGENIC AMINE RECEPTORS

A. Dopamine Receptors

Five dopamine receptors have been identified by molecular cloning (D_1, D_2, D_3, D_4, and D_5). The D_2 receptor has two splice variants (D_{2L} and D_{2S}) (15), whereas the D_4 receptor has a large number of isoforms (see (16) for review). Typical antipsychotic drugs have preferentially high affinity for D_2-dopamine receptors (17,18) and atypical antipsychotic drugs have relatively low affinity for D_2-dopamine receptors (19,20). Atypical antipsychotic drugs also bind to D_3- (21,22) and D_4- (23,24) dopamine receptors but, in general, have relatively low affinities for D_1- and D_5-dopamine receptors (Table 1). It has been proposed that D_2- affinities are lower (19,25), and hence dissociation rates (25) faster, for atypical antipsychotic drugs as a group. It can clearly be seen from Table 1, however, that atypical antipsychotic drugs have varying affinities for D_2 receptors with some drugs having low affinities (e.g., clozapine, quetiapine, olanzapine) and others having high affinities (e.g., ziprasidone, risperidone, amisulpride, aripiprazole). Although D_{2L} and D_{2S} isoforms subsume distinct functions (26), there are no apparent differences in terms of relative or absolute drug binding affinities (Table 1). D_{2L} has been shown to act mainly at postsynaptic sites while D_{2S} acts as a presynaptic autoreceptor

Table 1 Average Affinities of Representative Typical and Atypical Antipsychotic Drugs for Cloned Human Dopamine Receptors

Drug	Typical (T) or atypical (A)	D_1	D_{2L}	D_{2S}	D_3	D_4	D_5
Haloperidol	T	55	2.4	1.5	4	1.4	113
Chlorpromazine	T	58	6.7	NA	4.4	1.2	133
Clozapine	A	168	187	152	275	33	266
Quetiapine	A	1277	700	445	340	2029	1513
Olanzapine	A	35	31	29	49	11	74
Risperidone	A	523	1.65	4.8	14	16	563
Ziprasidone	A	330[a]	4.6	4.2	10	39	152
Aripiprazole	A	410[a]	2.3[a]	0.59[a]	7.5[a]	260[a]	1200[a]
Sertindole	A	210[a]	7	6	10	0.9	NA
Amisulpride	A	NA	1.3[b]	1.3[b]	2.3[a]	NA	NA

[a]Nonhuman receptor preparation.
[b]Information on D_{2L} and D_{2S} unavailable. NA, not available. Data represent K_i values in nM obtained from the NIMH PDSP K_i database for human cloned receptors. For values for which more than one dataset is available, the mean K_i value is reported (see http://kidb.bioc.cwru.edu/pdsp.php for complete links to references).

(26). Interestingly, the cataleptic effects of haloperidol are absent in D_{2L}-deficient mice. These results suggest that many of the functions of D_2-receptor antagonists are differentially mediated by D_{2L} and D_{2S} receptors. It has also been suggested that atypical antipsychotic drugs have preferentially higher affinities for D_4-dopamine receptors (23). As we have pointed out previously, D_4-dopamine receptor affinity does not distinguish between typical and atypical antipsychotic drugs (24). This is readily seen in Table 1 as several atypicals actually have higher affinities for D_2-dopamine than D_4-dopamine receptors (e.g., risperidone, ziprasidone, aripiprazole, quetiapine). Indeed, studies with D_4-dopamine receptor knock-out (KO) mice imply that blockade of D_4-dopamine receptors is likely to have psychotomimetic actions (27). This is because data obtained with D_4-KO mice demonstrate that cortical glutamatergic neurons are hyperexcitable (27). Additionally, there are now reports that drugs with selectively high affinities for D_4-dopamine receptors, e.g., fananserin, are not effective in schizophrenia (28).

D_3-dopamine receptors have also been suggested to be essential for atypical antipsychotic drug actions (21), although the lack of effect of clozapine on *c-fos* expression in D_3-KO mice (29) casts doubt on this assertion. Amisulpride is an interesting atypical antipsychotic drug that is relatively selective for D_2- and D_3-dopamine receptors (30,31,125), and its utility in treating schizophrenia has prompted the hypothesis that D_3-antagonists may be effective in treating schizophrenia.

As can also be seen from Table 1, typical and atypical antipsychotic drugs have uniformly low affinities for D_1- and D_5-dopamine receptors. Some relatively selective D_1-antagonists (e.g., SCH39166 (32) and CEE-03-310 (33)) were developed for treatment of schizophrenia, but had no apparent efficacy (Table 2). Table 2 also lists trials of D_3- and D_4-selective drugs for schizophrenia; none of these drugs has shown efficacy in human trials. Taken together, these results demonstrate that some degree of D_2-receptor blockade is likely necessary for effective antipsychotic drug actions in humans.

B. Serotonin Receptors

There are at least 15 distinct serotonin (5-hydroxytryptamine; 5-HT) receptors in the human genome (34) (35) and atypical antipsychotic drugs interact with many including the 5-HT_{1A} (36), 5-HT_{2A} (19), 5-HT_{2C} (37,38), 5-HT_6 (39,40) and 5-HT_7 (39) (Table 2). As has been reviewed elsewhere, most atypical antipsychotic drugs are characterized by having relatively higher affinities for 5-HT_{2A} receptors than for D_2-dopamine receptors (19,41–43) although this is clearly not universal, since atypical antipsychotic

Table 2 Representative Antipsychotic Drug Trials Using Novel Molecular Targets Other Than D_2-Dopamine Receptors

Drug	Target	Clinical trials	Outcome	Status	Ref.
CEE-03-310	D_1-dopamine	None	Dropped	Other applications	(33)
NNC 01-0687	D_1-dopamine	Phase I	Unknown	Unknown	(121)
SCH39166	D_1-dopamine	Open label	Ineffective	Unknown	(32)
SB-277011	D_3-dopamine	None	Unknown	Unknown	(122)
(+)-UH232	D_3-dopamine	Placebo controlled; double blind	Worsened	Unknown	(123)
Fananserin	D_4-dopamine	Placebo controlled; double blind	Worsened	Dropped	(28)
M100907	$5\text{-}HT_{2A}$	Double blind; placebo controlled	Improved; haloperidol superior to M100907	Dropped	(124)
SR46349B	$5\text{-}HT_{2A}$	Placebo controlled; double blind	Improved; haloperidol superior to SR46349B	Dropped	H. Y. Meltzer, personal communication
S-16924	$5\text{-}HT_{1A}$	NA	NA	Unknown	(60)
Gransitron	$5\text{-}HT_3$	Open label	No effect on akathisia	Unknown	(72)
Zacopride	$5\text{-}HT_3$	Single blind	No effect	Unknown	(71)
BuTAC	m_3-muscarinic	Animal models only	"Antipsychotic-like effects"	Unknown	(90)
EMD 57445	Sigma	Open label	No effect	Dropped	(109)
BMY14802	Sigma	Double blind	Worsened	Dropped	(108)
D-cycloserine	NMDA	Additive	Improved	Continues	(115)
Glycine	NMDA	Additive	Improved	Continues	(116)

drugs such as aripiprazole and amisulpride (Tables 1 and 3) have higher affinities for D_2-dopamine than 5-HT_{2A} serotonin receptors. Additionally, loxapine and amoxapine are two typical antipsychotic drugs with higher affinities for 5-HT_{2A} than for D_2 receptors, and are misclassified as "atypical" by the $5\text{-HT}_{2A}/D_2$ ratio criterion (19,44,45,125) but which are typical in terms of EPS liabilities and elevation of serum prolactin levels.

Although it has been clear for many years that a relatively high affinity for 5-HT_{2A} receptors is characteristic of many atypical antipsychotic drugs, it has not been appreciated until recently why preferential binding to 5-HT_{2A} receptors might be important. It is now known that 5-HT_{2A} receptors are highly concentrated in Layer V pyramidal neurons in the cortex (46–48). 5-HT_{2A} receptors are also found on dopaminergic neurons in the ventral tegmental area (49) and dopaminergic terminals in the prefrontal cortex (50). Finally, 5-HT_{2A} receptors have been found on GABA-ergic pallido-striatal projection neurons (51). 5-HT_{2A} receptor activation of cortical pyramidal neurons enhances cortical excitability (52,53) and disrupts working memory (54). It is conceivable that 5-HT_{2A} receptor blockade of cortical neuronal excitation enhances working memory. Furthermore, since 5-HT_{2A} agonists are hallucinogenic (43), it is conceivable that 5-HT_{2A} receptor blockade is involved in reducing positive symptoms of schizophrenia. In this regard (Table 2), two large-scale trials of relatively selective 5-HT_{2A} antagonists (M100907 and SR46349B) have demonstrated that monotherapy with 5-HT_{2A} antagonists significantly reduces symptoms of schizophrenia when compared with placebo, but not to the same degree as the conventional antipsychotic drug haloperidol (S. Potkin and H.Y. Meltzer, personal communications).

5-HT_{2A} receptors on ventral tegmental neurons and dopaminergic terminals are likely involved in modulating dopamine release. Thus, Yan has demonstrated (55) that activation of 5-HT_{2A} receptors augments dopamine (DA) release in the nucleus accumbens, while others have shown that ritanserin (a $5\text{-HT}_{2A/2B/2C}$ antagonist) reverses the dopaminergic-induced inhibition of midbrain DA neurons (56). Finally, Pehek and colleages (57) have demonstrated that M100907 attenuates stimulated DA release in the medial prefrontal cortex. Taken together, these results suggest that 5-HT_{2A} receptors likely modulate DA release in a salutary manner in schizophrenia and related disorders.

Atypical antipsychotic drugs have been known for many years to have actions at 5-HT_{1A} receptors (58), and it is now clear that many atypical antipsychotic drugs are partial 5-HT_{1A} agonists (36). Because 5-HT_{1A} receptor activation reduces Layer V pyramidal neuronal excitability (52), it is likely that combined partial agonism at 5-HT$_{1A}$ receptors and antagonism at 5-HT$_{2A}$ receptors helps to normalize cortical neuronal actions (59). One atypical antipsychotic drug with a relative selectivity toward 5-HT$_{1A}$ receptors has been developed (60), though it is important to realize that this compound (S-16924) interacts with a large number of other targets, including D$_2$-dopamine and 5-HT$_{2A}$ receptors (60). Because 5-HT$_{1A}$ receptors have been implicated in anxiety and depression (61) it has been suggested that partial agonism at 5-HT$_{1A}$ receptors might serve to "stabilize" serotonergic neuronal transmission and, thus, alleviate depression and anxiety in schizophrenia (59,125,126). It is unlikely that 5-HT$_{1A}$ agonism alone would be useful in treating schizophrenia.

The relevance of 5-HT$_{2C}$ receptor interactions for atypical antipsychotic drug actions is unknown. It has been known for over 10 years that selected typical and atypical antipsychotic drugs bind with high affinity to 5-HT$_{2C}$ receptors (37). 5-HT$_{2C}$ receptors are known to be involved in the regulation of appetite (62) and likely mediate the actions of fenfluramine as an appetite suppressant (63). Because 5-HT$_{2C}$ agonists suppress appetite and 5-HT$_{2C}$ knock-out mice are obese, some have suggested that the weight gain associated with antipsychotic drug use might be due to 5-HT$_{2C}$ receptor blockade (9,10). Indeed a recent study demonstrated that a polymorphism in the 5-HT$_{2C}$ receptor was associated with weight gain for two antipsychotic drugs (chlorpromazine and risperidone) (64). The notion that 5-HT$_{2C}$ antagonism induces weight gain is difficult to reconcile with the data that ziprasidone, an atypical that does not induce substantial weight gain, has high affinity for 5-HT$_{2C}$ receptors. Additionally, quetiapine is a drug associated with substantial weight gain which has virtually no affinity for 5-HT$_{2C}$ receptors (Table 3). Indeed our recent report (127) concluded that 5-HT$_{2C}$ antagonism did not predict weight gain among atypical antipsychotic drugs. Finally, animal studies have demonstrated that selective 5-HT$_{2C}$ antagonists to not induce weight gain (65).

5-HT$_{2C}$ receptors are also involved in regulating dentate gyrus functioning (66), suggesting that blockade of 5-HT$_{2C}$ receptors may disrupt certain types of hippocampal-based learning and memory. These studies suggest that 5-HT$_{2C}$ blockade may counteract any beneficial effects of atypical antipsychotic drugs on learning and memory. In this regard, Herrick-Davis and colleagues (67) suggested that atypical antipsychotic drugs as a group are characterized by inverse agonism of 5-HT$_{2C}$ receptors while typical antipsychotic drugs are neutral antagonists. Two other studies (38,68) showed, however, that both typical and atypical antipsychotic drugs are 5-HT$_{2C}$ inverse agonists. It will be interesting, then, to determine

Table 3 Average Affinities of Representative Typical and Atypical Antipsychotic Drugs at Selected Human Cloned 5-HT Receptors

	5-HT$_{1A}$	5-HT$_{1B}$	5-HT$_{1D}$	5-HT$_{2A}$	5-HT$_{2C}$	5-HT$_3$	5-HT$_6$	5-HT$_7$
Haloperidol	2,832	270	>5,000	50	4,475	>10,000	6,600	501
Chlorpromazine	3,115	1,489[a]	NA	12	6.1	1,032[a]	19	54[a]
Clozapine	140	390	580	13	7.5	110[a]	9.5	24
Quetiapine	320	2,050	>5,000	1,568	1,184	4,060[a]	33	290
Olanzapine	2,720	660	540	3.5	14	84[a]	10	119[a]
Risperidone	420	9.8	140	0.55	33	>10,000[a]	2,400	1.4[a]
Ziprasidone	12	1	5.1	1.4	4.1	2,830[a]	61	4.9[a]
Aripiprazole	5.6	833	63	4.6	181	628	574	10
Sertindole	280	520	78	0.35	0.7	3,180[a]	5.4[a]	28[a]
Amisulpride	>10,000	>10,000	>10,000	2,000	>10,000	>10,000	NA	NA

[a]Nonhuman receptor preparation.

Data represent K_i values in nM obtained from the NIMH PDSP K_i database for human cloned receptors or unpublished data from the PDSP. For values for which more than one dataset is available, the mean K_i value is reported (see http://kidb.bioc.cwru.edu/pdsp.php for complete links to references). For 5-HT$_{1E}$, 5-HT$_{1F}$, 5-HT$_{2B}$, 5-HT$_4$, 5-HT$_{5A}$ receptors, affinities of atypical antipsychotic drugs are generally greater than 1000 nM (PDSP database; unpublished data).

if drugs with potent $5\text{-}HT_{2C}$ agonism improve cognition and memory in schizophrenia.

$5\text{-}HT_3$ antagonists have been tested in schizophrenia because of the suggestion that $5\text{-}HT_3$ receptors might modulate dopamine release and facilitate latent inhibition in the rat (69,70). One open label study with zacopride, a selective $5\text{-}HT_3$ antagonist (71), for schizophrenia showed no effect. An additional study investigating whether $5\text{-}HT_3$ antagonists might diminish akathisia also showed no effect (72). It is not surprising that $5\text{-}HT_3$ antagonists are ineffective in schizophrenia because of (a) the relative paucity of $5\text{-}HT_3$ receptors in the brain, and (b) the low affinity of antipsychotic drugs for $5\text{-}HT_3$ sites.

Atypical antipsychotic drugs also have variable affinities for $5\text{-}HT_6$ and $5\text{-}HT_7$ receptors (Table 3). Indeed, one study suggests that clozapine preferentially labels a "5-HT6-like receptor" (73), while another suggests that chronic clozapine treatment down-regulates $5\text{-}HT_6$ receptors (74) in vitro. However, $5\text{-}HT_6$ receptors are not altered in schizophrenia, nor following antipsychotic drug administration to rodents (75). There is no evidence that $5\text{-}HT_6$ or $5\text{-}HT_7$ receptors are involved in antipsychotic drug action, although selective drugs targeting these receptors are in early stages of clinical development (76).

C. Adrenergic Receptors

It has been known for many decades that antipsychotic drugs have varying affinities for adrenergic receptors, in particular, α_1- and α_2-adrenergic receptor subtypes (77–80). There are now at least nine distinct adrenergic receptors in three families: α_1-, α_2-, and β-adrenergic; Table 4 lists the average affinities of atypical antipsychotic drugs at cloned human α_{1A}-, α_{1B}-, α_{2A}-, α_{2B}-, and α_{2C}-adrenergic receptors, since antipsychotic drugs do not generally have appreciable affinities for β-adrenergic sites.

In general, the affinities of atypical antipsychotic drugs for α_{1A}-adrenergic receptors parallel their propensities to induce orthostatic hypotension (80). Thus, clozapine, chlorpromazine and risperidone regularly induce orthostasis while others do not. Some investigators have proposed that adrenergic blockade contributes to the atypical profile of drugs like clozapine (81,82), though it is unlikely since typical antipsychotic drugs like chlorpromazine have such preferentially high affinities for α_1-adrenergic receptors.

Others have suggested that α_2-adrenergic receptors are involved in the "atypical" properties of drugs like clozapine (83). This is due in large part to a recent study which demonstrated that the cataleptic actions of raclopride

Table 4 Affinities of Typical and Atypical Antipsychotic Drugs for Selected Adrenergic Receptors

	α_{1A}	α_{1B}	α_{2A}	α_{2B}	α_{2C}
Haloperidol	12	8	1,130	480	550
Chlorpromazine	0.3	0.8	184	28	46
Clozapine	1.6	7	142	27	34
Quetiapine	22	39	3,630	747	29
Olanzapine	109	263	314	82	29
Risperidone	4.5	9	151	108	1.3
Ziprasidone	18	9	160	48	77
Aripiprazole	25	34	74	102	38
Sertindole	3.9^a	NA	640	450	450
Amisulpride	7,410	14,100	1,600	NA	NA

[a]Noncloned human receptor preparation.
Data represent K_i values in nM obtained from the NIMH PDSP K_i database for human cloned receptors or unpublished data from the PDSP. For values for which more than one dataset is available, the mean K_i value is reported (see http://kidb.bioc.cwru.edu/pdsp.php for complete links to references).

can be reversed by the α_2 antagonist idazoxan (83). Additionally, studies in humans have demonstrated that idazoxan can augment the actions of typical antipsychotic drugs (84). Again, this hypothesis is difficult to reconcile with the observation that many atypical antipsychotic drugs (quetiapine, olanzapine, ziprasidone, and sertindole) have very low affinities for α_2-adrenergic receptors (Table 4). It is likely that α_2-antagonism may contribute to the actions of selected atypical antipsychotic drugs, but by itself is not essential for "atypicality" or is neither necessary nor sufficient for "atypicality."

D. Muscarinic Receptors

For nearly 30 years it has been known that antipsychotic drugs interact to a variable extent with muscarinic receptors, and that their affinities for muscarinic receptors were approximately correlated with their propensities to induce EPS (85). It is now known that atypical antipsychotic drugs have varying affinities for the five cloned muscarinic receptors (m_1, m_2, m_3, m_4, m_5), as was first noted by (86) (Table 5). It is clear from Table 5 that antipsychotic drugs can have negligible (e.g., ziprasidone, risperidone, aripiprazole, amisulpride) or high affinities (e.g., clozapine, olanzapine) for various muscarinic receptors. Generally, atypical antipsychotic drugs are antagonists at muscarinic receptors, although some atypicals are

Table 5 Affinities of Atypical and Selected Typical Antipsychotic Drugs for Cloned Muscarinic Acetylcholine Receptors

	m_1	m_2	m_3	m_4	m_5
Haloperidol	>10,000	>10,000	>10,000	>10,000	>10,000
Chlorpromazine	25	180	67	40	42
Clozapine	3.1	48	20	11	11.2
Quetiapine	858	1,339	1,943	542	1,942
Olanzapine	24	79	51	998	9
Risperidone	>10,000	3,700	>10,000	2,900	>10,000
Ziprasidone	>10,000	>10,000	>10,000	>10,000	>10,000
Aripiprazole	6,776	3,507	4,677	1,521	2,327
Sertindole	>5,000[a]	>5,000[a]	>5,000[a]	>5,000[a]	>5,000[a]
Amisulpride	>5,000[a]	>5,000[a]	>5,000[a]	>5,000[a]	>5,000[a]

[a]Noncloned human receptor preparation.
Data represent K_i values in nM obtained from the NIMH PDSP K_i database for human cloned receptors or unpublished data from the PDSP. For values for which more than one dataset is available, the mean K_i value is reported (see http://kidb.bioc.cwru.edu/pdsp.php for complete links to references).

agonists at m4-muscarinic receptors (87,88). The significance of m_4 receptor activation for the actions of clozapine and related atypicals is unknown.

The m_3-muscarinic receptors have begun to be targets for atypical antipsychotic drug development. At present several compounds are in development, including (5R,6R)-6-(3-butylthio-1,2,5-thiadiazol-4-yl)-1-azabicyclo(90)octane (BuTAC) (90) and (5R,6R)-6-(3-propylthio-1,2,5-thiadiazol-4-yl)-1-azabicyclo(90)octane (PTAC) (91), both of which show unexpected antipsychotic drug actions in animal models. The status of these compounds is currently unknown.

In general, the ability of atypical antipsychotic drugs to bind to muscarinic receptors predicts the presence of anticholinergic side effects in humans (80), such as constipation and dry mouth (92,93). Constipation following clozapine treatment can be quite severe, and has led to death in at least one individual (94,95). In addition to the peripheral actions of anticholinergic medications, it is well known that these medications may impair cognition (96). It is likely that the anticholinergic actions of certain atypicals (e.g., clozapine, olanzapine) counteract the potential cognition-enhancing properties of these medications. It has also recently been noted that drugs such as clozapine and olanzapine augment acetylcholine release in the hippocampus and cortex (97,98). It is likely that the indirect cholinergic agonist actions of these medications counteract their anticholinergic effects.

Table 6 Affinities of Atypical and Selected Typical Antipsychotic Drugs for Cloned Histamine Receptors

	H_1	H_2	H_3	H_4
Haloperidol	4,160	>10,000	>10,000	>10,000
Chlorpromazine	31	174	>10,000	7
Clozapine	0.23	153	820[a]	510
Quetiapine	2.2	NA	NA	NA
Olanzapine	0.65	NA	NA	NA
Risperidone	27	NA	NA	NA
Ziprasidone	130	NA	NA	NA
Aripiprazole	23	NA	NA	NA
Sertindole	130	NA	NA	NA
Amisulpride	>10,000	NA	NA	NA

[a]Noncloned human receptor preparation.

Data represent K_i values in nM obtained from the NIMH PDSP K_i database for human cloned receptors or unpublished data from the PDSP. For values for which more than one dataset is available, the mean K_i value is reported (see http://kidb.bioc.cwru.edu/pdsp.php for complete links to references).

E. Histamine Receptors

Chlorpromazine, the first antipsychotic drug, was initially developed as a sedative antihistamine for use as a pre-anesthetic agent, mainly by virtue of its interactions with H_1-histamine receptors. It is now known that there are at least four distinct histamine receptors (H_1, H_2, H_3, H_4) and that atypical antipsychotic drugs have varying affinities for all of them (Table 6). In general, the ability of atypical antipsychotic drugs to bind to H_1-histamine receptors correlates with their propensities to induce weight gain (127), as has been suggested by others for many decades (99–102). As a group, atypical antipsychotic drugs do not have appreciable affinities for other histamine receptors, with the exception of clozapine which binds to H_3- and H_4-histamine receptors (103,104). At present no selective histamine receptor antagonists are being developed for use in schizophrenia.

F. Other Receptors and Channels

1. Sigma Receptor Antagonists

Since the discovery that many antipsychotic drugs bind to sigma receptors (105,106), it has been suggested that sigma receptor-selective compounds might be effective in treating schizophrenia (despite the fact that clozapine, for instance does not bind to sigma receptors with high affinity (107)). Several sigma antagonists have been tested in schizophrenia including rimcazole, BMY14802 (108) and, most recently, EMD 57445 (109). Despite the fact that sigma-1 antagonists, to date, have not been effective, there are still studies ongoing with sigma-1 antagonists.

2. Cannabinoid Receptor Antagonists

It has long been recognized that marijuana may exacerbate psychosis, and that cannabis may occasionally induce a toxic psychosis (110). Recently, it was reported that a polymorphism in the CB-1 locus for the CB-1 cannabinoid receptor is associated with "hebephrenic schizophrenia" in a Japanese sample (111). There is also preclinical evidence that a CB-1 antagonist (SR1417156) may have antipsychotic-like actions in certain animal models (112), though clinical studies have demonstrated no effect (H. Y. Meltzer, personal communication).

3. Glutamatergic Drugs

Atypical antipsychotic drugs do not interact to any appreciable extent with glutamatergic receptors, of which there are both ionotropic (e.g., NMDA, AMPA, Kainate) and metabotropic (e.g., mGluR) subfamilies. Because clozapine and other putative atypical antipsychotic drugs (e.g., M100907) block many of the behavioral effects of phencyclidine (PCP) and other NMDA antagonists (59,113), it has been suggested that NMDA agonists may be effective in treating schizophrenia (114). D-Cycloserine, an indirect glutamatergic agonist, has been reported to have an intermediate effect in schizophrenia (115), as has high-dose glycine (116).

It has also been suggested that metabotropic agonists may be effective in treating schizophrenia (117). This notion is based on the observation that Group II mGluR agonists attenuate the effects of hallucinogens on 5-HT$_{2A}$-mediated actions (59,118). Studies with mGluR agonists in schizophrenia are ongoing.

III. CONCLUSIONS

The main conclusion of this review is that multiple pharmacological mechanisms are likely to contribute to the actions of atypical antipsychotic drugs (Table 7). Thus, although a balanced antagonism of 5-HT$_{2A}$ serotonin and D$_2$-dopamine receptors provides a reliable template to produce "atypical" antipsychotic drugs, other targeting strategies are also

Table 7 Classification of Atypical Antipsychotic Drugs Based on Pharmacological Mechanism

	$5\text{-}HT_{2A}/D_2$	D_2/D_3	D_2 partial agonist	$5\text{-}HT_{2A}$ inverse agonists
Drug	Risperidone; ziprasidone; olanzapine; quetiapine; clozapine	Amisulpride; remoxipride	Aripiprazole	M100907; SR46349B
Extrapyramidal side effects	Varies from absent (clozapine; quetiapine) to high (risperidone)	Moderately low	Low to absent	None
Weight gain liabilities	Varies from low (ziprasidone) to high (clozapine, olanzapine)	Moderately low	Low	None
Anticholinergic/ orthostasis	Varies	Low	Low	Low/none

likely to be successful. These alternative strategies include D_2-dopamine receptor partial agonism and balanced D_2/D_3 antagonism. Finally, it is possible that atypical antipsychotic drugs may be developed that do not interact with either dopamine or 5-HT receptors, although at present there are no such drugs available with demonstrated efficacy at treating schizophrenia.

It is clear from the foregoing that a certain level of D_2-dopamine receptor antagonism is essential for antipsychotic actions in schizophrenia (Table 8). This is because, to date, all tested non-D_2-based therapies have proven either to worsen schizophrenia (e.g., sigma receptor antagonists), have no effect (e.g., CB-1 antagonists), or not be superior to conventional medications (e.g., 5-HT$_{2A}$ antagonists). A challenge for the next generation of atypical antipsychotic drugs will be to define how weak affinity for D_2-receptors can be attained while retaining efficacy. Atypical antipsychotic drugs, as a class, are quite heterogeneous. By strict pharmacological criteria, only clozapine and quetiapine (and perhaps aripiprazole) would be classed as atypical because these are the only known medications which are devoid of EPS and do not elevate serum prolactin levels. The other atypical antipsychotic drugs either induce EPS to some extent, typically in a dose-related manner, or elevate serum prolactin levels, or both. It is also clear that drugs such as clozapine probably have unique advantages as well, since clozapine has now been demonstrated to reduce suicide among schizophrenics (7,119,120). Indeed a recent direct comparison of clozapine and olanzapine treatment demonstrated that clozapine is superior to olanzapine for reducing suicide risk in schizophrenia (128). Additionally, although other atypical antipsychotic drugs may be effective in so-called "treatment-resistant schizophrenia," clozapine remains the "gold standard" for treating treatment-resistant patients. Unfortunately, clozapine has an exceedingly complex and robust pharmacology, since it interacts with high affinity with more than 20 GPCRs, acting as an inverse agonist at some (e.g., 5-HT$_{2A/2C}$) and partial agonist at others (e.g., H$_4$-histamine; 5-HT$_{1A}$). It is likely that the salutary actions of clozapine are due in large part to its robust pharmacology rather than interaction with a single receptor.

Finally, this chapter summarizes the available information on the receptor sites responsible for many of the major side effects of atypical antipsychotic drugs (Table 8). Thus, weight gain and sedation are likely due to interactions with H$_1$-histamine receptors. Interactions with α_1-adrenergic receptors are responsible for hypotension, while antimuscarinic actions induce constipation. Utilizing this information early in the course of drug discovery will likely facilitate the rational design of atypical antipsychotic drugs with greater efficacies and fewer side effects.

Table 8 Summary of Main Points for Clinicians

---

1. Atypical antipsychotic drugs vary in the degree of atypicality (e.g., lack of EPS; lack of serum prolactin elevations)
   a. Clozapine and quetiapine are highly "atypical"
   b. Olanzapine and ziprasidone are moderately "atypical"
   c. Risperidone's degree of "atypicality" varies depending on dose
2. No unitary pharmacological mechanism can be provided to explain the various actions of a drug like clozapine
3. It is likely that drugs devoid of D_2-antagonist properties will not have antipsychotic actions
4. The receptor pharmacology essential for "atypicality" can be differentiated from the side-effect profile pharmacology
   a. Weight gain is due to chance interaction with H_1-histamine receptors
   b. Orthostasis is due to α_1-adrenergic receptor blockade
   c. Constipation is due to muscarinic receptor blockade

ACKNOWLEDGMENTS

This work was supported in part by KO2MH01366, RO1MH57635, RO1MH618867, and NO2MH80002 to B. L. R.

REFERENCES

1. Kane J, et al. Clozapine for the treatment-resistant schizophrenic. Arch Gen Psychiatry 1988; 45:789–796.
2. Meltzer HY. Outcome in schizophrenia: beyond symptom reduction. J Clin Psychiatry 1999; 60(suppl 3)(2):3–7; discussion 8.
3. Jibson MD, Tandon R. New atypical antipsychotic medications. J Psychiatr Res 1998; 32(3–4):215–228.
4. Roth BL, Shapiro DA. Insights into the structure and function of 5-HT2 family serotonin receptors reveal novel strategies for therapeutic target development. Exp Opin Ther Targets 2001; 5:685–695.
5. Revicki DA. Cost effectiveness of the newer atypical antipsychotics: a review of the pharmacoeconomic research evidence. Curr Opin Investig Drugs 2001; 2(1):110–117.
6. Geddes J, et al. Atypical antipsychotics in the treatment of schizophrenia: systematic overview and meta-regression analysis. Brit Med J 2000; 321(7273): 1371–1376.
7. Meltzer HY. Suicidality in schizophrenia: a review of the evidence for risk factors and treatment options. Curr Psychiatry Rep 2002; 4(4):279–283.
8. Meltzer HY, McGurk, SR. The effects of clozapine, risperidone, and olanzapine on cognitive function in schizophrenia. Schizophr Bull 1999; 25(2):233–255.

9. Wetterling T. Bodyweight gain with atypical antipsychotics. A comparative review. Drug Saf 2001; 24(1):59–73.
10. McIntyre RS, McCann SM, Kennedy SH. Antipsychotic metabolic effects: weight gain, diabetes mellitus, and lipid abnormalities. Can J Psychiatry 2001; 46(3):273–281.
11. Fontaine KR, et al. Estimating the consequences of anti-psychotic induced weight gain on health and mortality rate. Psychiatry Res 2001; 101(3):277–288.
12. Stip E. Novel antipsychotics: issues and controversies. Typicality of atypical antipsychotics. J Psychiatry Neurosci 2000; 25(2):137–153.
13. Chouinard G, et al. A Canadian multicenter placebo-controlled study of fixed doses of risperidone and haloperidol in the treatment of chronic schizophrenia. J Clin Psychopharmacol 1993; 13:25–40.
14. Copolov DL, Link CG, Kowalcyk B. A multicentre, double-blind, randomized comparison of quetiapine (ICI 204,636, 'Seroquel') and haloperidol in schizophrenia. Psychol Med 2000; 30(1):95–105.
15. Monsma FJ Jr et al. Multiple D2 dopamine receptors produced by alternative RNA splicing. Nature 1989; 342(6252):926–929.
16. Sibley DR, Monsma FJ Jr Molecular biology of dopamine receptors. Trends Pharmacol Sci 1992. 13(2):61–69.
17. Seeman P, Lee T. Antipsychotic drugs: direct correlation between clinical potency and presynaptic action on dopamine neurons. Science 1975; 188(4194):1217–1219.
18. Creese I, Burt DR, Snyder SH. Dopamine receptor binding predicts clinical and pharmacological potencies of antischizophrenic drugs. Science 1976; 192(4238):481–483.
19. Meltzer HY, Matsubara S, Lee J-C. Classification of typical and atypical antipsychotic drugs on the basis of dopamine D-1, D-2 and serotonin2 pKi values. J Pharmacol Exp Ther 1989; 251:238–246.
20. Seeman PCRVT. HHM, Atypical neuroleptics have low affinity for dopamine D2 receptors or are selective for D4 receptors. Neuropsychopharmacology 1997; 16(2):93–135.
21. Sokoloff P, et al. Molecular cloning and characterization of a novel dopamine receptor (D3) as a target for neuroleptics. Nature 1990; 347(6289):146–151.
22. Seeman P, Van Tol HH. Dopamine receptor pharmacology. Trends Pharmacol Sci 1994; 15(7):264–270.
23. Van Tol HHM, et al. Cloning of the gene for a human dopamine D4 receptor with high affinity for the antipsychotic clozapine. Nature 1991; 350:610–614.
24. Roth BL, et al. D4 dopamine receptor binding affinity does not distinguish between typical and atypical antipsychotic drugs. Psychopharmacology (Berl) 1995; 120(3):365–368.
25. Kapur S, Seeman P. Does fast dissociation from the dopamine d(2) receptor explain the action of atypical antipsychotics?: A new hypothesis. Am J Psychiatry 2001; 158(3):360–369.
26. Usiello A, et al. Distinct functions of the two isoforms of dopamine D2 receptors. Nature 2000; 408(6809):199–203.

27. Rubinstein M, et al. Dopamine D4 receptor-deficient mice display cortical hyperexcitability. J Neurosci 2001; 21(11):3756–3763.

28. Truffinet P, et al. Placebo-controlled study of the D4/5-HT2A antagonist fananserin in the treatment of schizophrenia. Am J Psychiatry 1999; 156(3):419–425.

29. Carta AR, Gerfen CR. Lack of a role for the D3 receptor in clozapine induction of c-fos demonstrated in D3 dopamine receptor-deficient mice. Neuroscience 1999; 90(3):1021–1029.

30. Curran MP, Perry CM. Amisulpride: a review of its use in the management of schizophrenia. Drugs 2001; 61(14):2123–2150.

31. Schoemaker H, et al. Neurochemical characteristics of amisulpride, an atypical dopamine D2/D3 receptor antagonist with both presynaptic and limbic selectivity. J Pharmacol Exp Ther 1997; 280(1):83–97.

32. Karlsson P, et al. Lack of apparent antipsychotic effect of the D1-dopamine receptor antagonist SCH39166 in acutely ill schizophrenic patients. Psychopharmacology (Berl) 1995; 121(3):309–316.

33. Eder DN. CEE-03-310 CeNeS pharmaceuticals. Curr Opin Investig Drugs 2002; 3(2):284–288.

34. Roth B, et al. Multiplicity of serotonin receptors: useless diverse molecules or an embarrassment of riches? The Neuroscientist 2000; 6:252–262.

35. Kroeze WK, Kristiansen K, Roth BL. Molecular biology of serotonin receptors structure and function at the molecular level. Curr Top Med Chem 2002; 2(6):507–528.

36. Newman-Tancredi A, et al. Agonist and antagonist actions of antipsychotic agents at 5-HT1A receptors: a [35S]GTPgammaS binding study. Eur J Pharmacol 1998; 355(2–3):245–256.

37. Roth BL, Ciaranello RD, Meltzer HY. Binding of typical and atypical antipsychotic agents to transiently expressed 5-HT1C receptors. J Pharmacol Exp Ther 1992; 260(3):1361–1365.

38. Rauser L, et al. Inverse agonist actions of typical and atypical antipsychotic drugs at the human 5-hydroxytryptamine(2C) receptor. J Pharmacol Exp Ther 2001; 299(1):83–89.

39. Roth BL, et al. Binding of typical and atypical antipsychotic agents to 5-hydroxytryptamine-6 and 5-hydroxytryptamine-7 receptors. J Pharmacol Exp Ther 1994; 268(3):1403–1410.

40. Kohen R, et al. Cloning, characterization, and chromosomal localization of a human 5- HT6 serotonin receptor. J Neurochem 1996; 66(1): 47–56.

41. Kroeze WK, Roth BL. The molecular biology of serotonin receptors: therapeutic implications for the interface of mood and psychosis. Biol Psychiatry 1998; 44(11):1128–1142.

42. Roth BL, Meltzer H, Khan N. Binding of typical and atypical antipsychotic drugs to multiple neurotransmitter receptors. In: Advances in Pharmacology. San Diego: Academic Press, 1998:482–485.

43. Roth BL, et al. Activation is hallucinogenic and antagonism is therapeutic: role of 5-HT$_{2A}$ receptors in atypical antipsychotic drug actions. The Neuroscientist 1999; 5:254–262.

44. Kapur S, et al. Is amoxapine an atypical antipsychotic? Positron-emission tomography investigation of its dopamine2 and serotonin2 occupancy. Biol Psychiatry 1999; 45(9):1217–1220.

45. Kapur S, Zipursky RB. Do loxapine plus cyproheptadine make an atypical antipsychotic? PET analysis of their dopamine D2 and serotonin2 receptor occupancy [letter]. Arch Gen Psychiatry 1998; 55(7):666–668.

46. Willins D, Deutch A, Roth BL. Serotonin 5-HT2A receptors are expressed on pyramidal cells and interneurons in the rat cortex. Synapse 1997; 27:79–82.

47. Hamada S, et al. Localization of 5-HT2A receptor in rat cerebral cortex and olfactory system revealed by immunohistochemistry using two antibodies raised in rabbit and chicken. Brain Res Mol Brain Res 1998; 54(2):199–211.

48. Jakab R, Goldman-Rakic P. 5-Hydroxytryptamine2A serotonin receptors in the primate cerebral cortex: possible site of action of hallucinogenic and antipsychotic drugs in pyramidal cell apical dendrites. Proc Natl Acad Sci USA 1998; 95:735–740.

49. Nocjar C, Roth BL, Pehek EA. Localization of 5-HT(2A) receptors on dopamine cells in subnuclei of the midbrain A10 cell group. Neuroscience 2002; 111(1):163–76.

50. Miner LAH, et al. Ultrastructural localization of serotonin2A receptors in the middle layers of the rat prelimbic prefrontal cortex. Neuroscience 2002; In press.

51. Bubser M, et al. Distribution of serotonin 5-HT(2A) receptors in afferents of the rat striatum. Synapse 2001; 39(4):297–304.

52. Araneda R, Andrade R. 5-Hydroxytryptamine2 and 5-hydroxytryptamine1A receptors mediate opposing responses on membrane excitability in rat association cortex. Neuroscience 1991; 40(2):399–412.

53. Carr DB, et al. Serotonin receptor activation inhibits sodium current and dendritic excitability in prefrontal cortex via a protein kinase C-dependent mechanism. J Neurosci 2002; 22(16):6846–6855.

54. Williams GV, Rao SG, Goldman-Rakic PS. The physiological role of 5-HT2A receptors in working memory. J Neurosci 2002; 22(7):2843–2854.

55. Yan QS. Activation of 5-HT2A/2C receptors within the nucleus accumbens increases local dopaminergic transmission. Brain Res Bull 2000; 51(1):75–81.

56. Shi WX, Nathaniel P, Bunney BS. Ritanserin, a 5-HT2A/2C antagonist, reverses direct dopamine agonist-induced inhibition of midbrain dopamine neurons. J Pharmacol Exp Ther 1995; 274(2):735–740.

57. Pehek EA, et al. M100,907, a selective 5-HT(2A) antagonist, attenuates dopamine release in the rat medial prefrontal cortex. Brain Res 2001; 888(1): 51–59.

58. Nash JF, Meltzer HY, Gudelsky GA. Antagonism of serotonin receptor mediated neuroendocrine and temperature responses by atypical neuroleptics in the rat. Eur J Pharmacol 1988; 151(3):463–469.

59. Martin-Ruiz R, et al. Control of serotonergic function in medial prefrontal cortex by serotonin-2A receptors through a glutamate-dependent mechanism. J Neurosci 2001; 21(24):9856–9866.

60. Millan MJ, et al. S-16924 [(R)-2-[1-[2-(2,3-dihydro-benzo[1,4]dioxin-5-yloxy)-ethyl]- pyrrolidin-3yl]-1-(4-fluorophenyl)-ethanone], a novel, potential antipsychotic with marked serotonin1A agonist properties: III. Anxiolytic actions in comparison with clozapine and haloperidol. J Pharmacol Exp Ther 1999; 288(3):1002–1014.

61. Zhuang X, et al. Altered emotional states in knockout mice lacking 5-HT1A or 5-HT1B receptors. Neuropsychopharmacology 1999; 21(2 Suppl):52S–60S.

62. Tecott LH, et al. Eating disorder and epilepsy in mice lacking 5-HT2c serotonin receptors [see comments]. Nature 1995; 374(6522):542–546.

63. Vickers SP, et al. Reduced satiating effect of d-fenfluramine in serotonin 5-HT(2C) receptor mutant mice. Psychopharmacology (Berl) 1999; 143(3): 309–314.

64. Reynolds GP, Zhang ZJ, Zhang XB. Association of antipsychotic drug-induced weight gain with a 5-HT2C receptor gene polymorphism. Lancet 2002; 359(9323):2086–2087.

65. Kennett GA, et al. SB 242084, a selective and brain penetrant 5-HT2C receptor antagonist. Neuropharmacology 1997; 36(4–5):609–620.

66. Tecott LH, et al. Perturbed dentate gyrus function in serotonin 5-HT2C receptor mutant mice. Proc Natl Acad Sci USA 1998; 95(25):15026–15031.

67. Herrick-Davis K, Grinde E, Teitler M. Inverse agonist activity of atypical antipsychotic drugs at human 5-hydroxytryptamine2C receptors. J Pharmacol Exp Ther 2000; 295(1):226–232.

68. Weiner DM, et al. 5-Hydroxytryptamine2A receptor inverse agonists as antipsychotics. J Pharmacol Exp Ther 2001; 299(1):268–276.

69. Costall B, Naylor RJ, Tyers MB. The psychopharmacology of 5-HT3 receptors. Pharmacol and Ther 1990; 47:181–202.

70. Moran PM, Moser PC. MDL 73,147EF, a 5-HT3 antagonist, facilitates latent inhbition in the rat. Phamacol Biochem Behav 1992; 42:519–522.

71. Newcomer JW, et al. Zacopride in schizophrenia: a single-blind serotonin type 3 antagonist trial. Arch Gen Psychiatry 1992; 49(9):751–752.

72. Poyurovsky M, Weizman A. Lack of efficacy of the 5-HT3 receptor antagonist granisetron in the treatment of acute neuroleptic-induced akathisia. Int Clin Psychopharmacol 1999; 14(6):357–360.

73. Glatt CE, et al. Clozapine: selective labeling of sites resembling 5HT6 serotonin receptors may reflect psychoactive profile. Mol Med 1995; 1(4): 398–406.

74. Zhukovskaya NL, Neumaier JF. Clozapine downregulates 5-hydroxytryptamine6 (5-HT6) and upregulates 5-HT7 receptors in HeLa cells. Neurosci Lett 2000; 288(3):236–240.

75. East SZ, et al. 5-HT6 receptor binding sites in schizophrenia and following antipsychotic drug administration: Autoradiographic studies with [125I]SB-258585. Synapse 2002; 45(3):191–199.

76. Jones BJ, Blackburn TP. The medical benefit of 5-HT research. Pharmacol Biochem Behav 2002; 71(4):555–568.
77. Peroutka SJ, et al. Neuroleptic drug interactions with norepinephrine alpha receptor binding sites in rat brain. Neuropharmacology 1977; 16(9):549–556.
78. Peroutka SJ, Synder SH. Relationship of neuroleptic drug effects at brain dopamine, serotonin, alpha-adrenergic, and histamine receptors to clinical potency. Am J Psychiatry 1980; 137(12):1518–1522.
79. Cohen BM, Lipinski JF. In vivo potencies of antipsychotic drugs in blocking alpha1 noradrenergic and dopamine D-2 receptors: implications for drug mechanisms of action. Life Sci 1986; 39:2571–2586.
80. Richelson E, Souder T. Binding of antipsychotic drugs to human brain receptors focus on newer generation compounds. Life Sci 2000; 68(1):29–39.
81. Baldessarini RJ, et al. Do central antiadrenergic actions contribute to the atypical properties of clozapine? Brit J Psychiatry Suppl 1992; 169:12–16.
82. Carasso BS, Bakshi VP, Geyer MA. Disruption in prepulse inhibition after alpha-1 adrenoceptor stimulation in rats. Neuropharmacology 1998; 37(3): 401–404.
83. Hertel P, Fagerquist MV, Svensson TH. Enhanced cortical dopamine output and antipsychotic-like effects of raclopride by alpha2 adrenoceptor blockade. Science 1999; 286(5437):105–107.
84. Litman RE, et al. Idazoxan and response to typical neuroleptics in treatment-resistant schizophrenia. Comparison with the atypical neuroleptic, clozapine. Brit J Psychiatry 1996; 168(5):571–579.
85. Miller RJ, Hiley CR. Anti-muscarinic properties of neuroleptics and drug-induced parkinsonism. Nature (London) 1974; 248:546–547.
86. Bolden C, Cusack B. Richelson E. Antagonism by anitmuscarinic and neuroleptic compounds at the five cloned human muscarinic cholinergic receptors expressed in Chinese hamster ovary cells. J Pharmacol Exp Ther 1992; 260:576–580.
87. Zeng XP, Le F, Richelson E. Muscarinic m4 receptor activation by some atypical antipsychotic drugs. Eur J Pharmacol 1997; 321(3):349–354.
88. Zorn SH, et al. Clozapine is a potent and selective muscarinic M4 receptor agonist. Eur J Pharmacol 1994; 269(3):R1–R2.
89. Bonhaus DW, et al. [3H]BIMU-1, a 5-hydroxytryptamine3 receptor ligand in NG-108 cells, selectively labels sigma-2 binding sites in guinea pig hippocampus. J Pharmacol Exp Ther 1993; 267(2):961–970.
90. Rasmussen T, et al. The muscarinic receptor agonist BuTAC, a novel potential antipsychotic, does not impair learning and memory in mouse passive avoidance. Schizophr Res 2001; 49(1–2):193–201.
91. Bymaster FP, et al. Unexpected antipsychotic-like activity with the muscarinic receptor ligand (5R,6R)6-(3-propylthio-1,2,5-thiadiazol-4-yl)-1-azabicyclo [3.2.1]octane. Eur J Pharmacol 1998; 356(2–3):109–119.
92. Bhana N, et al. Olanzapine: an updated review of its use in the management of schizophrenia. Drugs 2001; 61(1):111–161.
93. Jann MW. Clozapine. Pharmacotherapy 1991; 11(3):179–195.

94. Drew L, Herdson P. Clozapine and constipation: a serious issue. Aust N Z J Psychiatry 1997; 31(1):149–150.
95. Levin TT, Barrett J, Mendelowitz A. Death from clozapine-induced constipation: case report and literature review. Psychosomatics 2002; 43(1):71–73.
96. Heinik J. Effects of trihexyphenidyl on MMSE and CAMCOG scores of medicated elderly patients with schizophrenia. Int Psychogeriatr 1998; 10(1):103–108.
97. Shirazi-Southall S, Rodriguez DE, Nomikos GG. Effects of typical and atypical antipsychotics and receptor selective compounds on acetylcholine efflux in the hippocampus of the rat. Neuropsychopharmacology 2002; 26(5):583–594.
98. Ichikawa J, et al. Atypical, but not typical, antipsychotic drugs increase cortical acetylcholine release without an effect in the nucleus accumbens or striatum. Neuropsychopharmacology 2002; 26(3):325–339.
99. Silverstone T, Schuyler D. The effect of cyproheptadine on hunger, calorie intake and body weight in man. Psychopharmacologia 1975; 40(4):335–340.
100. Doss FW. The effect of antipsychotic drugs on body weight: a retrospective review. J Clin Psychiatry 1979; 40(12):528–530.
101. Allison DB, et al. Antipsychotic-induced weight gain: a comprehensive research synthesis. Am J Psychiatry 1999; 156(11):1686–1696.
102. Wirshing DA, et al. Novel antipsychotics: comparison of weight gain liabilities. J Clin Psychiatry 1999; 60(6):358–363.
103. Schlicker E, Marr I. The moderate affinity of clozapine at H3 receptors is not shared by its two major metabolites and by structurally related and unrelated atypical neuroleptics. Naunyn Schmiedebergs Arch Pharmacol 1996; 353(3):290–294.
104. Kathmann M, Schlicker E, Gothert M. Intermediate affinity and potency of clozapine and low affinity of other neuroleptics and of antidepressants at H3 receptors. Psychopharmacology (Berl) 1994; 116(4):464–468.
105. Largent BL, et al. Novel antipsychotic drugs share high affinity for sigma receptors. Eur J Pharmacol 1988; 155(3):345–347.
106. Snyder SH, Largent BL. Receptor mechanisms in antipsychotic drug action: focus on sigma receptors. J Neuropsychiatry Clin Neurosci 1989; 1(1):7–15.
107. Schotte A, et al. Risperidone compared with new and reference antipsychotic drugs: in vitro and in vivo receptor binding. Psychopharmacology (Berl) 1996; 124(1–2):57–73.
108. Gewirtz GR, et al. BMY 14802, a sigma receptor ligand for the treatment of schizophrenia. Neuropsychopharmacology 1994; 10(1):37–40.
109. Muller MJ, et al. Antipsychotic effects and tolerability of the sigma ligand EMD 57445 (panamesine) and its metabolites in acute schizophrenia: an open clinical trial. Psychiatry Res 1999; 89(3):275–280.
110. Imade AG, Ebie JC. A retrospective study of symptom patterns of cannabis-induced psychosis. Acta Psychiatr Scand 1991; 83(2):134–136.

111. Ujike H, et al. CNR1, central cannabinoid receptor gene, associated with susceptibility to hebephrenic schizophrenia. Mol Psychiatry 2002; 7(5): 515–518.
112. Poncelet M, et al. Blockade of cannabinoid (CB1) receptors by 141716 selectively antagonizes drug-induced reinstatement of exploratory behaviour in gerbils. Psychopharmacology (Berl) 1999; 144(2):144–150.
113. Carlsson ML, et al. The 5-HT2A receptor antagonist M100907 is more effective in counteracting NMDA antagonist- than dopamine agonist-induced hyperactivity in mice. J Neural Transm 1999; 106(2):123–129.
114. Rowley M, Bristow LJ, Hutson PH. Current and novel approaches to the drug treatment of schizophrenia. J Med Chem 2001; 44(4):477–501.
115. Evins AE, et al. D-Cycloserine added to risperidone in patients with primary negative symptoms of schizophrenia. Schizophr Res 2002; 56(1–2):19–23.
116. Javitt DC, et al. Adjunctive high-dose glycine in the treatment of schizophrenia. Int J Neuropsychopharmacol 2001; 4(4):385–391.
117. Wickelgren I. A new route to treating schizophrenia? Science 1998; 281(5381):1264–1265.
118. Gewirtz JC, et al. Modulation of DOI-induced increases in cortical BDNF expression by group II mGlu receptors. Pharmacol Biochem Behav 2002; 73(2):317–326.
119. Meltzer HY. Suicide and schizophrenia: clozapine and the InterSePT study. International Clozaril/Leponex Suicide Prevention Trial. J Clin Psychiatry 1999; 60(suppl 12):47–50.
120. Meltzer HY, Okayli G. Reduction of suicidality during clozapine treatment of neuroleptic-resistant schizophrenia: impact on risk-benefit assessment. Am J Psychiatry 1995; 152(2):183–190.
121. Karle J, et al. NNC 01–0687, a selective dopamine D1 receptor antagonist, in the treatment of schizophrenia. Psychopharmacology (Berl) 1995; 121(3): 328–329.
122. Remington G, Kapur S. SB-277011 GlaxoSmithKline. Curr Opin Investig Drugs 2001; 2(7):946–949.
123. Lahti AC, et al. Effects of the D3 and autoreceptor-preferring dopamine antagonist (+)-UH232 in schizophrenia. J Neural Transm 1998; 105(6–7): 719–734.
124. de Paulis T. M-100907 (Aventis). Curr Opin Investig Drugs 2001; 2(1): 123–732.
125. Roth BL, Sheffler D, Potkin SG. Atypical antipsychotic drug actions: unitary or multiple mechanisms for "atypicality"? Clin Neurosci Res 2003; 3:108–117.
126. Roth BL, Hanizavareh SM, Blum AE. Serotonin receptors represent highly favorable molecular targets for cognitive enhancement in schizophrenia and other disorders. Psychopharmacology (Berl) Dec 2, 2003. e-pub ahead of print.
127. Kroeze WK, Hufeisen SJ, Popadak BA, et al. H1-histamine receptor affinity predicts short-term weight gain for typical and atypical antipsychotic drugs. Neuropsychopharmacology 2003; 28(3):519–526.

3

Neurophysiological Effects of Atypical Antipsychotic Drugs

Patricio O'Donnell

Albany Medical College,
Albany, New York, U.S.A.

I. INTRODUCTION

Antipsychotic drugs (APDs) act on a variety of brain receptors and regions. Determining which ones are responsible for improving schizophrenia symptoms has been largely controversial. The prevalent view is that APD clinical efficacy seems to be related to their ability to block dopamine (DA) D_2 receptors (1). Atypical antipsychotics are also D_2 antagonists, but they differ from classical APDs on a number of aspects: a) they block serotonin 5-HT$_2$ receptors with higher affinity than classical APDs (2,3), b) their D_2 receptor occupancy is typically less than 80% at clinically effective doses (4), and c) they seem to have some selectivity in the brain regions they affect. Perhaps assessing the electrophysiological actions of APDs may bring clues to elucidate why they are effective and what makes atypical APDs different. This chapter will review the neurophysiolgical actions of this class of drugs, taking into consideration both acute and chronic effects.

II. DOPAMINE SYSTEMS

There are several DA pathways in the brain, and their physiology has been extensively studied. The populations of DA neurons that may be important

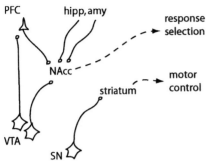

Figure 1 Parallel dopamine pathways. The ventral tegmental area (VTA) sends dopamine-containing projections to the nucleus accumbens (NAcc) and prefrontal cortex (PFC). In the NAcc, PFC output is integrated with limbic inputs arising from the hippocampus (hipp) and amygdala (amy). This integration is under tight dopaminergic control, and its outcome is an important factor in selecting behaviorally appropriate responses. The subtantia nigra (SN), on the other hand, projects to the dorsal aspect of the striatum, where it controls inputs arriving from motor cortical areas. This action is essential for proper motor control and movement initiation.

for APD actions are located in the midbrain, in particular in the substantia nigra pars compacta and in a region just medial to it, the ventral tegmental area (VTA). Neurons in the VTA project to the nucleus accumbens and prefrontal cortex (PFC), whereas DA neurons in the substantia nigra project to the striatum (Figure 1). A DA deficit in the latter is responsible for some of the symptoms occurring in Parkinson's disease, while the mesolimbic and mesocortical projections are thought to be involved in schizophrenia.

A. Dopamine Cell Electrophysiology and Dopamine Release

The basic physiological properties of DA cells have been extensively studied since Arvid Carlsson identified DA as a neurotransmitter and not simply a precursor for norepinephrine (5). Dopamine neurons can exhibit two basic firing modes: regular and bursting (6) (Figure 2). At rest, their electrical activity is dominated by intrinsic currents that render their membrane potential into a pacemaker oscillation (7). In these conditions, DA neurons fire regularly, yet at a slow rate. This slow firing causes occasional action potentials reaching DA terminals in target areas, which evoke a limited amount of DA release (termed "tonic" release). Excitatory inputs to the VTA and substantia nigra can enhance DA cell firing. Activation of NMDA receptors elicits a characteristic burst of action potentials in DA cells (8,9) that typically consists of 3–10 action potentials of decreasing amplitude and

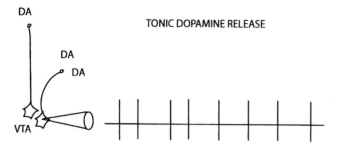

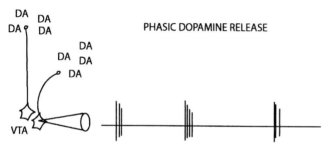

Figure 2 Tonic versus phasic dopamine release. Top: DA neurons can fire in a regular fashion, resulting in tonic levels of extracellular dopamine. The vertical markers crossing the horizontal line to the right represent individual action potentials recorded from a putative DA neuron. Bottom: when action potentials occur in bursts, the levels of DA released are much higher (phasic release).

increasing duration (10). NMDA glutamate receptors eliciting burst firing may be activated by inputs arriving from the PFC, the subthalamic nucleus, or the pedunculopontine nucleus (11,12). It has been shown that DA cell burst firing results in much larger DA release from terminals (13), suggesting that the effects of DA cell activity may be different when they fire in bursts versus when they are tonically active. It is conceivable that DA cell bursting and the relatively larger amount of DA it releases are important elements facilitating information processing in target areas (14,15) and enhancing synaptic plasticity, an action that will eventually contribute to learning and memory functions. Indeed, recordings of DA cell electrical activity in awake monkeys have shown that DA neurons fire bursts of action potentials when unexpected reward is presented to the animal, or in the presence of reward-predicting stimuli (16). Aversive stimuli have also been observed to activate DA projections (17). Thus, it is now accepted that DA cell bursting is a signal encoding saliency of external stimuli; some sort of an "alerting" system (14).

B. Control of Dopamine Release

A number of feedback mechanisms control DA cell firing and release. Most DA cells contain autoreceptors, which are primarily of the D_2 subtype. Some autoreceptors are located in the cell body and dendrites (18), and can be activated by dendritic release of DA when the cells fire action potentials, slowing down cell firing (19). Projection terminals in the striatum also contain autoreceptors. Activation of presynaptic autoreceptors reduces DA synthesis and release in the striatum and nucleus accumbens (20), and probably only release in the PFC (21). Whenever DA cells fire in pacemaker mode, there is a relatively small amount of DA being released. This is supposed to be the source of DA measured with extracellular detection methods (e.g., microdialysis), probably via diffusion away from terminals. Tonic levels of DA released by slow regular cell firing have been proposed to provide a constant activation of D_2 autoreceptors, down-regulating the release machinery. Thus, the amount of phasic DA released by bursts of action potentials is modulated by tonic DA levels (6).

C. Dopamine Systems in Schizophrenia

The nature of DA changes in schizophrenia has also been largely controversial. The DA hypothesis of schizophrenia originated in the finding that neuroleptics are DA antagonists (22). This was further supported by the observation that the binding affinity of APDs for DA correlates with their clinical efficacy (23). Later, this correlation was restricted to a subtype of DA receptors: the D_2 family (1) In addition, the DA-releasing agent amphetamine can elicit psychosis-like symptoms in normal subjects and worsen symptoms in schizophrenia patients (24). A complication of treating patients with Parkinson's disease with the DA precursor L-dopa is the development of psychotic episodes (25). Together, these facts gave rise to the widespread notion that there is DA hyperactivity in schizophrenia.

Some findings, however, have challenged the common assumption that schizophrenia is a disorder with enhanced DA activity. Post-mortem studies have been inconclusive in revealing increased DA levels in brains from schizophrenia patients (26); some even suggested the possibility of decreased DA levels, since DA turnover was reduced (27), particularly in patients with predominant negative symptoms (26). Furthermore, low doses of amphetamine can ameliorate symptoms in some patients (28), most notably negative symptoms if they are severe (29). These findings led some authors to speculate that at least in patients with prominent negative symptoms there may be a decrease (instead of an increase) in DA activity (30). How can these disparate views be reconciled? It is actually possible that both are correct.

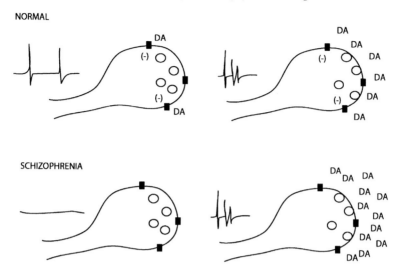

Figure 3 Coexistence of hypodopaminergic basal state and hyperdopaminergic responses in schizophrenia. Top: Cartoon representing a DA terminal. Tonic cell firing results in basal levels of DA that may down-regulate phasic release by acting on presynaptic autoreceptors. Arrival of a burst of action potentials (right) will cause a large amount of DA release, but not as large as it could be due to the autoreceptor modulation. Bottom: It has been suggested that DA systems in schizophrenia patients may have, as a consequence of hypofrontality, a reduced tonic level of DA. This would result in lower levels of autoreceptor-mediated inhibition of release. Thus, arrival of a burst of action potentials (right) will yield a much larger phasic release than in the normal condition.

Recent models propose that hypofrontality may result in hypodopaminergic states (31). Anthony Grace suggested that a reduced level of tonic DA cell firing may be present in schizophrenia (6), as a consequence of a PFC dysfunction (32,33). Such reduced activity will yield reduced tonic DA levels and low levels of autoreceptor occupancy. This would cause an up-regulation of release when DA cells fire in bursts, enhancing phasic DA release (Figure 3). Increased phasic release is likely to underscore positive symptoms, whereas negative symptoms are more related to alterations in glutamate transmission and perhaps reduced DA in the PFC (34).

III. ACUTE EFFECTS OF ANTIPSYCHOTICS

Because APDs are DA antagonists, one would expect that they dampen activity in the dopamine system, especially in the basal ganglia and PFC.

However, acute APD administration would also block D_2 autoreceptors and enhance the level of overall DA cell firing (35). In basal conditions, DA cells exhibit only occasional bursts of action potentials; the proportion of burst firing increases with acute haloperidol (36). Long-term administration of DA agonists has been shown to change the sensitivity of autoreceptors (37). Therefore, it is conceivable that the autoreceptor control of DA cell firing can be adjusted by antipsychotic drug-dependent continuous DA receptor blockade.

Overall, atypical and typical APDs exhibit similar acute effects on DA neurons; the differences seem to be in the DA pathways affected. Clozapine (Clozaril®) and quetiapine (Seroquel®) enhance DA cell firing in the VTA, but not in the substantia nigra (38). This effect seems to be stronger for VTA DA neurons projecting to the PFC (39). Olanzapine (Zyprexa®) and clozapine have been shown to block the inhibitory effects of amphetamine on DA cells (40). Again, this effect was stronger in the VTA than in the substantia nigra (40). All these findings indicate that atypical APDs may have preferential actions on mesolimbic and mesocortical DA projections.

IV. ATYPICAL ANTIPSYCHOTICS AND DEPOLARIZATION BLOCK OF DOPAMINE NEURONS

As stated above, all antipsychotic drugs, typical and atypical block DA receptors. Although not without controversy, this action is believed to result in the eventual inactivation of DA neurons in the mesolimbic and mesocortical projections (41). This effect, however, is only acquired following a relatively prolonged exposure to the drug (2 weeks or longer). Thus, this is an attractive mechanism to explain the clinical effects of APDs, since the therapeutic actions of APDs do not match the time course of postsynaptic DA receptor blockade, but do match the time course of these delayed effects on presynaptic activity (42). Clearly, the neurophysiological effects of atypical antipsychotic drugs may differ following an acute dose from long-term treatment.

When administered chronically, APDs can cause a drastic change in DA systems. In contrast to the enhanced firing rate and bursting of DA cells following an acute APD administration, long-term treatment results in a drastic reduction in the number of spontaneously active DA cells (6,35,41,43,44). This seems to be different from simple inactivation of neurons, since agents that would normally activate silent cells fail to engage DA neurons rendered silent by chronic APD treatment (35). In fact, DA cell activity can be restored by applying negative current or with DA agonists (45). This quiet state of DA neurons has been termed "depolarization block," and it is supposedly the result of excessive excitation of these neurons. When neurons are overly excited, they can depolarize to a point in which they cease firing. Because of this, depolarization block can be reversed by applying a GABA agonist or the DA agonist apomorphine (35). The mechanisms resulting in depolarization block are thought to involve an enhanced activation of feedback loops projecting to DA neurons, since striatal lesions (35) or cholecystokinin antagonists (46) abolish depolarization block. Thus, sustained DA receptor blockade by APDs could enhance the activity of basal ganglia–cortical loops, yielding an increased drive of electrical activity in the DA cell populations that causes excessive depolarization and the subsequent blockade of firing.

Different populations of DA neurons show depolarization block in response to atypical and typical APDs, and this is consistent with observations that these drug types exert their action on separate DA systems. While haloperidol can induce depolarization block in both the nigrostriatal and mesolimbic/mesocortical pathways, clozapine does so only in mesolimbic/mesocortical neurons, sparing the nigrostriatal pathway (38,43,47–49) (Figure 4). A similar regional specificity was reported for quetiapine (38) and olanzapine (50). In an excellent recent review, however, Ben Westerink (51) suggested that these different regional effects are not due to atypical APDs acting on a particular type of DA neurons, but to the moderate levels of D_2 receptor occupancy they achieve. Thus, prolonged treatment with compounds yielding a moderate (< 80%) D_2 receptor

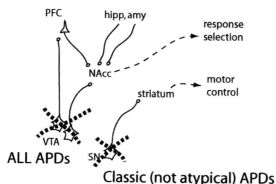

Figure 4 Atypical APDs cause depolarization block in mesolimbic and mesocortical neurons, but not in nigrostriatal dopamine projections. Classic APDs elicit depolarization block in DA neurons projecting to motor striatal regions, resulting in their higher propensity for EPS.

occupancy may cause depolarization block in VTA DA cells, whereas the greater than 80% D_2 occupancy typically attained with classical APDs renders nigrostriatal neurons also in depolarization block. In other words, atypical APDs may spare substantia nigra DA neurons precisely by virtue of the lower D_2 occupancy they cause.

Depolarization block can be evidenced by means other than electrophysiological recordings. A silencing of DA cells should cause a reduced level of DA in target areas. Indeed, chronic treatment with haloperidol decreases basal DA levels in the striatum measured with in vivo microdialysis (52). Furthermore, chronic treatment with clozapine reduces DA levels in the nucleus accumbens (53) and PFC (54). This effect of clozapine could not be observed in the caudate-putamen (53,54), an area in which haloperidol decreases DA levels (55). These results also support the idea of a selective regional action of atypical APDs. Although depolarization block by chronic APDs has been contested as being observed only in anesthetized animals (56), there is compelling behavioral evidence for this phenomenon (41). Both chronic haloperidol and clozapine attenuate reward performance in awake rats, an effect reversed by the DA agonist apomorphine (57). Thus, although depolarization block is a common mechanism for all APDs, atypical drugs may preferentially induce it in DA cells that project to the nucleus accumbens and PFC, avoiding the motor DA projections. Also, this phenomenon only emerges after a few weeks of treatment, a time course similar to that needed to obtain clinical effects. One of the key elements in the actions of atypical APDs, therefore, is their ability to set the mesolimbic and mesocortical projections into a new steady-state. While this might not restore "normal" function in the system, it might create a different level of activity in the target areas and eliminate the abnormal DA activity and reduce symptoms caused by hyperdopaminergic responses.

A number of new approaches are emerging regarding atypical APD treatment. One interesting recent addition to this class of drugs is aripiprazole (Abilify®). This is a new atypical APD, with partial agonist activity at D_2 receptors and antagonism at 5-HT$_{2A}$ receptors (58). Unlike other atypical APDs, aripiprazole administration can result in high D_2 receptor occupancy (up to 95%) without causing EPS; this is thought to result from its partial agonist activity (59). Very few studies have been conducted assessing electrophysiological actions of aripiprazole. The emerging picture is that this compound can reduce VTA DA cell firing by acting on autoreceptors (60). Thus, it may prevent the enhanced DA release evoked by burst firing. The partial agonist profile may cause the reduced ability to down-regulate the nigrostriatal pathway, resulting in a reduced EPS liability.

V. EFFECTS OF ATYPICAL ANTIPSYCHOTICS ON NMDA GLUTAMATE RECEPTORS

Negative symptoms can be ameliorated by atypical APDs, and this may be related to their ability to enhance a deficient glutamatergic cortical activity. In particular, hypofrontality in schizophrenia seems to be tied to low levels of glutamate NMDA receptor activity (31,34). This is evidenced in the ability of NMDA antagonists (such as phencyclidine or ketamine) to elicit psychotic symptoms in naïve subjects (61), and to evoke a relapse in schizophrenia patients in remission (62). Clozapine, but not haloperidol, can reverse changes in NMDA receptor activation brought about by subchronic administration of phencyclidine (63). Also, olanzapine and clozapine enhance NMDA currents in the PFC (64,65). In addition, glutamate release was found to be increased in the nucleus accumbens following chronic clozapine, but not haloperidol (66), an effect thought to result from enhanced cortical activity. These actions of atypical APDs in the PFC may be related to negative symptom improvement, as well as amelioration of cognitive deficits. Indeed, many behavioral effects produced by administration of NMDA receptor antagonists in rats can be reversed by clozapine and olanzapine (67). However, risperidone (Risperdal®), like typical APDs, failed to reverse the social withdrawal elicited by phencyclidine (67). On the basis of these findings, one could argue that most atypical APDs can enhance cortical NMDA receptor function and that this effect might add to their efficacy in patients with schizophrenia.

APDs can also augment NMDA receptor activity by tapping into their intracellular modulation by DA (68). Since blockade of D_2 receptors may enhance NMDA function, APD efficacy could be related to both DA blockade and a subsequent enhancement of NMDA function. In the PFC, NMDA responses can be enhanced by co-activation with D_1 DA receptors (69). Clozapine can enhance glutamatergic excitatory synaptic potentials in the PFC, and this effect can be blocked by a D_1 antagonist (70). Thus, D_1–NMDA interactions in the PFC could also be a target of atypical APDs, an action that may improve cognitive functions.

VI. CLINICAL NEUROPHYSIOLOGY OF ATYPICAL ANTIPSYCHOTIC DRUGS

Atypical APDs can also reverse electroencephalographic deficits in schizophrenia patients. EEG effects of acute olanzapine or clozapine include increasing theta rhythms, as seen with other medications that cause somnolence (71). A variety of alterations in evoked potentials and event-related potentials has also been detected in schizophrenia patients.

For example, P50 suppression is a reduction in EEG responses to pairs of clicks, and is taken as a measure of sensory gating. P50 suppression is normalized in schizophrenia patients receiving clozapine, olanzapine, or risperidone, but not in those receiving classical APDs (72,73). This finding suggests that atypical, not classical, APDs normalize sensory gating functions in schizophrenia. Clozapine also affects a number of neurophysiological measures of attention, known to be disrupted in schizophrenia. P300 and mismatch negativity are cognitive event-related potentials altered in schizophrenia patients. Clozapine, but not haloperidol, treatment increases P300 amplitude (74), but fails to improve mismatch negativity (74). Risperidone, on the other hand, shortens the latency of P300, without changing its amplitude (75). These results suggest that atypical APDs may improve the neurophysiological bases of attention; clozapine may enhance attention, while risperidone may differ in increasing the speed of information processing in schizophrenia patients.

The effects of APDs on sensorimotor gating can be tested in animals and human beings using the phenomenon of prepulse inhibition. An unexpected strong sensory input (e.g., a loud sound or a strong puff of air delivered to the face) typically results in a measurable startle reaction. If the startling stimulus is preceded by an attenuated stimulus (prepulse), the startling reaction is diminished. This phenomenon, called prepulse inhibition, is observed in normal subjects and can also be tested in experimental animals. Schizophrenia patients and their close relatives exhibit a clear deficit in prepulse inhibition (76). This deficit has been suggested to stem from an impaired ability to filter out irrelevant information. Altered prepulse inhibition is also a central component of developmental animal models. In rats with a neonatal ventral hippocampal lesion (77) and in animals reared in social isolation (78), prepulse inhibition is disrupted. The deficit in animals with a neonatal ventral hippocampal lesion is not observed following chronic treatment with atypical (but not classical) APDs (79). The glutamate hypothesis of schizophrenia is also supported by NMDA antagonists impairing prepulse inhibition (80–82). In addition, DA agonists also disrupt prepulse inhibition (83). Thus, this phenomenon requires proper levels of activity of NMDA and DA systems, both in the nucleus accumbens (80,84) and PFC (85).

All clinically effective APDs can reduce the disruptive effects of DA agonists in this model. This action has been shown for haloperidol and other classical APDs, although they do so weakly. Atypical APDs have a stronger effect reversing disrupted prepulse inhibition; this is true for clozapine (81,86), ziprasidone (Geodon®) (87), and olanzapine (88). The disruption of prepulse inhibition by NMDA antagonists is also reversed by atypical APDs (88), but not by haloperidol (89). Taking all these results together, it is not surprising that prepulse inhibition has been used as a screening tool for potential atypical antipsychotics (90,91). Most studies mentioned above are preclinical, however. Studies on the effects of APDs on prepulse inhibition in schizophrenia patients are now emerging. As predicted by animal data, patients receiving atypical APDs exhibit normal prepulse inhibition whereas this phenomenon is disrupted in patients receiving classical APDs (92,93). However, a recent study indicates that 3-month treatment with risperidone failed to improve prepulse inhibition (94). This discrepancy may be explained by risperidone being different from other atypical APDs in many respects, particularly in its lesser ability to increase NMDA function. Indeed, atypical APD effects on prepulse inhibition are much stronger for clozapine than for risperidone (93). These results indicate that sensorimotor gating and overall cognitive function can be improved to a greater extent by atypical APDs, although with some differences among the different drugs.

VII. OTHER ATYPICAL ANTIPSYCHOTIC ACTIONS

Atypical APDs have a variety of other neurophysiological effects. In the nucleus accumbens, cortical and limbic information can be integrated to select behavioral responses appropriate for the contextual conditions (15,95). An important element in this integration is the establishment of ensembles of active neurons. DA can gate these ensembles by sustaining membrane depolarization in a population of nucleus accumbens neurons (15). Such depolarizations can be synchronized among the neurons in these ensembles by virtue of direct cell-to-cell electronic transmission. Indeed, nucleus accumbens neurons exhibit gap junctions (96), which are channels directly connecting neurons that allow equalization of slow membrane potentials and sharing of second messengers. DA has been shown to modulate gap junction permeability in the nucleus accumbens (96). Chronic, but not acute, APD treatment increases electrical coupling in the nucleus accumbens; this effect is induced by both haloperidol and clozapine. On the other hand, haloperidol, but not clozapine, enhances coupling in the motor striatum (97). This suggests that at least clozapine (and probably other atypical APDs as well) can reinforce ensemble coding in limbic, but not motor basal ganglia circuits. This action may allow a restoration of impaired function and cortical throughput in this region.

Other transmitter systems are also affected by APD treatment. Olanzapine, for example, activates firing of neurons in the locus coeruleus, where the cell bodies of norepinephrine neurons are found (98). This region gives rise to a widespread array of noradrenergic projections to the cortex and other brain regions, and is supposed to be involved in attention and arousal. Thus, this effect of olanzapine has been proposed to be related to negative symptom improvement (98). Ziprasidone is different from other atypical APDs in its blockade of 5-HT$_1$ receptors (99).

VIII. CONCLUSION

Atypical and typical APDs share several electrophysiological actions. Since both drug classes are clinically effective, primarily against positive symptoms, it is likely that the shared effects are involved in their efficacy for this group of symptoms. The ability of both drug types to elicit depolarization block in the VTA may therefore be a critical component in improving positive symptoms. The differences between typical and atypical APDs, on the other hand, can explain the higher propensity of the former to cause EPS and the stronger effects of the latter on cognitive deficits. Classical APDs cause DA neurons in the substantia nigra to enter into depolarization block, and so affect motor control and cause EPS. Atypical APDs not only do not affect nigrostriatal projections, but they also can restore changes brought about by blockade of NMDA receptors. These effects are likely to account for their efficacy in improving negative symptoms and cognitive deficits. Overall, atypical APDs exert their actions in mesolimbic and mesocortical projections, affecting DA–glutamate function in the PFC and in the ventral striatum. Many of the preclinical studies to support these hypotheses have been primarily conducted with clozapine. The effects of other atypical APDs and their potential differences with clozapine remain to be comprehensively determined.

REFERENCES

1. Seeman P. Dopamine receptors and the dopamine hypothesis of schizophrenia. Synapse 1987; 1:133–152.
2. Stockmeier CA, DiCarlo JJ, Zhang Y, Thompson P, Meltzer HY. Characterization of typical and atypical antipsychotic drugs based on in vivo occupancy of serotonin2 and dopamine2 receptors. J Pharmacol Exp Ther 1993; 266:1374–1384.
3. Meltzer HY, McGurk SR. The effects of clozapine, risperidone, and olanzapine on cognitive function in schizophrenia. Schizophr Bull 1999; 25:233–255.
4. Kapur S, Seeman P. Does fast dissociation from the dopamine D2 receptor explain the action of atypical antipsychotics?: A new hypothesis. Am J Psychiatry 2001; 158:360–369.
5. Carlsson A, Lindqvist M, Magnusson T, Waldeck B. On the presence of 3-hydroxytyramine in brain. Science 1958; 127:471.

6. Grace AA. Phasic versus tonic dopamine release and the modulation of dopamine system responsivity: a hypothesis for the etiology of schizophrenia. Neuroscience 1991; 41:1–24.

7. Grace AA, Onn S-P. Morphology and electrophysiological properties of immunocytochemically identified rat dopamine neurons recorded in vitro. J Neurosci 1989; 9:3463–3481.

8. Overton P, Clark D. Iontophoretically administered drugs acting at the N-methyl-D-aspartate receptor modulate burst firing in A9 dopamine neurons in the rat. Synapse 1992; 10:431–440.

9. Chergui K, Charléty PJ, Akaoka H, et al. Tonic activation of NMDA receptors causes spontaneous burst discharge of rat midbrain dopamine neurons in vivo. Eur J Neurosci 1993; 5:137–144.

10. Grace AA, Bunney BS. Intracellular and extracellular electrophysiology of nigral dopaminergic neurons – 1. Identification and characterization. Neuroscience 1983; 10:301–315.

11. Chergui K, Akaoka H, Charléty PJ, Saunier CF, Buda M, Chouvet G. Subthalamic nucleus modulates burst firing of nigral dopamine neurones via NMDA receptors. Neuroreport 1994; 5:1185–1188.

12. Kitai ST, Shepard PD, Callaway JC, Scroggs R. Afferent modulation of dopamine neuron firing patterns. Curr Opin Neurobiol 1999; 9:690–697.

13. Gonon FG. Nonlinear relationship between impulse flow and dopamine released by rat midbrain dopaminergic neurons as studied by in vivo electrochemistry. Neuroscience 1988; 24:19–28.

14. O'Donnell. Ensemble coding in the nucleus accumbens. Psychobiology 1999; 27:187–197.

15. O'Donnell P. Dopamine gating of forebrain neural ensembles. Eur J Neurosci 2003; 17:429–435.

16. Schultz W, Dayan P, Montague PR. A neural substrate of prediction and reward. Science 1997; 275:1593–1599.

17. Horvitz JC. Mesolimbocortical and nigrostriatal dopamine responses to salient non-reward events. Neuroscience 2000; 96:651–656.

18. Groves PM, Wilson CJ, Young SJ, Rebec GV. Self-inhibition by dopaminergic neurons. Science 1975; 190:522–529.

19. Pucak ML, Grace AA. Evidence that systemically administered dopamine antagonists activate dopamine neuron firing primarily by blockade of somatodendritic autoreceptors. J Pharmacol Exp Ther 1994; 271:1181–1192.

20. Gonon FG, Buda MJ. Regulation of dopamine release by impulse flow and by autoreceptors as studied by in vivo voltammetry in the rat striatum. Neuroscience 1985; 14:765–774.

21. Wolf ME, Roth RH. Dopamine neurons projecting to the medial prefrontal cortex possess release-modulating autoreceptors. Neuropharmacology 1987; 26:1053–1059.

22. Carlsson A, Lindqvist M. Effect of chlorpromazine or haloperidol on formation of 3-methoxytyramine and normetanephrine in mouse brain. Acta Pharmacol Toxicol 1963; 20:140–144.

23. Creese I, Burt DR, Snyder SH. Dopamine receptor binding predicts clinical and pharmacological potencies of antischizophrenic drugs. Science 1976; 192: 596–598.

24. Angrist B, Santhananthan G, Wilk S, Gershon S. Amphetamine psychosis: behavioral and biochemical aspects. J Psychiat Res 1974; 11:13–23.

25. Jenkins RB, Groh RH. Mental symptoms in parkinsonian patients treated with L-DOPA. Lancet 1970; ii:177–179.

26. van Kammen DP, Bok van Kammen W, Mann LS, Seppala T, Linnoila M. Dopamine metabolism in the cerebrospinal fluid of drug-free schizophrenic patients with and without cortical atrophy. Arch Gen Psychiatry 1986; 43: 978–983.

27. Heritch AJ. Evidence for reduced and dysregulated turnover of dopamine in schizophrenia. Schizophr Bull 1990; 16:605–615.

28. Angrist BM, Peselow E, Rubinstein M, Corwin J, Rotrosen J. Partial improvement in negative schizophrenia symptoms after amphetamine. Psychopharmacology 1982; 78:128–130.

29. Sanfilipo M, Wolkin A, Angrist B, et al. Amphetamine and negative symptoms of schizophrenia. Psychopharmacology 1996; 123:211–214.

30. Weinberger DR. Implications of normal brain development for the pathogenesis of schizophrenia. Arch Gen Psychiatry 1987; 44:660–669.

31. Grace AA. Gating of information flow within the limbic system and the pathophysiology of schizophrenia. Brain Res Rev 2000; 31:330–341.

32. Csernansky JG, Murphy GM, Faustman WO. Limbic/mesolimbic connections and the pathogenesis of schizophrenia. Biol Psychiatry 1991; 30:383–400.

33. Davis KL, Kahn RS, Ko G, Davidson M. Dopamine in schizophrenia: a review and reconceptualization. Am J Psychiatry 1991; 148:1474–1486.

34. O'Donnell P, Grace AA. Dysfunctions in multiple interrelated systems as the neurobiological bases of schizophrenic symptom clusters. Schizophr Bull 1998; 24:267–283.

35. Bunney BS, Grace AA. Acute and chronic haloperidol treatment: comparison of effects on nigral dopaminergic cell activity. Life Sci 1978; 23: 1715–1728.

36. Grace AA, Bunney BS. The control of firing pattern in nigral dopamine neurons: Burst firing. J Neurosci 1984; 4:2877–2890.

37. Kamata K, Rebec GV. Nigral dopaminergic neurons: differential sensitivity to apomorphine following long-term treatment with low and high doses of amphetamine. Brain Res 1984; 321:147–150.

38. Goldstein JM, Litwin LC, Sutton EB, Malick JB. Seroquel: electrophysiological profile of a potential atypical antipsychotic. Psychopharmacology 1993; 112:293–298.

39. Melis M, Diana M, Gessa GL. Clozapine potently stimulates mesocortical dopamine neurons. Eur J Pharmacol 1999; 366:R11–R13.

40. Stockton ME, Rasmussen K. Olanzapine, a novel atypical antipsychotic, reverses d-amphetamine-induced inhibition of midbrain dopamine cells. Psychopharmacology (Berl) 1996; 124:50–56.

41. Grace AA, Bunney BS, Moore H, Todd CL. Dopamine cell depolarization block as a model for the therapeutic actions of antipsychotic drugs. Trends Neurosci 1997; 20:31–37.
42. Pickar D, Labarca R, Linnoila M, et al. Neuroleptic-induced decrease in plasma homovamillic acid and antipsychotic activity in schizophrenic patients. Science 1984; 225:954–957.
43. Chiodo LA, Bunney BS. Typical and atypical neuroleptics: differential effects of chronic administration on the activity of A9 and A10 midbrain dopaminergic neurons. J Neurosci 1983; 3:1607–1619.
44. Skarsfeldt T. Comparison of short-term administration of sertindole, clozapine and haloperidol on the inactivation of midbrain dopamine neurons in the rat. Eur J Pharmacol 1994; 254:291–294.
45. Grace AA, Bunney BS. Induction of depolarization block in midbrain dopamine neurons by repeated administration of haloperidol: analysis using in vivo intracellular recording. J Pharmacol Exp Ther 1986; 238: 1092–1100.
46. Wang RY, Jiang L-H, Ti X, Kasser RJ. Cholecystokinin and actions of antipsychotic drugs. In: Hughes J, Dockray G, Woodruff G, eds. The Neuro-peptide Cholecystokinin (CCK). Anatomy and Biochemistry, Receptors, Pharmacology, and Physiology. Chichester: Ellis Horwood, 1989:163–170.
47. White FJ, Wang RY. Differential effects of classical and atypical antipsychotic drugs on A9 and A10 dopamine neurons. Science 1983; 221:1054–1057.
48. Skarsfeldt T. Differential effects after repeated treatment with haloperidol, clozapine, thioridazine and tefludazine on SNC and VTA dopamine neurones in rats. Life Sci 1988; 42:1037–1044.
49. Todorova A, Dimpfel W. Multiunit activity from the A9 and A10 areas in rats following chronic treatment with different neuroleptic drugs. Eur Neuropsychopharmacol 1994; 4:491–501.
50. Stockton ME, Rasmussen K. Electrophysiological effects of olanzapine, a novel atypical antipsychotic, on A9 and A10 dopamine neurons. Neuropsycho-pharmacology 1996; 14:97–105.
51. Westerink BH. Can antipsychotic drugs be classified by their effects on a particular group of dopamine neurons in the brain? Eur J Pharmacol 2002; 455:1–18.
52. Lane RF, Blaha CD. Chronic haloperidol decreases dopamine release in striatum and nucleus accumbens in vivo: depolarization block as a possible mechanism of action. Brain Res Bull 1987; 18:135–138.
53. Chen J, Paredes W, Gardner EL. Chronic treatment with clozapine selectively decreases basal dopamine release in nucleus accumbens but not in caudate-putamen as measured by in vivo brain microdialysis: further evidence for depolarization block. Neurosci Lett 1991; 122:127–131.
54. Hernandez L, Hoebel BG. Chronic clozapine selectively decreases prefrontal cortex dopamine as shown by simultaneous cortical, accumbens, and striatal microdialysis in freely moving rats. Pharmacol Biochem Behav 1995; 52: 581–589.

55. Moore H, Todd C, Grace A. Striatal extracellular dopamine levels in rats with haloperidol-induced depolarization block of substantia nigra dopamine neurons. J Neurosci 1998; 18:5068–5077.

56. Mereu G, Lilliu V, Vargiu P, Muntoni AL, Diana M, Gessa GL. Failure of chronic haloperidol to induce depolarization inactivation of dopamine neurons in unanesthetized rats. Eur J Pharmacol 1994; 264:449–453.

57. Boye SM, Rompre PP. Behavioral evidence of depolarization block of dopamine neurons after chronic treatment with haloperidol and clozapine. J Neurosci 2000; 20:1229–1239.

58. McGavin JK, Goa KL. Aripiprazole. CNS Drugs 2002; 16:779–786.

59. Yokoi F, Grunder G, Biziere K, et al. Dopamine D2 and D3 receptor occupancy in normal humans treated with the antipsychotic drug aripiprazole (OPC 14597): a study using positron emission tomography and [11C]raclopride. Neuropsychopharmacology 2002; 27:248–259.

60. Momiyama T, Amano T, Todo N, Sasa M. Inhibition by a putative antipsychotic quinolinone derivative (OPC-14597) of dopaminergic neurons in the ventral tegmental area. Eur J Pharmacol 1996; 310:1–8.

61. Javitt DC, Zukin SR. Recent advances in the phenciclidine model of schizophrenia. Am J Psychiatry 1991; 148:1301–1308.

62. Luby ED, Cohen BD, Rosenbaum G, Gottlieb JS, Kelly R. Study of a new schizophrenomimetic drug – Sernyl. Arch Neurol Psychiatry 1959; 81: 363–369.

63. Arvanov VL, Wang RY. Clozapine, but not haloperidol, prevents the functional hyperactivity of N-methyl-D-aspartate receptors in rat cortical neurons induced by subchronic administration of phencyclidine. J Pharmacol Exp Ther 1999; 289:1000–1006.

64. Jardemark KE, Ai J, Ninan I, Wang RY. Biphasic modulation of NMDA-induced responses in pyramidal cells of the medial prefrontal cortex by Y-931, a potential atypical antipsychotic drug. Synapse 2001; 41:294–300.

65. Jardemark KE, Liang X, Arvanov V, Wang RY. Subchronic treatment with either clozapine, olanzapine or haloperidol produces a hyposensitive response of the rat cortical cells to N-methyl-D-aspartate. Neuroscience 2000; 100:1–9.

66. Yamamoto BK, Cooperman MA. Differential effects of chronic antipsychotic drug treatment on extracellular glutamate and dopamine concentrations. J Neurosci 1994; 14:4159–4166.

67. Corbett R, Camacho F, Woods AT, et al. Antipsychotic agents antagonize non-competitive *N*-methyl-D-aspartate antagonist-induced behaviors. Psychopharmacology 1995; 120:67–74.

68. Leveque JC, Macias W, Rajadhyaksha A, et al. Intracellular modulation of NMDA receptor function by antipsychotic drugs. J Neurosci 2000; 20:4011–4020.

69. Wang J, O'Donnell P. D$_1$ dopamine receptors potentiate NMDA-mediated excitability increase in rat prefrontal cortical pyramidal neurons. Cerebral Cortex 2001; 11:452–462.

70. Chen L, Yang CR. Interaction of dopamine D1 and NMDA receptors mediates acute clozapine potentiation of glutamate EPSPs in rat prefrontal cortex. J Neurophysiol 2002; 87:2324–2336.
71. Hubl D, Kleinlogel H, Frolich L, et al. Multilead quantitative electroencephalogram profile and cognitive evoked potentials (P300) in healthy subjects after a single dose of olanzapine. Psychopharmacology (Berl) 2001; 158:281–288.
72. Nagamoto HT, Adler LE, Hea RA, Griffith JM, McRae KA, Freedman R. Gating of auditory P50 in schizophrenics: unique effects of clozapine. Biol Psychiatry 1996; 40:181–188.
73. Light GA, Geyer MA, Clementz BA, Cadenhead KS, Braff DL. Normal P50 suppression in schizophrenia patients treated with atypical antipsychotic medications. Am J Psychiatry 2000; 157:767–771.
74. Umbricht D, Javitt D, Novak G, et al. Effects of clozapine on auditory event-related potentials in schizophrenia. Biol Psychiatry 1998; 44:716–725.
75. Iwanami A, Okajima Y, Isono H, et al. Effects of risperidone on event-related potentials in schizophrenic patients. Pharmacopsychiatry 2001; 34:73–79.
76. Braff DL, Geyer MA. Sensorimotor gating and schizophrenia. Human and animal model studies. Arch Gen Psychiatry 1990; 47:181–188.
77. Lipska BK, Swerdlow NR, Geyer MA, Jaskiw GE, Braff DL, Weinberger DR. Neonatal excitotoxic hippocampal damage in rats cause post-pubertal changes in prepulse inhibition of startle and its disruption by apomorphine. Psychopharmacology 1995; 132:303–310.
78. Geyer MA, Wilkinson LS, Humby T, Robbins TW. Isolation rearing of rats produces a deficit in prepulse inhibition of acoustic startle similar to that in schizophrenia. Biol Psychiatry 1993; 34:361–372.
79. Le Pen G, Moreau JL. Disruption of prepulse inhibition of startle reflex in a neurodevelopmental model of schizophrenia: reversal by clozapine, olanzapine and risperidone but not by haloperidol. Neuropsychopharmacology 2002; 27:1–11.
80. Reijmers LGJE, Vanderheyden PML, Peeters BWMM. Changes in prepulse inhibition after local administration of NMDA receptor ligands in the core region of the rat nucleus accumbens. Eur J Pharmacol 1995; 272:131–138.
81. Bakshi VP, Swerdlow NR, Geyer MA. Clozapine antagonizes phencyclidine-induced deficits in sensorimotor gating of the startle response. J Pharmacol Exp Ther 1994; 271:787–794.
82. Al-Amin HA, Schwarzkopf SB. Effects of the PCP analog dizocilpine on sensory gating: potential relevance to clinical subtypes of schizophrenia. Biol Psychiatry 1996; 40:744–754.
83. Swerdlow NR, Keith VA, Braff DL, Geyer MA. Effects of spiperone, raclopride, SCH 23390 and clozapine on apomorphine inhibition of sensorimotor gating of the startle response in rat. J Pharmacol Exp Ther 1991; 256:530–536.
84. Wan FJ, Geyer MA, Swerdlow NR. Accumbens D_2 modulation of sensorimotor gating in rats: assessing anatomical localization. Pharmacol Biochem Behav 1994; 49:155–163.

85. Ellenbroek BA, Budde S, Cools AR. Prepulse inhibition and latent inhibition: the role of dopamine in the medial prefrontal cortex. Neuroscience 1996; 75:535–542.

86. Swerdlow NR, Caine SB, Braff DL, Geyer MA. The neural substrates of sensorimotor gating of the startle reflex: a review of recent findings and their implications. J Psychopharmacol 1992; 6:176–190.

87. Mansbach RS, Carver J, Zorn SH. Blockade of drug-induced deficits in prepulse inhibition of acoustic startle by ziprasidone. Pharmacol Biochem Behav 2001; 69:535–542.

88. Bakshi VP, Geyer MA. Antagonism of phencyclidine-induced deficits in prepulse inhibition by the putative atypical antipsychotic olanzapine. Psychopharmacology 1995; 122:198–201.

89. Keith VA, Mansbach RS, Geyer MA. Failure of haloperidol to block the effects of phencyclidine and dizocilpine on prepulse inhibition of startle. Biol Psychiatry 1991; 30:557–566.

90. Rigdon G, Viik K. Prepulse inhibition as a screening test for potential antipsychotics. Drug Dev Res. 1991; 23:91–99.

91. Swerdlow NR, Geyer MA. Using an animal model of deficient sensorimotor gating to study the pathophysiology and new treatments of schizophrenia. Schizophr Bull 1998; 24:285–301.

92. Leumann L, Feldon J, Vollenweider FX, Ludewig K. Effects of typical and atypical antipsychotics on prepulse inhibition and latent inhibition in chronic schizophrenia. Biol Psychiatry 2002; 52:729–739.

93. Oranje B, Van Oel CJ, Gispen-De Wied CC, Verbaten MN, Kahn RS. Effects of typical and atypical antipsychotics on the prepulse inhibition of the startle reflex in patients with schizophrenia. J Clin Psychopharmacol 2002; 22:359–365.

94. Mackeprang T, Kristiansen KT, Glenthoj BY. Effects of antipsychotics on prepulse inhibition of the startle response in drug-naive schizophrenic patients. Biol Psychiatry 2002; 52:863–873.

95. Goto Y, O'Donnell P. Timing-dependent limbic-motor synaptic integration in the nucleus accumbens. Proc Natl Acad Sci USA 2002; 99:13189–13193.

96. O'Donnell P, Grace AA. Dopaminergic modulation of dye coupling between neurons in the core and shell regions of the nucleus accumbens. J Neurosci 1993; 13:3456–3471.

97. O'Donnell P, Grace AA. Different effects of subchronic clozapine and haloperidol on dye coupling between neurons in the rat striatal complex. Neuroscience 1995; 66:763–767.

98. Dawe GS, Huff KD, Vandergriff JL, Sharp T, O'Neill MJ, Rasmussen K. Olanzapine activates the rat locus coeruleus: in vivo electrophysiology and c-Fos immunoreactivity. Biol Psychiatry 2001; 50:510–520.

99. Sprouse JS, Reynolds LS, Braselton JP, Rollema H, Zorn SH. Comparison of the novel antipsychotic ziprasidone with clozapine and olanzapine: inhibition of dorsal raphe cell firing and the role of 5-HT1A receptor activation. Neuropsychopharmacology 1999; 21:622–631.

4

Behavioral Models of Atypical Antipsychotic Drug Action in Rodents

Mark E. Bardgett

Northern Kentucky University,
Highland Heights, Kentucky, U.S.A.

I. INTRODUCTION

The previous chapters in this book have discussed how atypical antipsychotic drugs interact with distinct receptors, produce unique patterns of gene expression in the central nervous system, and exert differential effects on neuronal firing rates. Ultimately, however, it is the actions of these drugs on behavior which may be the most predictive of their clinical value. A drug that interacts with the right receptor, turns on the right gene, and activates the right set of neurons will not garner much interest if it does not affect the right behavior. The purpose of this chapter is to present the preclinical behavioral tests which are used to predict antipsychotic drug action and to discriminate potential atypical antipsychotic drugs from typical ones. In presenting each test, the caveats and interpretative problems unique to each particular assay will be considered. This chapter will focus solely on work in rats and mice. While beyond the scope of this review, it should be noted however that the effects of antipsychotic drugs are sometimes tested in non-human primates.

II. WHAT IS AN ANIMAL MODEL OF ANTIPSYCHOTIC DRUG ACTION?

Before we can examine the clinical effects of antipsychotic drugs in humans, we must study their behavioral effects in animals. But the choice of behavioral tests is not easy because psychotic symptoms may be uniquely human. One can emulate the clinical symptoms of Parkinson's disease, namely muscular rigidity, tremor and impaired movement, in an animal model. In this case, the preclinical behavioral test for an anti-parkinsonian drug is its ability to reverse impaired movement and coordination in affected animals. Even in models of some psychiatric disorders, one can be reasonably assured that one is observing a similar phenomenon in a rodent. Anxiety is a good example. One can assume with some confidence that an otherwise healthy animal which remains huddled in a darkened enclosed area, is relatively inactive, and will not explore unfamiliar areas is anxious or fearful. The test of an anti-anxiety drug is then whether a drug produces an opposite effect in the animal: does it increase locomotor or exploratory activity? These behavioral models can be considered to be *face-valid* models, since similar behaviors are manifested in the clinical disorder and in the animal model.

So how does one emulate psychosis in a rat or mouse in order to test the effects of an antipsychotic drug? This question often provokes amusing responses from students, clinicians, and researchers alike. Because one cannot be sure if an animal has experienced a hallucination or delusion, much less, be able to measure such a thing, behavioral models of anti-psychotic drug action do not involve reversals of rat or mouse psychosis. As a result, the field of behavioral pharmacology lacks face-valid animal models of psychosis.

Nonetheless, behavioral pharmacologists have developed several behavioral models that have been proven to predict a drug's antipsychotic potential. One of the best preclinical predictors of antipsychotic activity in rodents is a drug's ability to reduce the hyperactivity produced by the stimulant drug, d-amphetamine. Granted, hyperactivity in a rodent and psychosis in a human are not the same thing, but drugs which reduce hyperactivity are potential candidates for reducing psychosis in humans (see below). Such an animal model possesses a more important form of validity in terms of drug development: *predictive validity* (23). Predictive validity has several meanings (23), but one definition involves the ability of a test to reliably discriminate a clinically effective drug from a non-effective one. A positive result in a single preclinical test that possesses predictive validity is typically not enough to establish a drug's potential antipsychotic efficacy. The case for potential clinical efficacy is always stronger if the drug shows positive effects in a series of other preclinical behavioral and biological assays possessing predictive validity.

Finally, it should be noted that some aspects of schizophrenia may already lend themselves to face-valid emulation at the level of animal behavioral testing and possess some level of predictive validity. One aspect of schizophrenia that may cause significant functional impairment for patients is reduced social interaction. At an animal level, researchers can take advantage of the rich social interactions often observed in laboratory animals and record the effects of drugs that either increase or decrease such interactions. Another aspect of schizophrenia that has received increasing attention is the memory impairment exhibited by many patients. Preclinical research can ascertain drugs that improve memory in laboratory animals in the context of pathological conditions believed to exist in people with schizophrenia. Thus, as the symptoms of schizophrenia, such as decreased social interaction or specific memory deficits become better appreciated, understood, and operationally defined (see below), more and better face-valid models of schizophrenia and atypical antipsychotic drug action will become available.

III. HOW IS ATYPICALITY DEFINED AND ESTABLISHED?

As discussed in the first chapter of this book, pharmacologists and psychiatrists make distinctions between typical and atypical antipsychotic drugs. Some of these distinctions are based upon differences in the activity of the two drug classes in preclinical behavioral models or in clinical use. To date, all clinically effective antipsychotic drugs, typical and atypical, block the D_2-type receptor for the neurotransmitter dopamine (DA) (although the potential antipsychotic drug, aripiprazole may act as a partial agonist at D_2 sites (32)). However, according to one pharmacological definition, atypical antipsychotic drugs have the additional feature of blocking the $5\text{-}HT_2$-type receptor for the neurotransmitter, serotonin (5-HT or 5-hydroxytryptamine). Others have argued for a different pharmacological definition of atypicality, perhaps most recently by Kapur and Seeman (29) who proposed that fast dissociation from the D_2 receptor is the distinguishing factor between typical and atypical drugs. These pharmacological distinctions between typical and atypical drugs may or may not fully explain their differential effects on physiology, animal behavior, and clinical symptoms.

Another criterion for atypicality is anatomy; that is, how a drug affects physiology in a brain region-specific manner. Animals that are injected daily for 2–3 weeks with clinically effective antipsychotic drugs exhibit reduced firing rates (depolarization blockade) of DA neurons found in the ventral

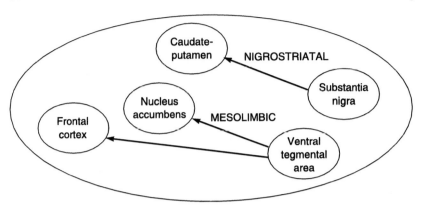

Figure 1 Schematic of mesolimbic and nigrostriatal dopaminergic projection systems in the mammalian brain. Neurons that produce DA project from the ventral tegmental area and release DA into synapses within the nucleus accumbens and prefrontal cortex. This projection is known as the mesolimbic pathway and, the action of antipsychotic drugs, both typical and atypical, within this pathway is likely to account for their antipsychotic effects. In animals, this pathway is responsible for locomotor activity and PPI. Neurons that produce DA also project from the substantia nigra and release DA into synapses within the caudate-putamen (or striatum). This projection is known as the nigrostriatal pathway and, the action of typical antipsychotic drugs within this pathway likely accounts for their motor side effects. In animals, this pathway is responsible for catalepsy, stereotypy, and oral dyskinesia.

tegmental area of the midbrain. These neurons have projections that terminate in forebrain regions such as the nucleus accumbens, frontal cortex, and limbic system. This projection is known as the mesolimbic projection (see Figure 1). In comparison, chronic treatment with typical antipsychotic drugs also produces depolarization blockade in DA neurons found in the substantia nigra of the midbrain. The DA-producing neurons in the substantia nigra project to the striatum (also known as the corpus striatum or caudate nucleus in the rat) and this projection is known as the nigrostriatal projection. The mesolimbic and nigrostriatal projections are important in understanding a second anatomical distinction of typical versus atypical drugs. Acute administration of all clinically effective antipsychotic drugs induces immediate early gene expression within the nucleus accumbens, while administration of typical drugs tends to induce immediate early gene expression in the striatum as well.

Of course, these distinctions would be moot if typical and atypical drugs did not differ at the clinical level. The most common clinical definition of an atypical antipsychotic drug is one that does not produce extrapyramidal side effects (see Chapter 1). However, other clinical distinctions have been proposed as defining criteria for atypicality: 1) lack of propensity for producing hyperprolactinemia (29), 2) effectiveness in patients who do not respond to typical antipsychotics, and 3) ability to improve negative or cognitive symptoms of schizophrenia (40).

Preclinical behavioral models of antipsychotic drug action can reliably predict several phenomena related to atypicality. First, they can be used to identify drugs with antipsychotic activity, regardless of the drug's status as typical or atypical. Second, recent studies (see below) suggest that they can be used to identify drugs that are effective in the treatment of negative and/ or cognitive symptoms. Finally, behavioral models are used to identify compounds that may or may not cause side effects.

By far, the most studied atypical antipsychotic drug is the dibenzapine drug, clozapine. This drug was first developed in the early 1970s. Its clinical profile was surprising since it did not produce extrapyramidal side effects yet was highly effective. In spite of this remarkable profile, clozapine was withdrawn from further development because it produced agranulocytosis in some patients. Its clinical use has been subsequently re-approved contingent upon a careful monitoring for agranulocytosis. The preclinical and clinical actions of clozapine have come to serve the defining features of an atypical drug. Among physicians and pharmacologists, there is probably little disagreement over the statement that the terms "atypical" and "clozapine-like" are synonymous (26). Thus, if one wants to determine if a drug is atypical in an animal model, one can compare the effects of the candidate drug to clozapine. This is how many newer antipsychotic drugs have received the distinction of atypical, including aripiprazole, risperidone, olanzapine, quetiapine, ziprasidone, and zotepine.

Another way to establish the atypical nature of a drug is to compare the activity of a candidate compound to a typical antipsychotic drug. Perhaps the most studied typical compound in this regard has been the butyrophenone drug, haloperidol. Haloperidol is a relatively selective D_2 receptor antagonist with little affinity for $5\text{-}HT_2$ receptors, and, up until the introduction of risperidone and olanzapine, one of the most widely prescribed antipsychotic drugs. Clinically, it is a potent antipsychotic but produces extrapyramidal side effects in many patients. Furthermore, due to its sedative qualities, it can exacerbate some of the negative and cognitive symptoms of schizophrenia. Thus, in animal models, the behavioral effects of a new antipsychotic drug can be compared to the effects of haloperidol to establish its atypicality. If a drug mimics haloperidol in a test of antipsychotic activity, but does not produce haloperidol-like effects in a test of side-effect propensity, then the candidate drug may be considered "atypical".

IV. EFFECTS OF ATYPICAL ANTIPSYCHOTIC DRUGS IN BEHAVIORAL MODELS OF POSITIVE SYMPTOMS

Antipsychotic drugs are mainly used in the treatment of schizophrenia, although they are also prescribed for acute mania (28) and for the agitation associated with Alzheimer's disease (47). Schizophrenia has often been characterized as a syndrome involving three symptom clusters: positive, negative, and cognitive. Positive or psychotic symptoms are the ones typically associated with schizophrenia, and include hallucinations (unfounded sensations or perceptions) and delusions (false beliefs). On the whole, most antipsychotic drugs, typical and atypical, effectively reduce these symptoms in a majority of people with schizophrenia. However, some people do not respond to currently available drugs and, thus, researchers continue to search for more efficacious drugs.

How does a behavioral pharmacologist determine if a drug may be efficacious in the treatment of positive or psychotic symptoms of schizophrenia? First, they identify a manipulation that may have *etiological validity*; that is, they identify a pathophysiological process that produces psychosis in humans, such as a specific neurochemical imbalance or neuroanatomical deficit. The researcher then emulates the same process in the animal by injecting a drug or performing a lesion, and records the effects of such manipulations on rodent behavior (23). There are a number of etiologically valid animal models that are currently used to test antipsychotic drugs. This review will focus on three of these models: the amphetamine, phencyclidine, and hippocampal lesion models. Studies over the past 40 years have demonstrated that two behaviors, locomotor activity and prepulse inhibition (PPI) are significantly altered in all of these models. Clinically effective antipsychotic drugs have been found to reverse the hyperactivity and PPI deficits observed in these models, as well as suppress a third behavior known as conditioned avoidance responding (CAR).

A. Hyperactivity Models of Positive Symptoms

1. Amphetamine-Induced Hyperactivity

One of the oldest animal models of schizophrenia is the amphetamine model (Table 1). d-Amphetamine and related compounds are indirect DA agonists that increase synaptic DA levels in the brain either by blocking DA reuptake or evoking DA release. Work in the late 1960s and early 1970s demonstrated that these drugs produced symptoms in people that were indistinguishable from paranoid schizophrenia. These findings, along with the knowledge that most clinically effective antipsychotic drugs blocked DA receptors, led many investigators to propose that the positive symptoms of schizophrenia are a

Table 1 Locomotor Activity Models with Predictive Validity for the Treatment of Positive Symptoms

Model	Mechanism	Psychological analog in humans	Behavioral effect in rodents	Effect of typical drug in model	Effect of atypical drug in model
Amphetamine	Increased DA release in mesolimbic system	Paranoid psychosis/ hallucinations	Hyperactivity	Reduces activity	Reduces activity/ more potent at low amph. doses
Spontaneous activity	Regulated by mesolimbic DA system	—	—	Reduces activity	Reduces activity
Apomorphine	Direct DA agonist	(Not well characterized)	Decreased activity at low doses/ increased activity and climbing at high doses	Reduces activity	Reduces activity
Phencyclidine (PCP), MK-801, ketamine	Blocks NMDA receptors	Produces positive and negative symptoms	Hyperactivity	Reduces activity	Reduces activity
Hippocampal lesion	Loss of hippocampal neurons	Cognitive Impairment	Hyperactivity	Partially reduces activity	Reduces activity

product of excessive DA levels in the brain. Known as the DA hypothesis of schizophrenia, it remains one of the best neurochemical accounts of schizophrenia.

If amphetamine causes psychotic symptoms in humans, then one might assume that a drug that reverses amphetamine-induced psychosis may be an effective antipsychotic agent. Applying the same logic to an animal model, if amphetamine produces a clear behavioral effect in a rodent, then a drug that reverses this effect may have utility as an antipsychotic drug in humans. This idea has been the basis of the amphetamine model of schizophrenia in animals. Amphetamine produces a number of behavioral effects in rodents. At very low doses (e.g., 0.25 mg/kg), it can improve some aspects of attention and memory (3), at low to moderate doses (e.g., 1.0–3.0 mg/kg), it produces hyperactivity (i.e., forward motion and motility (9)) and attentional dysfunction (3), and at moderate to high doses it produces a behavioral syndrome known as stereotypy (> 2.0 mg/kg (2,44)). This latter syndrome includes excessive repetition of grooming, licking, and gnawing. In most studies, there is considerable overlap in the behavioral effects produced by a given dose of amphetamine; it is especially common to observe hyperactivity and moderate levels of stereotypy in an animal given a moderate dose of amphetamine (~3.0 mg/kg (44)). The behavioral effects of amphetamine are observed almost immediately following a subcutaneous injection in rats and mice and dissipate after an hour.

While lacking in face validity, it has been the hyperactivity produced by amphetamine that has served as one of the better preclinical predictors of antipsychotic activity. (The stereotypy produced by amphetamine is predictive of side-effect liability – this issue will be addressed later.) Numerous studies have shown that nearly all clinically effective antipsychotic drugs reduce the hyperactivity produced by amphetamine. The hyperactivity observed after amphetamine injection is likely due to excessive DA levels in the mesolimbic system, mainly within the nucleus accumbens, since animals with experimentally-induced damage to mesolimbic neurons are not hyperactive after amphetamine injection (31) (Figure 1).

Both typical and atypical antipsychotic drugs reduce the hyperactivity produced by amphetamine and this effect has been linked to D_2 receptor blockade. The similar action of typical and atypical antipsychotics in the amphetamine model is consistent with their similar blockade of D_2 receptors and their similar antipsychotic effect in the clinic. However, more detailed investigations have uncovered subtle yet significant distinctions between typical versus atypical drugs in the amphetamine model. In a study reported by Arnt (2), the dose of an atypical antipsychotic (clozapine, risperidone, olanzapine, ziprasidone, quetiapine) required to inhibit the hyperactivity produced by a moderate dose of amphetamine (2.0 mg/kg) was roughly ten times higher than the dose required to inhibit the locomotor response to a lower dose of amphetamine (0.5 mg/kg). However, haloperidol was equipotent in reducing the hyperactivity produced by both moderate and low doses of amphetamine. Thus, it may be possible to distinguish atypical from typical drugs in the amphetamine model by comparing the ratio of drug doses needed to reduce the hyperactivity produced by low and moderate doses of amphetamine. The greater the ratio, the more likely that the drug will act as an atypical in other behavioral and biochemical tests. The neurochemical basis of the distinctive effect may be related to the ability of atypical drugs to antagonize 5-HT$_2$ receptors and the α_1-type receptors for the neurotransmitter, norepinephrine (NE) (2), in addition to antagonism of D$_2$ receptors. By blocking all three receptors at a low dose, atypical drugs reduce the hyperactivity produced by a low dose of amphetamine. However, it is likely that significant degree of D$_2$ receptor blockade alone is necessary to inhibit the hyperactivity produced by a moderate dose of amphetamine; a degree of blockade achieved only by a high dose of an atypical drug.

It should be noted that while drugs that act solely as 5-HT$_2$ and α_1 antagonists can inhibit amphetamine-induced hyperactivity, such drugs do not have antipsychotic effects in humans. Thus, an antipsychotic drug may be atypical if it binds to other receptors besides the D$_2$ receptor, but it will probably lack antipsychotic activity if it does not antagonize the D$_2$ receptor. Moreover, the suppressive effects of selective 5-HT$_2$ and α_1 antagonists on amphetamine-induced hyperactivity reveal a major shortcoming of the model: not all drugs which suppress activity, such as 5-HT$_2$ and α_1 antagonists, have antipsychotic properties in the clinic. Such false positives are a major obstacle in interpreting the data from activity models of antipsychotic drug action.

In addition to the amphetamine model, the effects of antipsychotic drugs on other forms of locomotor activity/hyperactivity have been considered. First, many studies have simply assessed drug effects on spontaneous locomotor activity. Spontaneous locomotor activity refers to the activity observed in rodents after they have been habituated to a testing chamber. When rodents are first placed into a testing chamber, they exhibit a high rate of activity and exploration during the first 20 minutes of testing and relatively lower rates of activity during the remaining testing period. When placed in the same chamber a day or two later, the animals exhibit less activity. The level of spontaneous activity is presumed to reflect DA levels in the mesolimbic pathway (40). Both typical and atypical antipsychotics reduce spontaneous activity. Atypical drugs such as clozapine and risperidone inhibit spontaneous activity at doses which also inhibit amphetamine-induced locomotion, while typical drugs, such as haloperidol, are 2–3 times more potent at inhibiting amphetamine-induced hyperactivity than spontaneous activity. Ogren (44) suggests that the differential effect of haloperidol on spontaneous versus amphetamine-elicited activity indicates that spontaneous activity involves not just DA but an amalgam of neurotransmitter systems. Finally, some have claimed that the effect of an antipsychotic drug on spontaneous activity is a preclinical indicator of sedation and not of antipsychotic activity. The validity of this claim, however, is questionable (23,44).

Finally, in addition to characterizing the effects of indirect DA agonists, such as amphetamine or methylphenidate on locomotion, researchers have also studied the effects of direct DA agonists on locomotion. The most studied compound in this regard is the mixed D_1/D_2 receptor agonist, apomorphine, which binds directly to each DA receptor. Many clinically effective antipsychotics reduce the hyperactivity induced by apomorphine, regardless of their status as typical or atypical. However, apomorphine has a quirky behavioral pharmacology since low doses of the drug suppress locomotor activity while high doses of the drug increase activity (44). This biphasic effect makes it relatively difficult to interpret the effects of an antipsychotic drug on the locomotor changes produced by apomorphine. It should finally be noted that apomorphine can induce climbing behavior in mice (i.e., the mice climb on the wire lids of their cages for extended periods of time). This type of behavior can be blocked by antipsychotics (41).

2. Phencyclidine-Induced Hyperactivity

It has been known for several decades that disassociative anesthetic drugs, such as ketamine and phencyclidine (PCP), can produce hallucinations and delusions. In more recent studies, the symptoms produced by these drugs have been compared to the negative and cognitive symptoms found in people with schizophrenia (46). However, it should also be noted that some aspects of the PCP syndrome are not consistent with the clinical presentation of schizophrenia (59). Until the late 1980s, the biochemical mechanism of these drugs was a mystery. Work since that time has shown that these drugs act as non-competitive antagonists at the NMDA-type receptor for the excitatory amino acid neurotransmitter, glutamate (45).

In animals, NMDA antagonists, most notably PCP and dizocilipine (or MK-801), have numerous effects that are clearly dose-dependent. At high doses, such drugs produce head weaving, ataxia, and sedation. At lower doses, animals display an intense hyperactivity that is observed about 10–20 minutes after injection and can last for nearly 2 hours (1,9). At even lower doses, the drugs produce learning and memory deficits (1). It is the hyperactivity produced by NMDA antagonists that has been used extensively as an animal model of psychosis and as an assay of antipsychotic drug activity.

The mechanism behind the heightened locomotor activity observed in PCP-treated rats is not clear. Using an immediate early gene assay to determine the effects of PCP and MK-801 on regional brain metabolism in rats, Jacobs et al. (27) found that each drug greatly increased neuronal activity in the motor cortex while having little or no effect on neuronal activity in the nucleus accumbens. This finding suggests that the hyperactivity found in rats after PCP treatment may be independent of mesolimbic DA function. On the other hand, Adams and Moghaddam (1) found that PCP treatment increased both extracellular DA and glutamate levels in the nucleus accumbens and prefrontal cortex. This result would implicate the mesolimbic pathway in the locomotor response to PCP. It should be noted, however, that the effects of PCP on locomotion and extracellular glutamate followed an identical time course, while the PCP-induced elevation in extracellular DA persisted long after the hyperactivity had subsided. Furthermore, drugs that reduce PCP-induced elevations in extracellular glutamate in the prefrontal cortex and nucleus accumbens can reduce the hyperactivity produced by PCP without affecting PCP-induced elevations in extracellular DA (42). This would suggest that some of the behavioral effects of PCP in rats are mediated by brain glutamate systems and not by brain DA levels. It may also imply that some forms of schizophrenia in humans are associated with altered glutamate function (46).

Many studies have shown that typical and atypical antipsychotics can inhibit the hyperactivity produced by NMDA antagonists in animals (see ref. (44) for review). There is little evidence that the effects of atypical drugs on PCP-induced hyperactivity differ from the effects of typical drugs. The ability of antipsychotic drugs to reduce the hyperactivity produced by PCP indicates that, despite the putative involvement of brain glutamate systems, the expression of the PCP-induced hyperactivity is nonetheless sensitive to D_2 antagonism. It has also been shown that the hyperactivity produced by NMDA antagonists can be reduced by drugs which exclusively block 5-HT$_2$ and α_1 receptors, suggesting that the hyperactivity produced by NMDA antagonists involves several neurotransmitter systems (13,38).

Finally, it should be mentioned that PCP and MK-801 are often viewed as interchangeable by behavioral pharmacologists, since both drugs increase activity in rats and mice. However, studies by Ogren and Goldstein (45) found that the ability of each drug to increase activity in rats is differentially affected by specific dopaminergic drugs, suggesting that the behavioral pharmacology of the two drugs is not identical. Furthermore, it has been shown that while the locomotor responses to PCP are age-dependent, similar responses to MK-801 are not (27). This provides further evidence that the putative similarities of PCP and MK-801 should be considered carefully.

3. Lesion-Induced Hyperactivity

Over the past 30 years, the most reliable findings to emerge from numerous neuroimaging studies of schizophrenia have been enlargement of the lateral ventricles (especially the temporal horn) and a mean reduction in the volume of temporal lobe structures such as the hippocampus (39,57). It should also be noted that some studies have found neuroanatomical and metabolic deficits in the frontal cortex and thalamus, among other regions. The hippocampus is a region of the limbic system located within the medial temporal lobe and has been implicated in the formation of new memories, especially ones related to personal experience (episodic memory) and spatial relationships (spatial memory). If and how reductions in hippocampal volume contribute to schizophrenia have been difficult to discern, since correlations between hippocampal alterations and psychopathology have been reported in some studies (48,57) but not in others (16).

If dysgenesis or damage in a specific brain region gives rise to the symptoms of schizophrenia, then the characterization of the behavioral effects of hippocampal damage in animals should provide insights into the treatment of schizophrenia. For example, if drugs can be identified that ameliorate the behavioral consequences of hippocampal damage in a rat, then these drugs may work to ameliorate the psychopathological consequences of hippocampal dysfunction in humans.

Several investigators have sought to develop an animal model of the hippocampal deficits reported in people with schizophrenia by experimentally inducing hippocampal damage in adult rats and mice. Under general anesthesia, animals in these models receive surgical infusions of neurotoxic compounds, such as kainic acid, ibotenic acid, or NMDA, directly into hippocampal tissue or in the surrounding ventricles. After a 2–3 week recovery period, the animals are tested in a variety of behavioral and biochemical assays. Their performance in each test is compared to animals that undergo surgery but receive infusions of sterile water or saline instead to control for the effects of the surgery alone (i.e., sham controls). The extent and degree of the hippocampal damage is verified in each animal following the completion of the behavioral experiment. It is important to keep in mind that the goal of these experiments should not be to create the complete destruction of the hippocampus, since the hippocampus is not missing in neuropsychiatric disorders. The goal should be to create a degree of cellular or volumetric loss on a scale consistent with the approximately 5–15% average reduction in hippocampal volume reported in schizophrenia (11,49).

Rats with kainic acid-type damage to the hippocampus demonstrate increases in locomotor activity within a 3-week period after surgery (8). In addition, the lesions potentiate the hyperactivity produced by exposure to a novel environment, amphetamine, and MK-801 (9). This hyperactivity may result from enhanced D_2 receptor function, since lesioned animals have a greater D_2 receptor density in the nucleus accumbens (8). Several studies have shown that typical antipsychotic drugs, such as haloperidol, reduce lesion-induced hyperactivity (see ref. (4) for review). Later research has shown that atypical antipsychotics, such as clozapine, risperidone, and olanzapine, also decrease the hyperactivity and hypersensitivity to amphetamine found in rats with kainic acid lesions (6,7).

While both typical and atypical antipsychotics reduce activity in rats with kainic acid lesions, such rats are consistently less sensitive to the suppressive effects of haloperidol relative to the effects of clozapine, risperidone, and olanzapine. In studies performed by Bardgett and colleagues (6,7), haloperidol failed to suppress amphetamine-induced hyperactivity in lesioned animals to the same extent that it suppressed activity in sham controls. However, clozapine reduced amphetamine-induced hyperactivity by a similar degree in both lesioned and control rats (7). A later study showed that the effects of risperidone and olanzapine are dose-dependent. Lesioned rats were slightly less sensitive to the locomotor suppressive effects of moderate doses of risperidone and olanzapine, but completely sensitive to the suppression produced by high doses of each drug (6). Accordingly, one potential preclinical test for atypical drugs may be the degree to which the candidate compound decreases locomotor activity in lesioned rats versus controls.

The observation that the hippocampus may be "damaged" in schizophrenia has led to speculation regarding the origin of these neuroanatomical changes. Some have argued that such changes may reflect a degenerative process that is concurrent with the onset of the syndrome, while others have adopted a neurodevelopmental account of these changes. According to these theorists, some type of neuronal insult must have occurred during gestation that altered the development of specific brain regions. This view has received significant empirical support from retrospective clinical and epidemiological studies and has driven some preclinical researchers to develop an analogous animal model. One interesting formulation has been a model developed by Lipska et al. (34), wherein a neurotoxin is injected into the ventral region of the rat hippocampus when the animals are 7 days old. These animals demonstrate normal activity until puberty, at which time they demonstrate increased spontaneous locomotor activity and enhanced locomotor sensitivity to amphetamine. The post-pubertal emergence of these behavioral changes in rats with neonatal ventral hippocampal damage is consistent with the delayed onset of schizophrenia in late adolescence. One possible caveat to the neonatal ventral hippocampal lesion model is the large size of the lesion. In some cases nearly half of the hippocampus is destroyed in such animals. The relevance of such a large lesion to the moderate reductions in hippocampal volume observed in schizophrenia is questionable.

Lipska and Weinberger (35) have assessed the effects of haloperidol in animals with neonatal ventral hippocampal lesions. The hyperlocomotion produced by such lesions is eliminated by 3 weeks of haloperidol treatment. However, rats with neonatal ventral hippocampal lesions are less sensitive than non-lesioned rats to the catalepsy produced by high doses of haloperidol (35). This finding is not unlike the reduced sensitivity of adult rats with kainic acid lesions to the locomotor suppressive effects of haloperidol. Taken together, it is possible that the neurobiological and behavioral actions of typical antipsychotics require hippocampal neurons while atypical drugs do not (6). This idea has obvious clinical implications for the treatment of patients where hippocampal dysfunction is suspected.

4. Summary

Suppression of hyperactivity is probably one of the most widely used, preclinical behavioral measures of antipsychotic drug action. In general, both typical and atypical antipsychotic drugs reduce the hyperactivity elicited by DA agonists, NMDA antagonists, or hippocampal lesions. However, some minor components in these models may be differentially sensitive to typical versus atypical drugs, such as how the latter class affects locomotor responses to low doses of amphetamine and how the former class does not reduce activity in lesioned animals to the same degree seen in non-lesioned rats.

One criticism of the suppressive effects of antipsychotic drugs on locomotor activity is that the drugs are simply sedating the animals. While there may be some truth to this claim, one must nonetheless bear in mind that the drug's ability to reduce locomotion in rodents is highly predictive of its ability to reduce psychosis in humans. This defense, however, raises yet another problem: many non-antipsychotic drugs can also reduce the locomotor effects of DA agonists, NMDA antagonists, or lesions. As discussed, a 5-HT_2 or α_1 receptor antagonist can reduce the hyperactivity produced by DA agonists and NMDA receptor antagonists. However, these drugs are not very effective antipsychotics. A clinician scanning the preclinical literature for potential new antipsychotic drugs must be wary of false positives in these hyperactivity tests. It can be concluded that most if not all clinically effective antipsychotic drugs, regardless of their typical/atypical status, reduce hyperactivity in animals; but it cannot be concluded that all drugs which reduce hyperactivity are clinically effective antipsychotic drugs. To support the contention that a candidate compound may be an effective antipsychotic drug, one must test the compound in other behavioral tests that are predictive of antipsychotic potential, such as PPI or CAR.

B. Prepulse Inhibition

Work initiated in the late 1970s demonstrated that people with schizophrenia demonstrate deficits in a sensorimotor process known as prepulse inhibition (PPI) (see ref. (59) for review). In animals and humans, PPI is demonstrated as follows: 1) the organism is exposed to a discrete presentation of a low intensity stimulus, most commonly a tone, which is known as the "prepulse", 2) about 100–200 milliseconds after the offset of the prepulse, a discrete high intensity stimulus is presented, which can be considered the "pulse", and 3) the startle response to this latter stimulus is measured. Most organisms will show a significant startle response to the pulse if it is presented alone. However, if the pulse is preceded by a prepulse, as described above, then the startle response to the pulse will be decreased; in other words the prepulse inhibits the startle response to the pulse. People with schizophrenia, however, fail to show the same level of PPI on average as do people without the disorder. The mesolimbic DA system, as well as the hippocampus, appear to be active components in the neural circuitry underlying PPI.

What is important about PPI is that it can be produced in both humans and laboratory animals, such as rats or mice. This means that if PPI deficits are found in animals, such deficits can serve as a face-valid model of the deficient PPI found in people with schizophrenia. Moreover, the types of experimental manipulations which can give rise to PPI deficits in animals are the same conditions that have been implicated in schizophrenia, such as excessive activity at DA receptors, NMDA receptor blockade, and hippocampal dysfunction (59). Furthermore, all clinically effective antipsychotic drugs reverse PPI deficits in animals, although atypicals may be more effective under some circumstances. It should also be noted that drugs that have psychoactive properties but are not antipsychotic do not improve PPI deficits in animals. In other words, there are fewer false positives in tests of PPI compared to locomotor testing. These aspects of PPI make it an attractive behavioral test to use as a preclinical predictor of antipsychotic drug action. However, perhaps the biggest caveat to the PPI deficit is its meaning within the framework of psychopathology in schizophrenia.

Most early studies of PPI in animals assessed the effects of the DA agonist, apomorphine, on PPI in rats. The increased activity at DA receptors produced by apomorphine was intended to emulate the putative increases in DA activity in schizophrenia. Nearly all of these studies found that apomorphine produces a PPI deficit without dramatically altering startle responses to the pulse alone. Most typical and atypical antipsychotic drugs reverse apomorphine-induced deficits in PPI. Moreover, research by Swerdlow and colleagues (60) determined a close positive correlation between the antipsychotic dose needed to reverse apomorphine-induced PPI deficits and the average daily dose used to treat people with schizophrenia. This result suggests that a drug's ability to reverse apomorphine-induced PPI deficits may be highly predictive of its antipsychotic potential.

Another interesting aspect of PPI as a model of antipsychotic drug action may be its potential for discriminating atypical drugs from typical ones. This feature is not observed in tests of apomorphine-induced PPI deficits. But if the PPI deficit is produced by PCP, ketamine, or neonatal ventral hippocampal lesions, clozapine, risperidone, olanzapine, and ziprasidone have been observed to reverse some or all of these deficits while haloperidol has been observed to be relatively ineffective (33,37,59). The only problem with this series of studies is that haloperidol has been the only typical drug employed. A more robust typical versus atypical distinction awaits the testing of other typical drugs in the NMDA antagonist and hippocampal lesion models. In addition, a recent study by Wiley and Kennedy (61) indicated that the effect of clozapine on PCP-induced PPI deficits may not always be reliable.

C. Conditioned Avoidance

Another preclinical test that is used to predict a given drug's antipsychotic potential is the conditioned avoidance response (CAR) test. In this test, animals are placed in a box with two compartments and a grid floor. Animals are trained that when a conditioned stimulus (a light or sound cue) is emitted, a mild footshock (the unconditioned stimulus) will follow within a few seconds. The animal can avoid this footshock by simply "shuttling" into the other compartment during the presentation of the conditioned stimulus. On the other hand, animals that do not "avoid" footshock by responding to the conditioned stimulus can still "escape" to the safe compartment during presentation of the mild footshock. Most studies first train the animals to avoid the footshock to a specific criterion, for example, nine avoidances on ten trials. Once the animals are trained to avoid the footshock, the animals are then treated with an antipsychotic drug immediately before the next test session and their performance is compared to the performance observed after saline injection or after treatment with additional doses of the antipsychotic drug. In most cases, an effective dose that reduces the number of avoidances by 50% is determined by testing several doses of the drug. In addition to the standard approach described above, some studies have been performed to assess the effect of an antipsychotic drug on the acquisition of the CAR response, while others have examined the effect of such drugs on the extinction of the CAR response.

It is doubtful that CAR in animals emulates any aspect of the clinical syndrome of schizophrenia. However, it is an animal model possessing predictive validity, given that most clinically effective antipsychotic drugs reduce performance in the CAR test (see ref. (44) for review). The drug doses required to reduce CAR performance vary from slightly to significantly higher than those required to block amphetamine-induced hyperactivity (44). There is limited evidence that one can discriminate a typical antipsychotic drug from an atypical one based on its effects on CAR. The doses of some typical drugs, such as haloperidol, needed to reduce CAR are near the dose needed to reduce amphetamine-induced hyperactivity. The doses of clozapine, risperidone, and olanzapine required to reduce CAR are, in some cases, 10-fold higher than that required to reduce amphetamine-induced hyperactivity. However, it should be noted that the reported effective dose has varied widely for studies of both typical and atypical drugs. These differences most likely stem from idiosyncratic variations in the methods used to test these drugs between laboratories. Nonetheless, because of the relatively higher doses of antipsychotics required to reduce CAR, some investigators have suggested that CAR suppression may be a preclinical predictor of clinical side-effect liability than antipsychotic efficacy.

One explanation for the suppressive effects of antipsychotic drugs in the CAR paradigm is that the drugs simply sedate animals and interfere with locomotor responding. However, as discussed by Ogren (44), most rats will continue to *escape* footshock at drug doses that clearly suppress shock *avoidance*. If the animals were simply sedated, their responsiveness to the footshock would be as equally impaired as their response to the conditioned cues. Perhaps a more problematic aspect of the suppressive effect of antipsychotics on CAR is the fact that the antipsychotics may be interfering with memory retrieval. As will be discussed below, one of the most debilitating functional aspects of schizophrenia is memory impairment. An antipsychotic drug that impairs learning and memory in an animal model is likely to worsen cognitive symptoms in people with schizophrenia. However, as will be presented later, some antipsychotics, despite their disruptive effects on CAR, may actually have cognitive benefits in the clinic.

V. EFFECTS OF ANTIPSYCHOTIC DRUGS IN ANIMAL MODELS OF NEGATIVE SYMPTOMS

Most preclinical behavioral research on antipsychotic drug action has focused upon antipsychotic drug action in assays of positive symptoms, such as those described above. The attention given to positive symptom models reflects, in part, a lack of good models for the negative and cognitive symptoms of schizophrenia. This is an unfortunate situation, because the remediation of negative and cognitive symptoms may have a greater functional impact on outcome in schizophrenia than the treatment of positive symptoms (40).

Negative symptoms of schizophrenia include flat or inappropriate affect, impaired volition or motivation, and a lack of social interactions. Alterations in affect are especially difficult to record in animals since lack of responding to an emotion-laden stimulus, such as pain, could be independent of a lack of emotion. For example, an animal may not respond to painful stimulus because it has a higher pain threshold, it is inattentive, or it is physically ill. This problem is obviously intertwined with the valid recording of changes in animal volition or motivation. While developing a face-valid model of flat affect or impaired volition has been difficult, some researchers have developed a potential face-valid model of social interaction deficits in schizophrenia.

Laboratory rodents are remarkably social creatures, and during the active phase of their daily cycle, they will groom their cage-mates, establish dominance hierarchies within their cages, and engage in rough-and-tumble play. Research over the past 10 years has shown that drugs that produce some negative symptoms in humans can suppress social interaction in rats. Work by Sams-Dodd (50) showed that daily injections of amphetamine, which does not produce negative symptoms in humans, did not induce social isolation in rats, although it did produce a behavioral syndrome marked by hyperactivity and stereotyped behaviors. However, daily injections of PCP for 5 days did reduce social behaviors, such as sniffing, grooming, and other forms of between-animal contact.

Further work by the same investigator revealed that treatment of rats with clozapine for 3 weeks reversed the social isolation produced by PCP (51). Interestingly, similar treatment with haloperidol did not produce the same effect. These findings are consistent with the clinical effects of clozapine and haloperidol, in that the former drug can improve negative symptoms while the latter drug is typically ineffective against these symptoms. Thus, the PCP-induced social isolation paradigm may be a useful preclinical paradigm for discriminating atypical from typical antipsychotic drugs, although more work is needed in this area.

More recently, the effects of neonatal ventral hippocampal lesions on social interaction have been considered. These lesions have been found to decrease social interaction and increase aggressive behavior in rats (10,52). However, clozapine does not improve social interaction in animals with this type of lesion (52). This finding suggests that the social isolation produced by PCP treatment is regulated by different neurochemical substrates than the social isolation produced by hippocampal lesions. If a drug can be found that reverses the effects of the hippocampal lesions on social isolation, such a result may point to a novel and potentially important therapeutic target for treating negative symptoms in people with schizophrenia.

VI. EFFECTS OF ANTIPSYCHOTIC DRUGS IN ANIMAL MODELS OF COGNITIVE SYMPTOMS

Clinicians and researchers alike have long recognized that schizophrenia is a syndrome involving cognitive impairment. Indeed, some have argued that the cognitive deficits are at the core of the disorder, with the positive and negative symptoms of schizophrenia being manifested as a cognitive "response" to gaps in attention, memory, and executive function. Recently, the issue of cognitive impairment in schizophrenia has received a great deal of attention, because such impairment predicts long-term outcome in people with schizophrenia and because clozapine, risperidone, and olanzapine have been observed to improve some aspects of cognitive dysfunction in schizophrenia (12).

Many aspects of cognitive function are reportedly altered in people with schizophrenia. In the area of learning and memory, there is some disagreement over whether deficits occur in specific domains or if they are reflective of a general cognitive impairment (20). In agreement with the former point of view, Saykin and colleagues (53) demonstrated that performance in several learning and memory tests was impaired in people with schizophrenia, but that spatial working memory was the most compromised. Modeling this spatial working memory deficit in animals has recently attracted the attention of preclinical investigators interested in developing drugs that can enhance cognitive function in schizophrenia.

Spatial working memory is a short-term memory for a specific location; for example, a memory for where one has just parked one's car or just placed one's coffee cup. In humans, it is sometimes tested in a paradigm known as delayed non-matching to sample. This test involves being shown the location of a shape on a computer screen (this is known as the sample) followed by a delay wherein the computer screen is blank. The original shape is then re-presented in its original location along with an identical shape presented in a different location. If the subject selects the shape in the different location, it is recorded as a correct choice; i.e., after a delay, the location that does not match the sample was chosen.

This same type of memory can be studied in rodents. Most often, it is studied in an apparatus known as a T-maze. Rats are trained to run down the stem of the T-maze and choose an arm of the T configuration (the goal arm) to obtain a reward. After the delay, the animal is returned to the beginning of the stem of the T-maze. If the animal chooses the arm opposite to the one just chosen, it is rewarded; if it returns to the same arm that was selected in the previous trial, it is not rewarded. Thus, the animal must remember where it obtained the reward on the last trial in order to locate the reward on the next trial. This test is sometimes referred to as a spatial delayed non-matching to sample task or delayed spatial alternation.

How is delayed spatial alternation performance affected by drugs or manipulations that produce schizophrenia-like symptoms? The literature on DA agonists in rats and mice is mixed regarding the effect of these drugs on spatial alternation. Much of the confusion likely stems from differences in doses between studies. A more consistent literature has emerged from animal studies on NMDA antagonists and hippocampal lesions. Studies have shown that PCP and MK-801 can impair delayed spatial alternation in rats (24,42), at doses which also increase locomotor activity. Other research has shown that moderate damage to the dorsal hippocampus can also reduce alternation rates to chance levels (5), as can neonatal lesions to the ventral hippocampus (36).

Animal studies assessing the effects of acute antipsychotic drug injection on spatial memory in normal animals have revealed that the drugs either do not affect or have an adverse effect on memory (17,58). However, several studies have assessed whether antipsychotic drug treatment can reverse the memory deficits produced by NMDA antagonists or by hippocampal damage. Hauber (24) first reported that low to moderate doses of clozapine could improve impairments in spatial alternation produced by MK-801. Bardgett and Griffith (5) have more recently shown that clozapine can improve spatial alternation impairments produced by moderate damage to the hippocampus. Interestingly, such an improvement was only observed after a 3-week regimen of daily clozapine injections prior to and during testing. Single injections of clozapine on the test days alone did not improve the lesion-induced deficit. Considered together, the data suggest that acute doses of clozapine may improve memory impairments produced by NMDA antagonists, but chronic treatment with clozapine is required to overcome memory impairment produced by a lesion. It should also be appreciated that, in the study by Bardgett and Griffith (5), clozapine greatly increased the time needed for the animal to choose an arm of the T-maze. This phenomenon most likely reflects the sedative effects of clozapine and suggests that, in rats with hippocampal damage, the cognitive benefits of clozapine may come at the cost of motor slowing.

VII. MODELING THE BEHAVIORAL SIDE EFFECTS OF ANTIPSYCHOTIC DRUGS IN ANIMALS

Most antipsychotic drugs are excellent at reducing positive symptoms. One of the next frontiers in the development of better antipsychotic drugs will be the discovery of drugs that are more efficacious in the treatment of negative and cognitive symptoms. Some of the newer atypical drugs, along with clozapine, have partially fulfilled this goal. Another major frontier in antipsychotic drug development will be the identification of drugs that have fewer side effects.

There are many side effects associated with antipsychotic drug treatment. The most notable side effects are extrapyramidal symptoms (EPS), which are manifested as akathesia, dystonia, and parkinsonism. These symptoms appear to be related to the blockade of D_2 receptors in the nigrostriatal DA pathway. It is worth noting that within this pathway, the substania nigra degenerates in Parkinson's disease and the striatum degenerates in Huntington's chorea. Given that movement disorder is the primary symptom in both diseases, it is not surprising that the motor deficits of antipsychotic drugs have been linked to a disruption of dopaminergic neurotransmission in these brain regions.

There have been two primary strategies for identifying antipsychotic drugs with potential EPS liability. Just after the discovery of the antipsychotic properties of chlorpromazine in the 1950s, it was found that high doses of this and other antipsychotic drugs caused rats to become "frozen" and immobile (44). This phenomenon is known as catalepsy and was once used to predict the antipsychotic potential of candidate drugs (see ref. (44) for review). However, it is now used as a face-valid model of the extrapyramidal side effects produced by antipsychotic drug treatment in humans.

There are several ways catalepsy can be recorded in rats and mice. One way is to simply place the forepaws of a rat on a horizontal bar. Most animals will either climb upon the bar or release it. However, after injection with a high dose of an antipsychotic drug, rats will remain motionless and hang indefinitely from the horizontal bar. Another test for catalepsy is to place a rat on an inclined wire mesh screen. Most rats will climb up or down the screen within seconds of being placed upon it. Rats treated with a high dose of an antipsychotic will remain in the same place for many seconds. As reviewed by Ogren (44), most typical antipsychotic drugs, such as haloperidol, chlorpromazine, and others induce catalepsy at relatively low doses. In comparison, the effects of the atypical antipsychotics on catalepsy appear to be more variable. Risperidone and olanzapine can produce catalepsy, albeit at doses 10-fold higher than those needed to reduce amphetamine-induced hyperactivity, and other atypicals, such as clozapine and aripiprazole (56) do not produce it at all.

The other primary strategy for identifying drugs with potential EPS liability is to determine a compound's capacity to reduce DA agonist-induced stereotypy. As discussed previously, high doses of amphetamine and apomorphine produce stereotyped behavior in rats and mice, primarily repetitive licking, chewing, and sniffing. These effects are believed to be mediated by excessive dopaminergic release in the nigrostriatal pathway. While the face validity of this model is not immediately clear, stereotypy models do have appreciable predictive validity in the identification of drugs with EPS liability. Drugs with potent inhibitory effects on stereotypy are more likely to cause EPS symptoms in humans, while less potent drugs have fewer EPS side effects. By studying the effects of a given antipsychotic dose on both DA agonist-induced hyperactivity and stereotypy, behavioral pharmacologists have been able to make clear distinctions between typical and atypical antipsychotic drugs. A given dose of a typical antipsychotic drug tends to be equipotent at reducing both DA agonist-induced hyperactivity and stereotypy. But most atypical drugs are much more potent at reducing DA agonist-induced hyperactivity than stereotypy (see ref. (44) for review). Unfortunately, the mechanism that underlies the differential effects of most antipsychotics on agonist-induced locomotion and stereotypy is not completely understood. The $5-HT_2$ receptor antagonism found in some atypical drugs may counter the physiological and behavioral consequences of D_2 receptor blockade (44). Another equally valid theory is that the anticholinergic action of some atypical drugs in the caudate-putamen balances the antidopaminergic effects of these drugs (26,44).

Finally, researchers have been developing animal models of another antipsychotic-related side effect: tardive dyskinesia (TD). This side effect is observed in individuals after a long course of antipsychotic drug treatment and involves involuntary hyperkinetic movements of the face and tongue. Some investigators have suggested that TD is a consequence of elevated synaptic DA or of a sensitized dopaminergic system in the brain (26,55). Studies in rats have shown that chronic daily treatment of rats with fluphenazine, trifluroperazine, or haloperidol produces a syndrome of oral dyskinesias (14,54). These antipsychotic-induced oral dyskinesias may serve as a face-valid model of TD. It is notable that none of the atypical drugs (clozapine, olanzapine) produce oral dyskinesia in rats (21,22). The 5-HT$_{2A}$ antagonism produced by some atypical drugs may prevent the occurrence of TD, since low doses of specific 5-HT$_{2A}$ antagonists reduced the oral dyskinesia produced by haloperidol (43).

VIII. BENCH TO BEDSIDE ISSUES

The modeling of a uniquely human psychiatric disorder such as schizophrenia in the rat or mouse is fraught with interpretative difficulties. The same problems haunt the rational development of animal models of antipsychotic drug action. Despite these problems, behavioral models have provided important and necessary information for the development of many newer and better antipsychotic drugs. Furthermore, some of the problems that have marked preclinical behavioral research on antipsychotic drug action in the past may be avoidable in the future.

One persistent problem has been choosing the best dose to study. In doing so, one must realize that dosing in people (mg per day) is different from dosing in animals (mg per body weight). A typical clinical daily dose of haloperidol (10 mg/day) is roughly 0.125 mg/kg of body weight for an 80 kg person. This dose is fairly close to the dose of haloperidol needed to reduce amphetamine-induced hyperactivity in a rat by 50%. However, many animal studies involve doses of haloperidol that are clearly higher than this dose – some doses are as high as 1.0 mg/kg of body weight. In reviewing the preclinical research, one must be aware that such doses may have limited relevance to the effects of clinical doses. Secondly, most laboratory animals have much higher metabolic rates than do humans and the half-life of most antipsychotics is necessarily shorter in laboratory animals. Thus, dosing decisions in animal studies need to consider species differences in half-lives and tissue concentrations, as well as doses based on body weight.

A final comment on dosing regards receptor occupancy. Neuro-imaging studies have suggested that for a typical antipsychotic drug to be clinically effective, it must bind to 70–80% of the D$_2$ receptor sites in the striatum (18,19). However, the dose of haloperidol required to occupy 75% of striatal D$_2$ receptor sites in rats varies, due to methodological differences, between 0.06 mg/kg (30) and 0.35 mg/kg of body weight (15). This type of variation is not the only problem with the D$_2$ occupancy standard – some atypical drugs, notably clozapine, are clinically effective even when D_2 occupancy is below 50%. In summary, there is no single accepted strategy for determining an optimal dose to use in animal studies. However, data generated from studies involving excessively high doses of antipsychotic drugs may have limited clinical applicability.

Another issue that has been problematic in the design and interpretation of animal studies is the length of treatment. Most preclinical studies of antipsychotic drug action involve behavioral or biological responses to a single (or acute) drug injection. However, such a response may have limited relevance to antipsychotic activity since clinical efficacy is typically achieved only after 3–6 weeks of continuous treatment. Thus, animal studies demonstrating behavioral changes that emerge only after chronic treatment may offer better insights into the mechanisms of clinical efficacy. However, there is a significant paucity of data in regards to the behavioral effects of chronic antipsychotic treatment in animals – the work on animal models of TD and the cognitive benefits of chronic but not acute clozapine in lesion animals serving as exceptions within the existing literature.

Finally, an issue raised by Geyer and Markou (23) deserves attention. In the quest for a better antipsychotic with fewer side effects, most researchers compare the behavioral activity of a new drug to clozapine or haloperidol. The assumption is that if the activity of the drug is the same as clozapine in most assays, then it is a better drug. But this approach may ignore another possibility – that better drugs with fewer side effects could exert a profile of behavioral and biological activity distinct from clozapine. Thus, preclinical research should not be limited to looking for clozapine-like drugs. It should be mindful that the best antipsychotic drug might have a unique behavioral pharmacology of its own. In order to discover such drugs, new behavioral models of antipsychotic drug action may be required.

IX. SUMMARY OF INTERVENTIONS AND HYPOTHESIZED MECHANISMS OF THERAPEUTIC ACTION

Many animal models exist which can reliably predict the antipsychotic action of both typical and atypical antipsychotic drugs. Most of these models involve an experimental manipulation that is intended to mimic the pathophysiology of schizophrenia and related disorders and an observation of its behavioral consequences. Such models include drug injections that increase DA levels or block NMDA-type glutamate receptors, or other manipulations, such as hippocampal lesions or isolation rearing (59). The most notable behavioral consequences of these experimental treatments include locomotor hyperactivity and impaired PPI.

Behavioral pharmacologists use these behavioral changes to screen for possible antipsychotic activity in candidate compounds. Typically, if a drug reverses experimentally-induced changes in activity and PPI, as well as decreases CAR, without simply sedating the animal, then the drug meets the behavioral criteria as a potential antipsychotic drug. Of course, a better case can be made for antipsychotic potential if, in addition to such behavioral effects, the receptor binding, electrophysiological, and gene induction profiles of a given compound are also consistent with the effects of reference antipsychotic drugs. Overall, there are not striking distinctions between the effects of typical and atypical drugs in many behavioral assays of antipsychotic activity. The similar effects of either drug class fit with their similar ability to reduce psychotic symptoms. The ability of drugs to reduce locomotor hyperactivity, PPI deficits, and CAR is most likely a reflection of their antagonistic action at D_2 receptors within the mesolimbic dopaminergic pathway.

More recently, behavioral pharmacologists have become increasingly interested in modeling the negative and cognitive symptoms of schizophrenia. The development of these models should permit the preclinical identification of compounds with unique efficacy in the treatment of both symptoms. One existing behavioral model for negative symptoms has involved measures of social interaction in rats and mice. Clozapine appears to be one of the few antipsychotics that can increase interaction, although few other drugs have been tested. Further testing of other typical and atypical compounds in this paradigm will be needed before it can be fully accepted as a valid animal model of negative symptoms.

Several studies have now addressed the effects of potential antipsychotic drugs on memory function in rats and mice. Most of the memory impairments have been produced by pharmacological blockade of NMDA-type glutamate receptors, and such impairments have been ameliorated by clozapine. This latter effect has also been recently described in animals with hippocampal lesions. Again, more work is needed to identify the cognitive effects of other known reference drugs as well as the effects of potentially new antipsychotic drugs. The receptor mechanisms and brain regions responsible for the activity of clozapine in these assays are not known, but may involve antagonism of 5-HT$_2$ or alpha$_2$ receptors or partial agonist activity at some muscarinic cholinergic receptor subtypes (25,40).

Finally, behavioral models of antipsychotic drug action have been used to identify drugs with differing motor side-effect liabilities. For the most part, this process has involved simply determining if a potential drug causes catalepsy or if chronic drug treatment results in oral dyskinesias. The former phenomenon is an acute effect produced by DA receptor blockade in the caudate-putamen while the latter phenomenon may be related to antipsychotic-induced increases in DA levels or up-regulation of D_2 receptors within the same brain region. Another assay of extrapyramidal side-effect liability is the ability of a given drug to reduce DA agonist-induced stereotypy. This ability has also been linked to DA receptor blockade in the caudate-putamen. These behavioral models of side-effect liability allow one to make clear distinctions between typical and atypical antipsychotic drugs. If a drug produces catalepsy or blocks stereotypy at a dose which is similar to the dose needed to reverse locomotor hyperactivity or PPI deficits, then the drug is likely to produce motor side effects in the clinic. However, if the dose needed to produce catalepsy and inhibit stereotypy is significantly higher than that required to affect hyperactivity or PPI, then the drug is unlikely to produce motor side effects. Several mechanisms may account for an atypical drug's lack of motor side-effect liability: antagonistic activity at $5\text{-}HT_2$ receptors or at cholinergic receptors (44), fast dissociation from D_2 receptors (29), or partial agonist activity at these same receptors (56).

X. CRITERIA FOR EVALUATING A BEHAVIORAL MODEL

When reviewing a drug's activity in behavioral models of antipsychotic drug action, several issues need to be considered (Table 2). First, the most important feature of a behavioral model is not whether it emulates the symptom in question (i.e., has face validity), but whether it can be used to reliably predict whether or not a given drug will have antipsychotic activity in the clinic. Second, one must always be on guard for false positives and false negatives in behavioral assays. Some drugs that are poor antipsychotics may reduce amphetamine-induced locomotor hyperactivity. The best way to

Table 2 Criteria for Evaluating a Behavioral Model

Predictive validity: Does a drug's effect on a specific animal behavior, regardless of the behavior, reliably predict a specific clinical effect?

False positives and negatives: The best indicator of a drug's potential clinical utility is its activity in not one, but several behavioral models.

Drug dose: Be cautious of studies using very low or high doses of known or potential antipsychotic drugs.

Duration of treatment: Most behavioral models assay the acute effects of potential drugs, but such studies may have limited relevance to the delayed clinical efficacy of antipsychotic drug treatment. Behavioral studies may have greater clinical relevance when they isolate behavioral changes observed after chronic drug treatment.

judge the potential efficacy of a new drug is to determine its activity in several behavioral (and biological) assays. Obviously, the chances that a drug has antipsychotic activity are greater if it also reduces the activity produced by other DA agonists and NMDA antagonists, as well as reversing PPI deficits and reducing CAR. Third, behavioral studies of subclinical or supraclinical doses of antipsychotic drugs probably bear little relevance to the clinical mechanisms of these drugs. To further complicate matters, the pharmacokinetics of a given drug dose will obviously be different in rodents in comparison to humans; thus the interval between drug injection and behavioral assessment is an important consideration. Finally, the issue of treatment duration is an important one. Behavioral studies of rats receiving chronic (greater than 2 weeks) antipsychotic treatment may offer more valid insights into the clinical effects of these drugs relative to acute treatment studies.

XI. SUMMARY

Behavioral models are a necessary component in the preclinical development of antipsychotic drugs. Despite their general lack of face validity in modeling symptoms of schizophrenia, these assays have been particularly effective in identifying drugs with antipsychotic activity. Behavioral testing has also been a reliable indicator of side-effect liability and, from these tests, clear-cut distinctions between typical and atypical drugs have emerged. The development and validation of preclinical paradigms which model the negative and cognitive symptoms are sorely needed and stand as the next frontier for behavioral pharmacologists interested in antipsychotic drug development. Such models may allow researchers to identify compounds that not only treat the positive symptoms of schizophrenia but can ameliorate the functionally debilitating aspects of the disorder.

REFERENCES

1. Adams B, Moghaddam B. Corticolimbic dopamine neurotransmission is temporally dissociated from the cognitive and locomotor effects of phencyclidine. J Neurosci 1998; 18:5545–5554.
2. Arnt J. Differential effects of classical and newer antipsychotics on the hypermotility induced by two dose levels of D-amphetamine. Eur J Pharmacol 1995; 283:55–62.
3. Aultman JM, Moghaddam B. Distinct contributions of glutamate and dopamine receptors to temporal aspects of rodent working memory using a clinically relevant task. Psychopharmacology 2001; 153:353–364.

4. Bardgett ME, Csernansky JG. Antipsychotic drug action after lesions to the hippocampus or prefrontal cortex. In: Csernansky JG, ed. Antipsychotics. Berlin: Springer, 1996:267–288.
5. Bardgett ME, Griffith MS. Daily clozapine treatment improves spatial memory deficits produced by hippocampal damage in rats. Schizophr Res 2003; 60(suppl):56.
6. Bardgett ME, Humphrey WM, Csernansky JG. The effects of excitotoxic hippocampal lesions in rats on risperidone- and olanzapine-induced locomotor suppression. Neuropsychopharmacology 2002; 27: 930–938.
7. Bardgett ME, Jackson JL, Taylor BM, Csernansky JG. The effects of kainic acid lesions on locomotor responses to haloperidol and clozapine. Psychopharmacology 1998; 135:270–278.
8. Bardgett ME, Jackson JL, Taylor GT, Csernansky JG. Kainic acid decreases hippocampal neuronal number and increases dopamine receptor binding in the nucleus accumbens: an animal model of schizophrenia. Behav Brain Res 1995; 70:153–164.
9. Bardgett ME, Jacobs PS, Jackson JL, Csernansky JG. Kainic acid lesions enhance locomotor responses to novelty, saline, amphetamine, and MK-801. Behav Brain Res 1997; 84:47–55.
10. Becker A, Grecksch G, Bernstein HG, Hollt V, Bogerts B. Social behaviour in rats lesioned with ibotenic acid in the hippocampus: quantitative and qualitative analysis. Psychopharmcology 1999; 144:333–338.
11. Becker T, Elmer K, Schneider F, Schneider M, Grodd W, Bartels M, Heckers S, Beckmann H. Confirmation of reduced temporal limbic structure volume on magnetic resonance imaging in male patients with schizophrenia. Psychiatry Res 1996; 67, 135–143.
12. Bilder RM, Goldman RS, Volavka J, Czobor P, Hoptman M, Sheitman B, Lindenmayer J-P, Citrome L, McEvoy J, Kunz M, Chakos M, Cooper TB, Horowitz TL, Liberman JA. Neurocognitve effects of clozapine, olanzapine, risperidone, and haloperidol in patients with chronic schizophrenia or schizoaffective disorder. Am J Psychiatry 2002; 159:1018–1028.
13. Carlsson ML, Marin P, Nilsson M, Sorensen SM, Carlsson A, Waters S, Waters N. The 5-HT2A receptor antagonist M11907 is more effective in counteracting NMDA antagonist- than dopamine agonist-induced hyperactivity in mice. J Neural Trans 1999; 106:123–129.
14. Clow A, Jenner P, Theodorov A, Mardsen CD. Striatal dopamine receptors become supersensitive while rats are given trifluoperazine for six months. Nature 1979; 278:59–61.
15. Csernansky JG, Wrona CT, Bardgett ME, Early TS, Newcomer JW. Subcortical dopamine and serotonin turnover during acute and subchronic administration of typical and atypical neuroleptics. Psychopharmacology 1993; 110:145–152.
16. Csernansky JG, Wang L, Jones D, Rastogi-Cruz D, Posener JA, Heydebrand G, Miller JP, Miller MI. Hippocampal deformities in schizophrenia characterized by high dimensional brain mapping. Am J Psychiatry 2002; 159:2000–2006.

17. Didriksen M. Effects of antipsychotics on cognitive behaviour in rats using the delayed non-match to position paradigm. Eur J Pharmacol 1995; 281: 241–250.

18. Farde L, Wiesel FA, Hallidin C, Sedvall G. Central D_2-dopamine receptor occupancy in schizophrenic patients treated with antipsychotic drugs. Arch Gen Psychiatry 1988; 45:71–76.

19. Farde L, Nordstrom AL, Wiesel FA, Pauli S, Hallidin C, Sedvall G. Positron emission tomographic analysis of central D_1 and D_2 receptor occupancy in patients treated with classical neuroleptics and clozapine: relation to extrapyramidal side effects. Arch Gen Psychiatry 49:538–544.

20. Faustman WO, Hoff AL. Effects of antipsychotic drugs on neuropsychological measures. In: Csernansky JG, ed. Antipsychotics. Berlin: Springer, 1996: 445–478.

21. Gao XM, Hashimoto T, Cooper TB, Tamminga CA. The dose-response characteristics of rat oral dyskinesias with chronic haloperidol or clozapine administration. J Neural Trans 1997; 104:97–104.

22. Gao XM, Sakai K, Tamminga CA. Chronic clozapine or sertindole treatment results in reduced oral chewing movements in rats compared to haloperidol. Neuropsychopharmcology 1998; 19:428–433.

23. Geyer MA, Markou A. Animal models of psychiatric disorders. In: Bloom FE, Kupfer DJ, eds. Psychopharmacology: The Fourth Generation of Progress. New York: Raven Press, 1995.

24. Hauber W. Clozapine improves dizocilipine-induced delayed alternation impairment in rats. 1993; 94:223–233.

25. Hertel P, Fagerqusit MV, Svensson TH. Enhanced cortical dopamine output and antipsychotic-like effects of raclopride by α_2 adrenoreceptor blockade. Science 1999; 286:105–107.

26. Iversen SD, Iversen LL. Behavioral Pharmacology. 2nd edn. New York: Oxford University Press, 1981.

27. Jacobs PS, Taylor BM, Bardgett ME. Maturation of locomotor and Fos responses to the NMDA antagonists, PCP and MK-801. Dev Brain Res 2000; 122:91–95.

28. Julien RM. A Primer of Drug Action. 9th edn. New York: Worth, 2001.

29. Kapur S, Seeman P. Does fast dissociation from the dopamine D_2 receptor explain the action of atypical antipsychotics?: A new hypothesis. Am J Psychiatry 2001; 158:360–369.

30. Kapur S, Wadenberg M-L, Remington G. Are animal studies of antipsychotics appropriately dosed?: Lessons from the bedside to the bench. Can J Psychiatry 2000; 45:241–246.

31. Kelly PH, Seviour PW, Iversen SD. Amphetamine and apomorphine responses in the rat following 6-OHDA lesions of the nucleus accumbens septi and corpus striatum. Brain Res 1975; 94:507–522.

32. Kikuchi T, Tottori K, Uwahodo Y, Hirose T, Miwa T, Oshiro Y, Morita S. 7-(4-[4-(2,3-Dichlorophenyl)-1-piperazinyl]butyloxy)-3,4-dihydro-2(1H)-quino-linone (OPC-14597), a new putative antipsychotic drug with both presynaptic

dopamine autoreceptor agonistic activity and postsynaptic D2 receptor antagonistic activity. J Pharmacol Exp Ther. 1995; 274:329–336.

33. Le Pen G, Moreau JL. Disruption of prepulse inhibition of startle reflex in a neurodevelopmental model of schizophrenia: reversal by clozapine, olanzapine and risperidone but not by haloperidol. Neuropsychopharmacology 2002; 27:1–11.

34. Lipska BK, Jaskiw GE, Weinberger DR. Postpubertal emergence of hyperresponsiveness to stress and to amphetamine after neonatal excitotoxic hippocampal damage: a potential animal model of schizophrenia. Neuropsychopharmacology 1993; 9:67–75.

35. Lipska BK, Weinberger DR. Delayed effects of neonatal hippocampal damage on haloperidol-induced catalepsy and apomorphine-induced stereotyped behaviors in the rat. Dev Brain Res 1993; 75:213–222.

36. Lipska BK, Aultman JM, Verma A, Weinberger DR, Moghaddam B. Neonatal damage of the ventral hippocampus impairs working memory in the rat. Neuropsychopharmacology 2002; 27:47–54.

37. Mansbach RS, Carver J, Zorn SH. Blockade of drug-induced deficits in prepulse inhibition of acoustic startle by ziprasidone. Pharmacol Biochem Behav 2001; 69:535–542.

38. Mathe JM, Nomikos GG, Hildebrand BE, Hertel P, Svensson TH. Prazosin inhibits MK-801 induced hyperlocomotion and dopamine release in the nucleus accumbens. Eur J Pharmacol 1996; 309:1–11.

39. McCarley RW, Wible CG, Frumin M, Hirayasu Y, Levitt JJ, Fischer IA, Shenton ME. MRI anatomy of schizophrenia. Biol Psychiatry 1999; 45:1099–1119.

40. Meltzer HY, McGurk SR. The effects of clozapine, risperidone, and olanzapine on cognitive function in schizophrenia. Schizophr Bull 1995; 25:233–255.

41. Migler BM, Warawa EJ, Malick JB. Seroquel: behavioral effects in conventional and novel tests for atypical antipsychotic drugs. Psychopharmacology 1993; 112:299–307.

42. Moghaddam B, Adams BW. Reversal of phencyclidine effects by a group II metabotropic glutamate receptor agonist in rats. Science 1998; 281:1349–1352.

43. Naidu PS, Kulkarni SK. Effect of 5-HT1A and 5-HT2A/2C receptor modulation on neuroleptic-induced vacuous chewing movements. Eur J Pharmacol 2001; 428:81–86.

44. Ogren SO. The behavioural pharmacology of typical and atypical antipsychotic drugs. In: Csernansky JG, ed. Antipsychotics. Berlin: Springer, 1996:225–266.

45. Ogren SO, Goldstein M. Phencyclidine- and dizocilpine-induced hyperlocomotion are differentially mediated. Neuropsychopharmcology 1994; 11:167–177.

46. Olney JW, Farber NB. Glutamate dysfunction and schizophrenia. Arch Gen Psychiatry 1995; 52:998–1007.

47. Pollock BG, Mulsant BH. Use of antipsychotic drugs in the elderly. In: Csernansky JG, ed. Antipsychotics. Berlin: Springer, 1996:505–530.

48. Rajarethinam R, DeQuardo JR, Miedler J, Arndt S, Kirbat R, Brunberg JA, Tandon R. Hippocampus and amygdala in schizophrenia: assessment of the

relationship of neuroanatomy to psychopathology. Psychiatry Res 2001; 108:79–87.

49. Rossi A, Stratta P, Mancini F, Gallucci M, Mattei P, Core L, Di Michele V, Casacchia M. Magnetic resonance imaging findings of amygdala-anterior hippocampus shrinkage in male patients with schizophrenia. Psychiatry Res 1994; 52, 43–53.

50. Sams-Dodd F. Distinct effects of d-amphetamine and phencyclidine on the social behaviour of rats. Behav Pharmacol 1995; 6:55–65.

51. Sams-Dodd F. Phencyclidine-induced stereotyped behavior and social isolation in rats: a possible animal model of schizophrenia. Behav Pharmacol 1996; 7:3–23.

52. Sams-Dodd F, Lipska BK, Weinberger DR. Neonatal lesions of the rat ventral hippocampus result in hyperlocomotion and deficits in social behaviour in adulthood. Psychopharmacology 1997; 132:303–310.

53. Saykin A, Gur RC, Gur RE, Mozley D, Mozley L, Resnick SM, Kester B. Stafiniak P. Neuropsychological function in schizophrenia: selective impairment in learning and memory. Arch Gen Psychiatry 1991; 48:618–624.

54. See RE, Ellison G. Intermittent and continuous haloperidol regimens produce different types of oral dyskinesias in rats. Psychopharmacology 1990; 100: 404–412.

55. See RE, Kalivas PW. Tolerance and sensitization to the effects of antipsychotic drugs on dopamine neurotransmission. In: Csernansky JG, ed. Antipsychotics. Berlin: Springer, 1996: 203–224.

56. Semba J, Watanabe A, Kito S, Toru M. Behavioural and neurochemical effects of OPC-14597, a novel antipsychotic drug, on dopaminergic mechanisms in rat brain. Neuropharmacology. 1995; 34:785–791.

57. Shenton ME, Kikinis R, Jolesz FA, Pollak SD, LeMay M, Wible CG, Hokama H, Martin J, Metcalf D, Coleman M, McCarley RW. Abnormalities of the left temporal lobe and thought disorder in schizophrenia. A quantitative magnetic resonance imaging study. N Engl J Med. 1992; 327:604–612.

58. Skarsfeldt T. Differential effect of antipsychotics on place navigation of rats in the Morris swim maze. A comparative study between novel and reference antipsychotics. Psychopharmacology 1996; 124:126–133.

59. Swerdlow NR, Braff DL, Bakshi VP, Geyer MA. An animal model of sensorimotor gating deficits in schizophrenia predicts antipsychotic drug action. In: Csernansky JG, ed. Antipsychotics. Berlin: Springer, 1996:289–312.

60. Swerdlow NR, Braff DL, Taaid N, Geyer MA. Assessing the validity of an animal model of sensorimotor gating deficits in schizophrenic patients. Arch Gen Psychiatry 1994; 51:139–154.

61. Wiley JL, Kennedy KL. Evaluation of the efficacy of antipsychotic attenuation of phencyclidine-disrupted prepulse inhibition in rats. J Neural Transm 2002; 109:523–535.

5

Metabolic Regulation and Atypical Antipsychotic Drugs

Pierre Chue

University of Alberta,
Edmonton, Alberta, Canada

I. INTRODUCTION

The metabolic effects of antipsychotic drugs (APs) have become a focus of clinical attention influencing the choice and use of AP (1). With conventional antipsychotic drugs (CAPs), the focus of tolerability and safety concerns had been with neurological side effects such as extrapyramidal symptoms (EPS) and tardive dyskinesia (TD). Other tolerability and safety issues, notably diabetes mellitus (DM), weight gain, and dyslipidemia received less attention with CAPs, even though their occurrence had been reported with them. In contrast, the atypical antipsychotic drugs (AAPs) are associated with a much lower burden of movement disorders than CAPs, and consequently the focus has shifted to an examination of these metabolic issues as well as discussion concerning the most appropriate investigations and level of monitoring required with the use of AAPs in psychiatric populations (2,3).

II. DIABETES

There are increasing data describing a hierarchy of liability of diabetic association with the AAPs. However, most of these studies are either in the form of retrospective cohort and chart reviews (4–7), or analyses of prescription data (8–12). As a consequence of methodology, these studies likely underestimate the true prevalence of DM, particularly early glucose dysregulation, since they depend upon the diagnosis of DM either having been made and/or treatment initiated. Furthermore, any real differences between the APs are often confounded by lack of control for such factors as baseline weight and change, ethnicity, family history, treatment duration and history, diagnosis and phase of illness, smoking status, and concomitant medications including other APs. Furthermore, findings from studies based upon random glucose values (often extrapolated from clinical trial data) or even fasting plasma glucose (FPG) should be interpreted with caution, since these investigations lack sufficient sensitivity particularly to detect early stages of glucose dysregulation when compared to a standard oral glucose tolerance test (OGTT) (13).

A number of chart review studies have looked at the differences between AAPs. In a naturalistic retrospective chart review of 126 patients receiving an AAP in an academically affiliated state hospital over a 30-month period, baseline FPG levels were available for 21 patients, and 14 patients subsequently completed a diabetic evaluation (4). New onset acute impaired glucose tolerance (IGT) was reported to have developed in 11 of the 14 patients treated with clozapine, olanzapine, or quetiapine. Six of the 11 patients required insulin therapy (four received transient treatment) and five patients developed diabetic ketoacidosis (DKA). Of these five patients, two (a 49-year-old African-American male and a 31-year-old African-American female) were on olanzapine, two were on clozapine and one on quetiapine. Mean and median time to onset of DKA was 81 and 33 days respectively. Changes in GTT were not related to weight gain and generally occurred in the first 6 weeks of treatment. Mean and median weight gains in patients with new onset DM were 7.27 and 3.64 kg, respectively. The charts on 405 patients with schizophrenia in the primary care clinic of a schizophrenia treatment and research center were reviewed in another study (5). Fifty-five patients (13%) had been diagnosed with type 2 DM: (16%), fluphenazine (4%), haloperidol (6.6%), olanzapine (11%), risperidone (6%), and other antipsychotics (7.3%).

Clozapine was compared to olanzapine in a retrospective chart review of patients treated with either drug for 4 months or more (6). Mean length of treatment was 3.6 years on clozapine ($n = 29$) and 1.4 years on olanzapine ($n = 136$). Changes in body mass index (BMI) and FPG were measured. Six of 16 patients on clozapine (38%) with normal pre-treatment FPG developed elevations of FPG during treatment. Seven of 39 patients on olanzapine (18%) with normal pre-treatment FPG developed elevations of FPG during treatment. Sixty-nine percent of patients on clozapine and 50%

of patients on olanzapine showed weight gain of more than 7% above baseline. BMI increased from 25.53 to 29.35 (16%) in patients on clozapine and from 28.08 to 30.80 (9.7%) in patients on olanzapine. For both drugs, neither weight gain nor BMI change correlated with age, gender, dose, duration of treatment, or starting weight. Glucose elevations were not correlated with weight gain.

The frequency of DM across age groups and different APs was examined using a multiple logistic regression analysis over a 4-month period, and odds ratios (ORs) calculated at a 95% confidence interval (95%CI) (7). Of the 38,632 veterans studied, 15,984 received CAPs, and 22,648 received AAPs; clozapine ($n = 1207$), olanzapine ($n = 10,970$), quetiapine ($n = 955$), or risperidone ($n = 9902$). A higher percentage of the AAP cohort compared with the CAP cohort in the under 40 (8.74% versus 6.21%; $p = 0.007$), 40–49 (15.89% versus 13.93%, $p = 0.002$), and 50–59 (22.73% versus 20.56%; $p = 0.003$) age groups were diagnosed with DM. By medication prescribed, risk of DM was also increased for clozapine (OR = 1.251; 95%CI = 1.070–1.462), olanzapine (OR = 1.107; 95%CI = 1.038–1.180), and quetiapine (OR = 1.313; 95%CI = 1.113–1.547), but not risperidone (OR = 1.049; 95%CI = 0.982–1.120). Patients on AAPs were more likely to be female, have other psychiatric diagnoses, be African-American, not be on veteran support, and have fewer hospitalizations. Some patients on AAPs also received CAPs in the same period but were only included in the AAP group for analysis (94% of patients remained on the same drug through the 4 months of study). Sample sizes were disparate and there were no data on concomitant medications.

A number of prescription claims-based studies have looked at the differences between AAPs. Claims data for 7933 patients diagnosed with psychotic disorders within health plans in the US were analyzed (8). The frequency of new onset type 2 DM in untreated patients and among patients treated with risperidone, olanzapine, clozapine, high potency, and low potency CAPs was compared using episodes of treatment as the basis of observation. Logistic regression models developed to compare the ORs of reporting DM based on 12 months of exposure determined the values to be 2.44 (±2.10) for olanzapine, 6.72 (±4.71) for clozapine, 1.99 (±1.95) for high potency CAPs, 3.21 (±2.27) for low potency CAPs and 0.79 (±2.39) for risperidone. Older age, observation period length, and greater use of non-antipsychotic psychotropic medications were also significant predictors of DM. Although this study controlled for concomitant (non-antipsychotic) medications, patients could be on multiple APs and diabetic risk was ascribed to both drugs, and only 17.2% of patients had a diagnosis of schizophrenia. Patients were assessed at different time points and the data extrapolated to 12 months. Among patients receiving clozapine, schizophrenia was the commonest diagnosis (57%) and the duration of AP treatment was the longest (9.4 ± 5.5 months). Concurrent use of other APs was greater in the olanzapine group and the daily dose of olanzapine was higher than that of the other APs; dose was a predictor of DM for olanzapine only.

Another study examined a prescription claims database identifying patients on AP monotherapy who also received prescriptions for anti-diabetic agents (9). Hazard ratios (HRs) calculated using a Cox proportional hazard regression model were: 1.7 for quetiapine (95%CI = 1.2–2.4; $n = 4,186$), 3.0 for olanzapine (95%CI = 2.6–3.5; $n = 13,863$), 3.1 for haloperidol (95%CI = 2.6–3.7; $n = 8476$), 3.3 for clozapine (95%CI = 1.4–8.0; $n = 277$), 3.4 for risperidone (95%CI = 3.1–3.80; $n = 20,633$), and 4.2 for thioridazine (95%CI = 3.2–5.5; $n = 3133$). There was no statistically significant difference in risk of developing DM between the AAP and CAP cohorts (HR = 0.966; 95%CI = 0.8–1.1; $p = 0.6$), or between olanzapine and risperidone cohorts; the risperidone cohort compared to the haloperidol cohort was associated with an increased risk (HR = 1.2; 95%CI = 1.0–1.5; $p = 0.04$). The mean age for the AAP cohort was 60 years and for the CAP cohort was 64 years. No diagnostic information was available and the general population cohort comprised healthy non-psychotic individuals. The average duration of treatment for an AAP (except clozapine) was 90 days. Although mean age and gender were controlled, the individual cohorts varied considerably in age distribution with risperidone of the AAPs having the greatest percentage of subjects of age greater than 65 years (56%). Thus not only were sample sizes disparate, but the data are confounded by diagnostic issues and potentially by an age and treatment duration effect.

A population-based, nested, case-control study of 19,637 schizophrenic patients from the U.K. General Practice Database found that patients taking olanzapine had a significantly increased risk of developing DM compared to non-users of antipsychotics (OR = 5.8; 95%CI = 0.0–16.7), and those taking CAPs (OR = 4.2; 95%CI = 1.5–12.2) (10). Patients taking risperidone had a non-significant increased risk of developing DM compared to non-users of antipsychotics (OR = 2.2; 95%CI = 0.9–5.2), and those taking CAPs (OR = 1.6; 95%CI = 0.7–3.8). Women showed a higher incidence rate than men (5.3 versus 3.5/1000 person years), and the incidence rate for both sexes within 3 months of a prescription was 10.0/1000 person years for olanzapine (95%CI = 5.2–19.2), 5.4/1000 person years for risperidone (95%CI = 3.0–9.8), and 5.1/1000 person years for CAPs (95%CI = 4.5–5.8).

To directly compare the risk of DM among patients treated with olanzapine or risperidone, two cohorts totaling 33,946 patients were identified from the Quebec Medicare database (11). One cohort consisted of patients who had received at least one prescription of olanzapine ($n = 19,153$) and the other cohort consisted of patients who had received at least one prescription of risperidone but not olanzapine ($n = 14,793$). In the olanzapine cohort 319 patients developed DM compared to 217 in the risperidone cohort. When age, gender, and haloperidol use were controlled for using proportional hazard analysis, there was a 20% increased risk of diabetes with olanzapine relative to risperidone (95%CI = 0–43%; $p = 0.05$). Furthermore, after adjusting for the duration of treatment, the first 3 months of olanzapine treatment was associated with an increased risk of diabetes of 90% (95%CI = 40–157%; $p < 0.0001$). Women taking olanzapine had a 31% (95%CI = 5–65%) higher risk of developing DM compared to women on risperidone, and women taking olanzapine had a 68% (95%CI = 32–169%) higher risk of developing DM compared to men on olanzapine. Diagnosis was controlled for, but as with all of the prescription claims-based studies, there were no data on baseline BMI and weight change.

Lambert et al. (12) conducted a matched case-control study (3102 cases, 8271 age and gender-matched controls) from the California Medicaid claims data of patients with schizophrenia. Exposure to olanzapine (OR = 1.3; 95%CI = 1.17–1.45), clozapine (OR = 1.42; 95%CI = 1.2–1.69), or quetiapine (OR = 1.45; 95%CI = 1.11–1.9), but not risperidone (OR = 1.10; 95%CI = 0.98–1.24) increased the risk significantly of developing type 2 DM. African-American (and unknown) ethnicity were also risk factors as were concomitant medications.

Other studies have looked at the direct effect of APs on insulin and glucose metabolism. The effect of an oral 50 g dextrose challenge on plasma glucose (PG) and insulin levels was examined in patients with schizophrenia ($n = 32$) treated with risperidone, olanzapine, or clozapine, and in healthy controls ($n = 31$) (14). PG varied significantly across treatment groups at baseline; both clozapine and olanzapine patients had higher PG levels at baseline compared to controls ($P = 0.002$ and $P = 0.007$ respectively) and to risperidone patients ($P = 0.05$ and $P = 0.02$ respectively). At 75 min after glucose challenge, clozapine and olanzapine patients had higher PG levels than controls; clozapine patients also had higher insulin levels than controls, but this was not statistically significant. Although the oral dextrose challenge was lower than the 75 g used in a standard OGTT, the trends are not only consistent with most data in this area, but it is likely that the differences shown with olanzapine and clozapine would have been even greater with the larger dextrose dose. The authors further investigated the potential for different APs to influence glucose regulation independent of differences in adiposity (15). Modified OGTTs were

performed in schizophrenic patients ($n = 48$) receiving clozapine, olanzapine, risperidone, or CAPs, and untreated healthy controls ($n = 31$) matched
for age and adiposity. Subjects with DM were excluded. Blood samples were
obtained at 0 (fasting), 15, 45, and 75 min post glucose load. Significant
time × treatment group interactions for PG ($F(12,222) = 4.89$, $p < 0.001$)
and insulin ($F(12,171) = 2.10$, $p = 0.02$) were found. Effects of treatment
group on PG were significant at all time points, with olanzapine-treated
patients having significant glucose elevations at all time points (1.0–1.5
S.D.), in comparison to controls as well as patients receiving CAPs.
Clozapine-treated patients had significant glucose elevations at fasting and
75 min (1–1.5 S.D.) compared to controls and patients receiving CAPs.
Risperidone-treated patients had similar elevations in fasting and post-
load glucose levels, but only in comparison to healthy controls. The
authors postulated that clinically significant hyperglycemia could occur
during AP treatment independent of adiposity owing to insulin resistance
(IR) effects.

In contrast to the previous studies, an analysis was conducted of
random blood glucose data pooled from 78 clinical trials (16). The
incidences and estimated time-to-event rates (Kaplan–Meier analyses) were
calculated for treatment-emergent potential IGT (160 mg/dL) and potential
DM (200 mg/dL) in patients without indicators of hyperglycemia at baseline, and for treatment with olanzapine ($n = 4,574$), clozapine ($n = 200$),
risperidone ($n = 267$), haloperidol ($n = 888$), or placebo ($n = 445$). The
estimated rates of treatment-emergent IGT or DM (from 2.7–15.4% over
0.5 to 2 years) were higher than expected for all treatment groups and
placebo. Time-to-event time was not different between olanzapine,
risperidone, haloperidol, or placebo, but was significantly greater with
olanzapine compared to clozapine. Risk factors included age, an increase in
adiposity during treatment, and maximum absolute body weight. However,
as previously discussed random PG estimation is of very limited value as a
measure of potential DM.

There are a few studies looking specifically at indices of DM and IR
including the homeostasis model of insulin resistance (HOMA-IR) and lipid
metabolism changes including total cholesterol (TCHOL), triglycerides
(TGs), low-density cholesterol (LDL-C), and high-density cholesterol
(HDL-C) between the AAPs (17,18), following switches from olanzapine,
risperidone, or CAPs to ziprasidone (19), and olanzapine to risperidone
(20). A study of 85 chronic schizophrenics on AP monotherapy for at least
3 months (mean = 3.3 years) and controlling for confounding factors, found
statistically significant differences for FPG and TGs between clozapine-
and CAP-treated patients, and hyperinsulinemia and clinical obesity in
olanzapine-treated patients (17).

There have been case reports dating back to 1994 in the psychiatric literature linking clozapine with hyperglycemia, *de novo* DM, DKA, worsening of previously controlled DM, and increased risk of gestational diabetes (21–38). Furthermore, a number of these case reports describe resolution or improvement of DM on reduction or discontinuation of clozapine and recurrence of DM when rechallenged with the drug (26,27,38,39). The published case reports are dicussed in other reviews (40–43), and are summarized in Table 1 (21,22,24–35,38,39,44,45). In summary, more cases have been reported for males and non-Caucasians, and most, but not all patients had experienced significant weight gain. Time of onset of DM after clozapine initiation varied from 6 days to 2 years and dose of clozapine ranged from 100 mg to 900 mg/day.

Ethnicity is a risk factor for IR and may therefore be relevant in terms of predisposition to AP-associated DM. In a study of 23 individuals of mixed and Curaçao descent on clozapine in the Netherlands, hyperglycemia was detected in 10 patients and DM in two patients (46). In 16 patients, PG had been checked before the initiation of treatment and thus, the authors recommended routine determination of PG levels before and after treatment with clozapine particularly in mixed populations with subjects of African origin. Similarly, in a case of a 25-year-old Chinese male who demonstrated hyperglycemia, hypertriglyceridemia, and periodic paralysis repeatedly when challenged with doses of clozapine above 150 mg/day, these symptoms either disappeared on discontinuation or ameliorated with dose reduction (38). However, mental state deteriorated with dose reduction and the patient was eventually stabilized on a combination of haloperidol (20 mg/day) and clozapine (25 mg/day) with normalization of metabolic parameters. In contrast, in a 58-year-old male with type 2 DM on clozapine (600 mg/day) and benperidol (30 mg/day), the PG peaks of 135–140 mg/dL coincided with a reduction in his movement disorder (47). Pregnancy is associated with gestational DM, and a case report is described of a 28-year-old woman with a history of hyperglycemia who required oral hypoglycemics after commencing clozapine and later went on to require insulin during pregnancy; delivery was complicated by shoulder dystocia (36).

Other studies examining the association of DM with clozapine have looked at a direct effect on insulin action as well as indirectly through weight gain. In 45 patients with schizophrenia being treated with clozapine, seven cases with DM and three cases with impaired fasting glucose (IFG) were identified; 49% of the sample met the criteria for obesity (BMI > 30) (48). Total glucose intolerance (DM and IFG) was statistically associated with obesity, but not with age, race, or family history of DM. In contrast, an analysis of claims data from the Iowa Medicaid program (1990–1998) of 3013 patients with schizophrenia did not identify any significant differences

Table 1 Summary of Case Reports of Clozapine-Induced Glucose Dysregulation

Ref.	Concomitant medications	Clozapine dose	Age/race/ sex	Obesity, weight change, BMI (kg/m²)	Personal history	Family history	Time to onset of DM
21	None	300 mg	30/B/M	NR	HbA$_{1C}$ 11%	Negative	5 months
29	Ranitidine, benztropine	900 mg	41/B/M	NR	Negative	NR	2 months
26	Lithium, benztropine	250 mg	34/B/F	NR	Negative	Type 1 DM	6 weeks
31	NR	350 mg	42/NR/M	Obese	Negative	Type 2 DM	4 weeks
25	Lithium, verapamil, bethanechol	500 mg	46/B/M	NR	Hypertension	DM (type NR)	5 weeks
30	—	NR	37/C/M	NR	Negative	Negative	11 weeks
22	Carbamazepine	200 mg	31/C/M	BMI = 29/I kg	Negative	Negative	3 months
35	None	325 mg	30/B/M	NR	Negative	Negative	3 months
34	—	NR (low dose)	57/NR/F	NR	Negative	NR	
28	Ephedrine	425 mg	32/B/M	11% over IBW/4 kg increase over 5 weeks	Negative	Type 1 & 2 DM	8 weeks
28	Risperidone (taper), hydrochlorthiazide, lithium	450 mg	44/B/M	42% over IBW/1.4 kg increase over 5 weeks	Hypertension	Negative	5 weeks
28	Glyburide	200 mg	51/C/M	No change	Type 2 DM	NR	2 weeks

	Concomitant medications	Dose	Age/Race/Sex	Weight			Duration
28	Lisinopril, glyburide	900 mg	51/B/M	NR/no Change	Type 2 DM Hypertension	NR	4 months
44	Prazosin, H2 blockers, prednisone	900 mg	45/NR/M	53% over IBW, 23 kg in 6 years	Negative	Negative	17 months
44	Metoprolol, lisinopril, nitroglycerin, fludrocortisone	NR	54/NR/M	7% over IBW, 19 kg in 7 years	Hyperglycemia	Negative	4 years
32	—	150 mg	47/B/M	9% over IBW/11 kg (11%) increase over 8 weeks	IGT	Negative	2 months
32	—	400 mg	32/B/M	No obesity/26 kg (37%) increase over 18 months	Negative	Negative	18 months
32	—	100 mg	43/B/M	13% over IBW/3 kg (4%) increase over 20 weeks	Negative	Type 2 DM	6 months
32	—	200 mg	41/B/M	38% over IBW/ No weight change from baseline	Negative	Negative	5 weeks
33	—	120 mg	48/C/M	NR	NR	NR	Unclear
23	—	NR	40/B/M	NR	Negative	Negative	6 days
24	—	300 mg	50/C/M	NR	NR	NR	10 days
27	—	400 mg	50/C/F	NR	Negative	Negative	1 month
45	—		24/O/F				1 week
38	—	125 mg	25/C/M	NR	NR	NR	12 months
39	Perphenazine		40/C/M	NR	NR	NR	

NR, not reported; B, Black; C, Caucasian; O, Oriental; M, male; F, female; IBW, ideal body weight.

in overall incidence rates for DM, hyperlipidemia, or hypertension between clozapine-treated ($n = 552$) and CAP-treated groups ($n = 2461$) (49). However, a sub-analysis of younger patients (20–34 years) did find that clozapine was associated with a significantly increased relative risk (RR) of DM (RR = 2.5; CI 1.1–5.2) and hyperlipidemia (RR = 2.4; CI 1.1–5.2), but not hypertension (RR = 0.9; CI 0.4–0.2).

A comparison of 63 patients treated with clozapine with 67 patients treated with CAPs (haloperidol, zuclopenthixol, fluphenazine, perphenazine) was conducted in Sweden (50). Random PG tests were followed by an OGTT; none of the patients had evidence of DM before treatment. Of the patients treated with clozapine, 21 (33%) had hyperglycemia defined as PG > 6.6 mmol/L and 13 (22%) patients were classified as having DM or IGT. Of the patients treated with CAPs, 13 (19%) had hyperglycemia and six (9%) patients were classified as having DM or IGT. The findings were not statistically significant due to the small sample size. Subjects in the clozapine group were significantly younger, had a shorter duration of disease, and had been treated for a shorter period than subjects in the control group, but the two groups did not differ with respect to BMI or prevalence of DM in first degree relatives. Females were more often diagnosed with DM or IGT when treated with clozapine than when treated with CAPs. Although not statistically significant, the concentration of the metabolite, desmethylclozapine, was higher in patients with hyperglycemia. The influence of duration of treatment was shown in a 5-year naturalistic study of 102 out-patients with schizophrenia or schizoaffective disorder (51). Thirty patients of 82 completing the study (36%) were diagnosed with DM. Weight gain, gender, concomitant use of valproate, and total daily dose of clozapine were not significant risk factors for developing DM. However, weight gain was characteristic of patients who developed type 1 DM. Eleven patients were excluded from the study because of either a known history of DM ($n = 5$) or a FPG greater or equal to 140 ng/mL ($n = 6$). Of the five patients with a known history, two were on insulin and three on oral hypoglycemics. Both the insulin-treated patients required an almost two-fold increase in insulin requirements, and two of the patients on oral agents went on to require insulin after clozapine initiation. Age was significantly correlated with the development of DM. Although the small number of non-Caucasian patients precluded an analysis based on ethnicity, two of the African-American and two of three Hispanic patients had abnormal FPG and required treatment. The lack of dose effect is interesting and may be related to the poor correlation between dose and serum level with clozapine (serum levels of clozapine or desmethylclozapine were not measured in this study). This was further investigated in 28 patients treated with CAPs and 13 patients treated with clozapine (52). It was found that fasting plasma insulin (FPI) levels correlated positively with serum concentrations of clozapine, whereas no correlation was found between FPI and serum concentrations of perphenazine or zuclopenthixol. Correlations were also noted between insulin-like growth factor (IGF-1) and insulin-like growth factor binding protein (IGFBP-1) and clozapine. The normal PG levels in the clozapine group support the theory that clozapine induces concentration-dependent IR with secondary increased insulin secretion. In addition, lower growth hormone (GH) secretion in the clozapine group was detected. This impaired GH secretion together with the clozapine-induced IR was suggested to be one of the mechanisms behind weight gain during clozapine therapy; thus, clozapine may also be associated with DM indirectly through weight gain. It has also been suggested that clozapine-induced suppression of Ca^{2+}-dependent K^+ efflux may be responsible for reduced insulin secretion by β-pancreatic islet cells, leading to hyperglycemia (30). Another study examined PG, insulin, and C-peptide levels in three female and three male clozapine-treated patients (titrated to 450 mg/day from 12.5 mg/day in 6 weeks); all with negative family history of DM and no concomitant medications (53). Clozapine increased concentrations of PG, insulin, and C-peptide concentrations compared to baseline at 3 weeks (200 mg/day) and 6 weeks (450 mg/day). The authors concluded that clozapine's effect on glucose regulation was due to the development of IR.

Wang et al. (54) completed a case-control study of 7227 cases of newly diagnosed DM and 6780 controls, all with psychiatric disorders and enrolled in a U.S. state Medicaid program. Clozapine use was not associated with an increased risk of developing DM (OR = 0.98; CI = 0.74–1.31), in contrast to chlorpromazine (OR = 1.3; CI = 1.05–1.22), or perphenazine (OR = 1.34; CI = 1.11–1.62). However, clozapine-treated patients represented only 1.3% of the cases and 1.7% of the controls, and it was unclear as to whether AP treatment was exclusively monotherapy.

With olanzapine, there has been an increasing number of case reports since 1996 linking it with hyperglycemia, *de novo* DM, DKA, worsening of previously controlled DM, and increased risk of gestational diabetes (32,55–62). Similar to clozapine studies, a number of these case reports describe resolution or improvement of DM on reduction or discontinuation of olanzapine and recurrence of DM when rechallenged with the drug (57,59,63). The published case reports are discussed in other reviews (32,40,42), and are summarized in Table 2 (32,39,55,56–58,61,63–77).

As with clozapine, there appear to be risk factors for the development of DM with olanzapine that overlap with the risk factors for IR. There were more males and most, but not all patients had experienced significant weight gain. However, there were more Caucasians than non-Caucasians, but this may reflect the difference in use of olanzapine compared to clozapine. Time

Table 2 Summary of Case Reports of Olanzapine-Induced Diabetes or Glucose Dysregulation

Ref.	Concomitant medications	Olanzapine dose (mg/day)	Age/race/sex	Obesity, weight change, BMI (kg/m²)	Personal history	Family history	Time to onset of DM
32	—	25	38/B/M	Obese, 42% over IBW, 14 lbs (5%) increase over 12 weeks	Negative	Negative	3 months
32	—	25	56/C/M	Obese, 27% over IBW, no weight change from baseline	Negative	Negative	3 months
39	—	10	42/C/F	Negative	Negative	Type 2 DM	24 weeks
39	—	10	40/C/F	4.5–6.8 kg increase	Negative	Negative	17 months
39	—		41/C/F	NR	Negative	Negative	20 weeks
39	—		47/C/M	13.6 kg increase	Negative	Type 2 DM	5 weeks
39	—	10	43/C/M	11.4 kg increase	Negative	Negative	24 weeks
39	—	10	39/C/M	2.7 kg decrease	Negative	Type 2 DM	14 weeks
39	—	10	38/C/M	No change	Negative	Type 2 DM	12 weeks
56	—	10	45/B/M	25% increase	Type 2 DM	NR	4 weeks
57	—	20	32/B/M	NR	Negative	Negative	6 weeks
61	—		25/C/F	NR	Negative	NR	3 months
61[a]	Metoprolol, benzafibrate	20	24/C/NR	BMI = 22.3	Negative	NR	15 days
61		20	19/C/F	BMI = 26	Borderline GTT	Negative	3 months
58	—	30	50/B/M	9.5 kg increase	Negative	Negative	8 months
55	—	10	31/C/M	4 kg decrease	Negative	Negative	3 months
63[b]	Mirtazapine, sodium divalproex	10	31/B/M	12 kg increase, BMI = 32	Negative	DM (type unknown)	18 weeks
63[c]	Sodium divalproex, propanolol	15	44/C/M	BMI = 26	Negative	DM (type unknown)	4 months
64	None	20	31/NR/M	BMI = 29	Negative	NR	3 weeks

65[d]	None	15	40/C/F	35 kg increase during pregnancy	Negative	Positive	26 weeks
66	Venlafaxine, sodium valproate, atorvastatin, propanolol	20	38/C/M	BMI = 36.7, 14 kg increase	Negative	Negative	12 months
67	Fluoxetine	10	54/B/F	13 kg increase	Type 2 DM	NR	12 days
68	NR	NR	28/B/M	BMI = 34	NR	NR	3.5 months
68	NR	NR	44/C/M	BMI = 39	NR	NR	6.5 months
68	NR	NR	39/C/M	BMI = 36	NR	NR	19.5 months
69	Gabapentin, venlafaxine, lansoprazole, isosorbide	25	51/C/M	7% over IBW	Negative	NR	6.5 months
70	Cloprednole	2.5	79/C/W	BMI = 21	IGT	NR	6 weeks
71	NR	20	55/NR/M	BMI = 28 (7 kg decrease)	Negative	Type 2 DM	4 months
71	NR	NR	41/NR/M	BMI = 40 (4 kg decrease)	Negative	Negative	3 months
72	Sodium valproate, buspirone	20	15/B/M	BMI = 34	Negative	Type 2 DM	12 months
73	—	20	19/B/M	No change	Negative	Negative	4 weeks
74	Venlafaxine, risperidone	15	16/H/F	14 kg increase	Negative	Type 2 DM	6 months
75	—		48/M	BMI = 28	Negative	NR	2 months
76	Sodium valproate, carbamazepine, hydrochlorothiazide/triamterene, conjugated estrogens		46/B/F		Negative		
77	Sodium valproate	10	27/B/M	BMI = 27 after 10 months	Negative	Negative	29 months

NR, not reported; B, Black; C, Caucasian; O, Oriental; H, Hispanic; M, male; F, female; IBW, ideal body weight. [a,c]Patients died. [b]Exacerbation on rechallenge despite 18 kg weight loss (BMI = 25 kg/m²). [d]Gestational DM.

of onset of DM after olanzapine initiation varied from 8 days to 2 years and dose of olanzapine ranged from 5 mg to 30 mg/day. Confounding factors such as concomitant medications and smoking history were not recorded for most cases. Two of these cases were associated with a fatal outcome; the first in a 24-year-old female after 15 days of olanzapine treatment (61), and the second was in a 31-year-old male re-initiated on olanzapine for a 3-week period (64).

In a study of 47 patients from two clinical trials investigating the efficacy of olanzapine in medication-refractory schizophrenia, five patients (10%) had elevations of PG from baseline, of which three patients (6.4%) met the criteria for DM (these three patients all had a personal or family history of DM) (65). A subsample data set of 34 patients had statistically higher maximum glucose values during treatment with olanzapine, although generally not in the clinically significant range (with the exception of the five cases identified) and unrelated to olanzapine dose (which ranged from 20 to 40 mg/day), or clinically significant weight gain (mean $= 3.8 \pm 9.3$ kg). There was a trend for black and Hispanic patients to have a greater rise in glucose than white or Asian patients (although ethnicity was apparently determined by surname). The authors concluded that the risk of hyperglycemia with olanzapine was comparable to expected prevalence rates in U.S. adults over 20 years of age. However, it should be noted that this study was not primarily designed to evaluate hyperglycemia with olanzapine and, thus, glucose evaluations were not necessarily fasting and concomitant medications, including lithium, were allowed.

Koller and Doraiswamy (78) identified 237 patients with olanzapine-associated DM or hyperglycemia (including 15 deaths) from the U.S. MedWatch Surveillance System and case report literature. The mean patient age was 40.7 ± 12.9 years, the male:female ratio was 1.8, and 73% of cases had appeared within 6 months of starting therapy. An addendum identified a further 52 cases (including 10 deaths); the authors concluded that the frequency of newly diagnosed DM in the 0–44 year age group was twice as high among olanzapine-treated patients (66%) than in the general population (33%), however there was no comparison to other atypicals or a psychiatric population.

There are significantly fewer reports linking risperidone to DM compared to olanzapine despite earlier introduction to the market, as well as one study demonstrating an improvement in IR and pancreatic islet cell function following a switch from olanzapine to risperidone (20). Risperidone has been reported to not exacerbate DM in one patient with pre-existing type 1 DM (79). A study involving the evaluation of HbA$_{1C}$ after 6–9 months treatment with risperidone in a Veterans Administration Medical Center showed no significant changes except in patients with pre-existing DM

($n = 4$), in whom there was a significant increase in HbA_{1C} and an increase in oral hypoglycemics (80). A case is reported of a white HIV-positive male on risperidone, fluoxetine, and trazodone with negative family history admitted in DKA (81). He was eventually discharged on quetiapine and insulin. It is unlikely that the concomitant medications played a role, but asymptomatic HIV illness may have been a factor since this has been reported in itself to result in hyperglycemia (82). In the treatment of psychosis with risperidone in 11 geriatric patients, two patients were reported to have developed type 2 DM (83). In contrast, a report on the use of risperidone in elderly patients with chronic psychosis and medical illnesses, including three with DM did not find that any of the patients showed any worsening of the medical problems (84). Similarly, a study of geriatric patients with chronic psychoses and concurrent medical illnesses including three with DM, found no exacerbation of DM with risperidone (85).

There have been two case reports to date concerning quetiapine (86, 87). In the first, a 42-year-old white male with no prior history except for hypertriglyceridemia, developed new onset DM following 1 month of quetiapine (200 mg/day). Concomitant medications included lithium, gabapentin, and venlafaxine. In the second, a 30-year-old man of Ethiopian descent (BMI = 32.3) developed DM after 16.5 weeks of treatment. However, he was also receiving fluphenazine, loxapine, and sodium valproate during this period. In an open label, non-randomized trial, 65 patients on clozapine monotherapy, all of whom had gained weight (mean weight gain 6.5 kg), including 13 who had developed DM, were started on quetiapine (88). These patients were subsequently followed for 10 months with evaluations of weight and glucose control. The dose of clozapine was reduced during combination therapy with satisfactory control of the schizophrenia. Interestingly, metabolic status improved, as shown by a reduction in weight in all patients (0.45 kg–18.6 kg; mean = 4.2 kg) and PG in 20%. Three of the patients eventually required no intervention for their DM. The authors concluded that the combination produced satisfactory control of the underlying psychiatric condition, and that quetiapine allowed lowering of the clozapine dose and improvement in weight and glucose control. However, some individual changes in weight were very small and the effect of reduction in clozapine and consequent lowering of serum levels cannot be discounted.

Data concerning ziprasidone are limited, three 6-week randomized open label trials evaluated outcome in stable patients with schizophrenia following a switch from CAPs ($n = 93$), olanzapine ($n = 88$), or risperidone ($n = 41$) to ziprasidone (40–160 mg/day) (19). A significant improvement in TCHOL and TGs was noted in patients switched from olanzapine and risperidone ($P \leq 0.05$). For patients switched from olanzapine, a significant reduction in weight (mean change $= 1.6$ kg) and BMI was also observed ($P \leq 0.05$). An open label study of 37 patients switched from different (undisclosed) AP monotherapies found significant reductions in non-fasting TCHOL ($P < 0.001$) and TG levels ($P = 0.018$), independent of changes in BMI (89). Thus far, in mostly clinical trial populations, it would appear that ziprasidone has minimal clinical effects on glucose regulation.

The mechanisms by which APs are associated with glucose dysregulation are also not yet clearly elucidated (90). The etiology is complex and likely to be multifactorial, with different factors of importance for different drugs additionally influenced by the relationship between DM and schizophrenia and the general risk factors for DM and IR. The effects on glucose regulation appear to be related to particular patterns of CNS receptor blockade and direct metabolic effects on systemic organs as well as indirect effects via weight gain. Chemical structure may possibly play a role since olanzapine (a thienobenzodiazepine) and clozapine (a dibenzodiazepine) share some similarity of structure; however, it is not clear whether this is a more important factor than receptor antagonism profiles.

The complexity of this area is highlighted in the results of a study in rats given a D_2 agonist (bromocriptine), a D_2/D_3 agonist (quinpirole), or a D_3 agonist (7-hydroxy-2-(di-n-propylamino)tetralin, 7-OH-DPAT) (91). Administration of 7-OH-DPAT produced a decrease in plasma insulin and an increase in glucose levels, which were blocked by pre-treatment with a D_2/D_3 antagonist (raclopride); quinpirole caused an increase in glucose only and bromocriptine had no effect. The role of adrenaline was hypothesized to be important in mobilizing blood sugar from the liver since the plasma levels of glucagon remained constant in these experiments. According to Saller and Kreamer (92) sympathoadrenal activation results in an increase in PG levels that is mediated by D_2 receptors. Furthermore, it is known that CAPs that are associated with hyperglycemia such as chlorpromazine, can increase adrenaline release from the adrenals as well as blocking α-adrenergic receptors (93,94). Pancreatic islets contain α_2- and β_2-adrenergic receptors, and α_2-receptor stimulation inhibits insulin release in contrast to stimulation of β_2 and vagal muscarinic receptors, which enhances insulin release (95). However, pancreatic effects on glucose tolerance are offset by effects of hepatic glucose production, which is increased by β_2-stimulation and decreased by α_2-stimulation, while hepatic glycogen synthesis is reduced by β_2-stimulation and increased by α_2-stimulation. Not only do the AAPs possess different antagonisms at α_2-adrenergic receptors, but the overall result may be either hyperglycemia or hypoglycemia.

In contrast to the results from Uvnas-Moberg et al. (91), bromocriptine when given with SKF 38393 (D_1 agonist) has been shown to normalize hyperphagia, body fat, hyperglycemia, and hyperlipidemia in ob/ob mice (96,97). It is suggested that sympatholytic dopamine agonists may act via the hypothalamic–neuroendocrine axis to correct autonomic control of pancreatic islet function (98). In humans, bromocriptine compared to placebo, significantly reduced FPG and HbA_{1C} through enhanced maximally stimulated insulin-mediated glucose disposal in a 16-week double-blind study in 22 obese, type 2 diabetics (99).

It has also been proposed that glucose regulation is mediated via D_3 and 5-HT_{1A} receptors separately, but with a putative common mechanism involving oxytocin (91). Oxytocinergic neurons of the paraventricular nucleus (PVN) of the hypothalamus project to the dorsal motor nucleus of the vagus (DMX) (100) and local application of oxytocin into the DMX lowers insulin via a vagal mechanism (101). 7-OH-DPAT increases oxytocin levels and stimulation of 5-HT_{1A} and $5\text{-HT}_2/5\text{-HT}_{1C}$ receptors induces oxytocin release in male rats (102).

The possibility that these drugs may affect glucose homeostasis directly through their impact on serotonin receptors has been suggested (32). However, the data in this area are complex and contradictory. No significant effects on plasma insulin, glucagon, or glucose were seen in rats after treatment with the selective agonist N-(3-trifluoromethylphenyl) piperazine HCl (TFMPP), the $5\text{-HT}_{2A/2C}$ agonist 1-(2,5-dimethoxy-4-iodophenyl)-2-aminopropane (DOI), or the 5-HT_3 agonist 1-(m-chloro-phenyl)-biguanide HCl (m-CPBG) (91). However, DOI has been shown to induce hyperglycemia via central inhibition of insulin release, and a peripherally acting $5\text{-HT}_{2A/C}$ agonist (α-methyl-5-HT) also produced hyperglyemia (103). The effect of DOI was significantly blocked by ketanserin (a $5\text{-HT}_{2A/2C/\alpha 1}$ antagonist) (104). Ritanserin (a $5\text{-HT}_{1C}/5\text{-HT}_{2A/B/C}$ antagonist) also blocked, to a lesser extent, DOI-induced hyperglycemia (103) although it did not demonstrate any effects on glucose regulation when administered alone (105). Idazoxan (an α_2-antagonist) significantly blocked hyperglycemia induced by DOI, but a selective β-antagonist (ICI 118.551) had no effect (103). 5-HT_{1A} receptor agonists such as 8-hydroxy-2-(di-n-propylamino)tetralin (8-OH-DPAT) and buspir-one produce an increase in plasma glucose levels and a decrease in plasma insulin levels (103,106). This effect is suggested to be due to sympathoa-drenal activation and is blocked by hexamethonium and idazoxan; the decrease in insulin may be mediated via activation of α_2-adrenergic receptors on pancreatic β-cells through adrenaline secretion (107,108). Other studies have presented contrasting data that suggest agonism of 5-HT_{1A} receptors causes hypoglycemia (109), and of the AAPs, ziprasidone possesses some 5-HT_{1A} receptor agonism, but in fact appears to have no significant effects on glucose metabolism, possibly due to its actions at other receptors.

It has also been hypothesized that IR and hyperglycemia are associated with hyperprolactinemia, and that prolactin's diabetogenic properties result from the impairment of insulin's antilipolytic action (110,111). However, other studies have concluded that under physiological conditions prolactin does not appear to play an important role in the regulation of glucose in man (112,113). In support of this, AAPs such as risperidone and amisulpiride, are associated with hyperprolactinemia but do not appear to be more frequently associated with DM. In contrast, AAPs such as clozapine and olanzapine have little effect on prolactin but are more frequently associated with DM.

Another possible mechanism may involve inhibition of specific glucose transport (GLUT) proteins that are responsible for maintaining cellular levels of glucose (114). The brain expresses two forms of these proteins, GLUT1 and GLUT3. Clozapine and fluphenazine induced a 100–300% increase in GLUT3 and a 100% increase in GLUT1 (115). In contrast, haloperidol reduced the levels of GLUT1 and GLUT3 and only marginally inhibited 3H-2-deoxyglucose uptake into rat phaeochromocytoma (PC12) cells compared to clozapine and fluphenazine. Ardizzone et al. (116) demonstrated that risperidone and clozapine inhibited glucose transport measured by uptake of 3H-2-deoxyglucose in a dose-dependent manner (desmethylclozapine was more potent than the parent drug and clozapine-N-oxide was inactive). Clozapine and fluphenazine further inhibited glucose transport in the rat muscle (L6) cells, suggesting that APs may variably influence GLUT proteins both peripherally and in the CNS. Finally, the structural analogs of clozapine – loxapine and amoxapine – inhibited glucose transport with amoxapine being the least potent (an association with DM has been reported for both drugs (117)).

Pancreatitis may lead to disturbance of glucose metabolism and there have been isolated reports with clozapine (118–120) and risperidone (121), but the majority of cases are described with olanzapine although it can be difficult to make the diagnosis in the presence of DKA (78,122). Direct damage to pancreatic islet cells has been proposed as a mechanism of action of olanzapine-induced DM (59), but the contribution of disturbances of liver function described with olanzapine and clozapine may also play a role (123,124).

In summary, a hierarchy of diabetic association of the AAPs is emerging in which clozapine and olanzapine appear the most likely to be associated with induction or exacerbation of glucose dysregulation. Whilst this is frequently, but not exclusively in the presence of certain risk factors (principally risk factors for the development of IR), the use of particular AAPs in certain psychiatric populations appears to carry further increased risk. There is some overlap with the hierarchy of weight gain association, but it is also clear that glucose dyregulation can occur before discernible weight gain. Thus, early and specific changes in glucose and insulin metabolism are likely to be the cause of this phenomenon.

III. WEIGHT GAIN

Treatment with many psychotropic drugs is associated with weight gain leading to increased risk of cardiovascular disease, certain cancers, and DM (124). The weight complications of AAPs in particular, have attracted increasing attention (125). The negative impact on quality of life, treatment adherence, and health-care resource utilization are particularly salient given that the risk factors for AAP weight gain include younger age and female gender (126,127). With respect to the AAPs, olanzapine and clozapine are associated with the greatest weight gain, while ziprasidone and molindone appeared to cause the least (128,129). However, there are few comparative data for the AAPs and most of the information is derived from short-term clinical trials (130). A literature review by Wetterling (131) found that the average body weight gain was 2.3 kg/month for olanzapine, 1.7 kg/month for clozapine, 1.8 kg/month for quetiapine, 2.3 kg/month for zotepine, 1.0 kg/month for risperidone, and 0.8 kg/month for ziprasidone. Similarly, a retrospective chart review of patients receiving AP monotherapy for at least 2 weeks with clozapine, risperidone, sulpiride, or zotepine reported weight gain of 3.1, 1.5, 1.9, and 4.3 kg respectively (132). Taylor and McAskill (133) conducted a systematic review and concluded that from the available data, amisulpiride and ziprasidone were likely to be associated with the least weight gain.

However, many studies of short duration do not necessarily capture these data since the rate (trajectory) of weight gain, and the time to reach a steady weight (weight plateau) are very different between the drugs, e.g., up to 48 months with clozapine (51) and up to 36 weeks for olanzapine (134). Thus, early assessments of weight gain may be misleading since the full extent of weight change may not be seen until after many months of treatment. Similarly, data extracted from pooled clinical trials and open-label extensions may not necessarily reflect weight gain effects in real-world clinical populations over the long term particularly with respect to concomitant medication effects.

The potential mechanisms of AP-associated weight gain were comprehensively reviewed by Basile et al. (135). Dysregulation of energy homeostasis, satiety, and activity levels acting through central (hypothalamic) and peripheral (gastrointestinal) mechanisms and involving leptin and insulin signaling, neuropeptide Y (NPY), 5-HT_{2A} and 5-HT_{2C}

receptors, β_3-adrenergic and α_{1A}-adrenergic receptors, tumor necrosis factor α, histamine H_1 receptors, and dopamine D_1 receptors have been proposed.

Leptin is secreted by adipocytes and is the product of the obesity gene *ob*; it signals the size of peripheral fat stores to the brain and mediates catabolic pathways (136). Of the AAPs, clozapine and olanzapine are associated with the greatest and most frequent increases in leptin, possibly through disruption of central leptin pathways in the hypothalamus resulting in leptin insensitivity and subsequent hyperleptinemia. (52,137–140). An increase in serum leptin levels was reported in clozapine-treated patients leading to a doubling of leptin levels in eight out of 12 patients in the first 2 weeks of treatment (maximal relative increase over baseline was 536%) (137). Another study found leptin levels to be elevated in 21% of patients on clozapine and 57% of patients on olanzapine (138). Furthermore, olanzapine-treated patients had significantly higher insulin levels despite no difference in BMI, suggestive of a direct effect on insulin secretion. In addition, the normally existing gender difference in leptin levels (females having higher circulating levels than males) was not found in either the olanzapine or clozapine groups. Herrán et al. (141) found a correlation between weight increases and increases in leptin levels; patients treated with olanzapine had the highest leptin levels and with risperidone the lowest. Clozapine and olanzapine are also reported to increase insulin levels leading to an increase of food intake and body weight (52,53,139,140). Neuropeptide Y plays a complex and central role in energy homeostasis and its expression is influenced by insulin and APs, although the significance of the long-term effects of APs on NPY is not clearly understood (135,142,143).

Atypical antipsychotics such as clozapine possess a profile of antagonism of 5-HT$_{2A}$ and particularly 5-HT$_{2C}$ receptors that has been shown to increase food intake in rats (144), while agonists at these receptors such as fenfluramine and mCPP lead to weight loss. However, there are contradictory data at this time concerning the interaction of the serotonin system and AAPs. Thus, ziprasidone possesses a very high affinity for the 5-HT$_{2C}$ receptor as well as partial agonist activity at the 5-HT$_{1A}$ receptor, but does not appear to be associated with weight gain.

The adrenergic system is the primary efferent pathway mediating sympathetic responses such as basal metabolic rate (BMR), thermogenesis, etc., where α_1- and β_3-adrenergic receptors represent the first key messengers in the mitochondrial uncoupling proteins (UCP1-3) pathway (135). Both α- and β-adrenergic blockade is associated with weight gain and the AAPs exhibit varying antagonism at α_1- and α_2-adrenoreceptors. In an analysis of potential pharmacogenetic factors predictive of patient susceptibility to clozapine-induced weight gain, trends were observed for genetic polymorphisms of β_3-adrenoreceptor and α_{1A}-adrenoreceptor genes as well as for tumor necrosis factor α and 5-HT$_{2C}$ receptor genes (135). The authors are also currently examining the role of the M$_3$ muscarinic acetylcholine receptor at which clozapine acts as a partial agonist.

Increased levels of TNF-α are associated with IR, hyperinsulinemia, and hypertriglyceridemia. A number of studies have demonstrated early activation of the TNF-α system, occurring before weight gain, with olanzapine and clozapine (145–147). However, increased TNF-α levels have also been reported with CAPs, amitriptyline, and paroxetine (148, 149), and it has been postulated that at very high BMIs, TNF-α may play a catabolic role accounting for less weight gain in obese individuals on APs compared to those with a low baseline BMI at the initiation of treatment (135).

Antagonism of histamine H$_1$ receptors increases food intake and weight gain is prominent with anti-histaminic drugs such as tricyclic antidepressants, clozapine, and olanzapine. The relationships of the histaminergic system are not well elucidated, but it appears that histamine stimulates noradrenaline release and thus, may play a role in the regulation of BMR as well as intranuclear oxytocin (150) which has been shown to be important in the etiology of drug-induced DM (91). In a retrospective analysis of clinical trial data, Wirshing et al. (129) identified a relationship between the weight gain experienced by patients with schizophrenia and the in vitro H$_1$ receptor binding properties of clozapine, olanzapine, and quetiapine. Additionally, many potent H$_1$ antagonists are not only sedative, but also tend to have appetite stimulating effects that potentially lead to disruption of both satiety regulation and energy expenditure (151). Olanzapine-associated weight gain has been related to a decrease in energy expenditure (152). The role of histamine H$_2$ receptors in weight regulation is even less clear, with H$_2$ receptor antagonists appearing to mitigate weight gain, but limited benefits are described with the use of nizatidine and cimetidine in the treatment of AP-associated weight gain (153).

Asthenic body type was historically characterized as the typical body habitus of schizophrenia before medication (154) and AP treatment may in itself, have an impact on weight regulation that is commonly in the direction of weight gain, but may include weight loss or weight neutrality. A high potency CAP such as haloperidol that is a relatively selective and strong D$_2$ antagonist appears to be associated with a lesser risk of weight gain, in contrast to lower potency APs that in general, possess a broader profile of receptor antagonism and weaker D$_2$ antagonism. Of note, both D$_2$ agonists and antagonists are associated with a dose-dependent biphasic response in which low doses stimulate food intake and high doses are inhibitory (155). Dopamine agonists such as bromocriptine and amantadine have been shown to reduce body fat and food intake (156,157), and clozapine-induced hyperphagia in female mice showed reversal after treatment with SKF 38393 or quinpirole (158). There are few studies of dopamine agonists in AP-treated patients and while there is a potential theoretical risk of exacerbation of psychosis, amantadine was useful in one small study in attenuating weight gain associated with olanzapine without worsening of mental state (159).

Finally, behavioral changes accompanying AP treatment may modify potential weight gain. Thus, Frankenburg et al. (160) found that a reduction in smoking, and not increased appetite or sedation, made a significant contribution to the weight gain occurring with clozapine.

As with AAPs and DM, special populations such as children may be particularly susceptible to weight gain effects (161), thus weight gain of up to 8.8 kg was noted in three of five children (aged 6–11 years) treated with olanzapine for a mean duration of 32 days (162). Similarly 60 adolescents treated for 6 months with risperidone, CAPs, or no AP showed weight changes of 8.64 kg, 3.03 kg, and −1.04 kg respectively (163).

IV. DISTURBANCE OF LIPID METABOLISM

Disturbances of lipid metabolism have been noted with respect to the APs, notably clozapine, olanzapine, and perhaps quetiapine. Elevated TGs and LDL-C are a concern because of the increased risk of cardiovascular disease particularly in the context of DM and weight gain, and compounded by the very high prevalence of smoking in many psychiatric populations. Clozapine has been associated with an increase in TG levels, with reversal on switching to risperidone (164). Marked elevation of TG has been reported in male patients on clozapine compared to male patients on haloperidol, with the difference being less significant in female patients (165). It was hypothesized that this was due to a direct effect on lipoprotein lipase, but hyperinsulinemia also down-regulates this enzyme, which is involved in LDL-C metabolism, resulting in an increase in TG. A 6-week study comparing risperidone to clozapine in 20 patients found TCHOL, TGs, and PG were all significantly increased with clozapine compared to baseline (166). Clozapine's effects on TCHOL and PG were also significant compared to risperidone. Significant weight gain was noted in both clozapine responders and non-responders, and risperidone responders. Long-term data are consistent in this area, with clozapine-treated patients showing a significant and persistent increase in TGs over a 60-month study period (51). Differences between AAPs were further suggested in the results of the metabolic profile of 44 male smokers treated for 18 months (± 8 months). (167). The authors found 32% of the olanzapine-treated patients developed hyperinsulinemia, elevated apolipoprotein-B, and LDL-C (atherogenic triad) compared to 5% of risperidone-treated patients. Meyer (3) reported on 14 cases of severe hypertriglyceridemia (>600 mg/dL) associated with olanzapine and quetiapine treatment, including seven cases with serum TG levels >1000 mg/dL (four olanzapine and one quetiapine) were reported. Four of these patients also developed new onset DM and nine cases occurred in the first 8 months of commencing therapy. Weight changes were modest, 5.5 kg and 3.9 kg for the olanzapine and quetiapine groups respectively, and there was no correlation between weight gain and the severity of hypertriglyceridemia. Two other studies of olanzapine-treated patients of 16 months and 3 months found significant increases in TGs of 40% and 37% respectively (168,169). Mean weight change in 25 patients in the latter study was 5.45 kg and changes in body weight and TG levels were correlated. Similarly, Melkersson et al. (140) found increases in body weight, leptin, and lipids in 14 olanzapine patients treated for 3 months. Despite the relatively small numbers of patients and short time frame of most of these studies, it is nonetheless apparent that there are early and significant changes in lipid metabolism with certain APs that have important implications in terms of physical health. However, it has also been suggested that alterations in serum lipids may affect the plasma distribution of AAPs and have some relevance in their therapeutic actions, particularly for clozapine and olanzapine (169,170).

V. ENDOCRINE DISTURBANCES

Prolactin is a single chain 198 amino acid polypeptide hormone secreted by the lactotrophs of the anterior pituitary gland in which dopamine (prolactin inhibitory factor) is inhibitory and serotonin stimulates release (171). Serum prolactin levels are influenced by both physiological and pathological factors; high levels may result in galactorrhea and sexual dysfunction in both men and women, and amenorrhea and infertility in women. Women experience more frequent and greater prolactin elevation with CAPs and AAPs than men, and at a lower daily dose (172). Of the AAPs, chronic administration of risperidone and amisulpiride is associated with sustained prolactin elevation while clozapine, olanzapine, and quetiapine tend to have minimal or transient effects (173). However, with acute administration clozapine, risperidone, and olanzapine all caused a doubling of prolactin levels 6 hours post dose in 18 male patients (174). A study of 20 schizophrenic females switched from risperidone to olanzapine was associated with a decrease of mean prolactin from 132.2 ± 59.1 ng/mL to 23.4 ± 22.7 ng/mL after 8 weeks (173). Kleinberg et al. (175) analyzed prolactin data from 2725 patients treated with risperidone or haloperidol and found that there was no correlation between prolactin serum levels and prolactin-related adverse events for either men or women despite both drugs producing a dose-dependent increase in prolactin. Furthermore there was no correlation between risperidone dose and adverse events except in men at doses of more than 12 mg/day.

Sexual dysfunction is a complex area to evaluate with a multifactorial etiology that includes the effects of many different medications super-imposed upon factors pertaining to psychiatric and physical disease. In men treated with APs, factors including higher doses, greater anticholinergic or antiadrenergic side effects, and particularly hyperprolactinemia were associated with sexual dysfunction (176). For women in the same study, sexual dysfunction correlated with higher doses and prolactin levels. Sulpiride and flupenthixol tended to be associated with arousal problems compared to chlorpromazine which was more likely to be associated with anorgasmia. Of note, the use of AAPs possessing potent α_1-adrenergic antagonism inhibits detumescence in men leading to potential priapism and decreased ejaculatory volume (177). Although it is not widely used because of QTc prolongation, sertindole has the greatest α_1-adrenergic activity of the AAPs (178), however other AAPs, particularly when used in combination may lead to sexual dysfunction through this mechanism (179). Decreased sexual dysfunction with maintenance clozapine treatment was observed in a study of 60 male out-patient schizophrenics compared to maintenance treatment with CAPs (180). This was not correlated with differences in the severity of psychotic symptoms and although prolactin levels were lower for the clozapine-treated subjects, this was not significant. In contrast, Hummer et al. (181) in an in-patient study after 6 weeks of treatment found no difference in the frequency of sexual dysfunction between haloperidol and clozapine, but a correlation was observed between clozapine plasma levels and sexual adverse events for male subjects receiving clozapine.

There are few data concerning other endocrine disturbances and AAPs; however, quetiapine may be associated with elevation of TSH levels and there are case reports concerning the development of hypothyroidism (182).

V. SUMMARY

In summary, it is clear that AAPs differ significantly in their potential for metabolic adverse effects, thus any recommendations with respect to their use in individual patients will depend on the ratio of anticipated efficacy versus likely side effects (183). The mechanisms by which AAPs are associated with DM, weight gain, dyslipidemia, and endocrine disturbances are not yet clearly elucidated, but appear to be primarily related to the different profiles of CNS receptor actions. At present, there is limited predictability in these areas given the paucity of well controlled and directly comparative data (184). Therefore, clinical experience with the patient in terms of treatment history, presence of potential risk factors for specific adverse events, and knowledge of the chosen drug's effects are significant determinants in the choice of AP. It is also important to consider the longer-term risks associated with metabolic changes, particularly the development of DM and obesity (185) that may also influence the psychiatric illness being treated. The risk-to-benefit analysis for each AP must be taken into account for these long-term effects particularly when they are difficult to reverse. Early detection contingent upon regular and appropriate monitoring is recommended given that persons with schizophrenia are at significantly greater risk of cardiovascular morbidity and mortality from stroke, heart failure, ventricular arrhythmia, and diabetes (186). Psychiatrists need to be aware of the potential for metabolic changes occurring with the AAPs and ensure that patients are well informed and that an adequate medical follow up is in place. Finally, Kapur and Remington (187) have suggested that a more sophisticated approach to the management of schizophrenia may lie in the targeting of particular symptom domains with selective drugs that can be combined and titrated on an individual basis, with a view to maintaining efficacy throughout the course of the illness. Thus, given the complex and lifelong treatment required for the optimal control of schizophrenia, the use of AAPs is likely to be determined as much by tolerability as by efficacy.

REFERENCES

1. Collaborative Working Group on Clinical Trial Evaluations. Adverse effects of the atypical antipsychotics. J Clin Psychiatry 1998; 59:17–22.
2. Casey DE. Atypical antipsychotics: enhancing healthy outcomes. Arch Psychiatric Nursing 2002; 3:S12–S19.
3. Meyer JM. Effects of atypical antipsychotics on weight and serum lipid levels. J Clin Psychiatry 2001; 62:40–41.
4. Wilson DR, D'Souza L, Sarkar N, Newton M. New-onset diabetes and ketoacidosis with atypical antipsychotics. Schizophr Res 2003; 59:1–6.
5. Zoler ML. Antipsychotics linked to weight gain, diabetes. Clin Psychiatry News 1999; 27:20–21.
6. Casey DE. Weight gain and glucose metabolism with atypical antipsychotics. Presented at the 38th Annual Meeting of the American College of Neuro-psychopharmacology, Acapulco, Mexico, December 12–16, 1999.

7. Sernyak MJ, Leslie DL, Alarcon RD, Losonczy MF, Rosenheck RA. Association of diabetes mellitus with use of atypical neuroleptics in the treatment of schizophrenia. Am J Psychiatry 2002; 159:561–566.
8. Gianfrancesco FD, Grogg AL, Mahmoud RA, Wang RH, Nasrallah HA. Differential effects of risperidone, olanzapine, clozapine, and conventional antipsychotics on type 2 diabetes: findings from a large health plan database. J Clin Psychiatry 2002; 63:920–930.
9. Buse JB, Cavazzoni P, Hornbuckle K, Hutchins D, Breier A, Jovanovic L. A retrospective cohort study of diabetes mellitus and antipsychotic treatment in the United States. J Clin Epidemiol 2003; 56(2):164–170.
10. Koro CE, Fedder DO, L'Italien GJ, Wiess SS, Magder LS, Kreyenbuhl J, Revicki DA, Buchanan RW. Assessment of independent effect of olanzapine and risperidone on risk of diabetes among patients with schizophrenia: population based nested case-control study. Brit Med J 2002; 325:243–248.
11. Caro J, Ward A, Levington C, Robinson K. The risk of diabetes during olanzapine use compared with risperidone use: a retrospective database analysis. J Clin Psychopharmacol 2002; 63:1135–1139.
12. Lambert B, Chou C-H, Chang K-Y, Iwamoto T, Tafesse E. Assessing the risk of antipsychotic-induced type II diabetes among schizophrenics: a matched case control study. Presented at the 15th Congress of the European College of Neuropsychopharmacology, Barcelona, Spain, Oct 5–9, 2002.
13. Wolever T. Dietary carbohydrates in the insulin resistance syndrome. Can J CME 2001; 13:121–135.
14. Newcomer JW, Fucetola R, Haupt DW. Abnormalities in glucose regulation during antipsychotic treatment. Presented at the 38th Annual Meeting of the American College of Neuropsychopharmacology, Acapulco, Mexico, December 12–16, 1999.
15. Newcomer JW, Haupt DW, Fucetola R, Melson AK, Schweiger JA, Cooper BP, Selke G. Abnormalities in glucose regulation during antipsychotic treatment of schizophrenia. Arch Gen Psychiatry 2002; 59:337–345.
16. Beasley CM, Berg PH, Dananberg J, Kwong KC, Taylor CCM, Breier A. Treatment-emergent potential impaired glucose tolerance and potential diabetes with olanzapine compared to other antipsychotic agents and placebo. Presented at the 56th Annual Convention of the Society of Biological Psychiatry, New Orleans, LA, May 3–5, 2001.
17. Chue P, Welch R. Investigation of the metabolic effects of antipsychotics in patients with schizophrenia. Presented at the 51st Annual Meeting of the Canadian Psychiatric Association, Montreal, Canada, November 15–19, 2001.
18. Cohn T. Antipsychotic medication and insulin resistance. Presented at the 154th Annual Meeting of the American Psychiatric Association, New Orleans, LA, May 5–10, 2001.
19. Daniel DG, Weiden PJ, O'Sullivan R. Improvement in indices of health status in outpatients with schizophrenia following a switch to ziprasidone from conventional antipsychotics, olanzapine or risperidone. Presented at the 154th

Annual Meeting of the American Psychiatric Association, New Orleans, LA, May 5–10, 2001.

20. Berry S, Mahmoud R. Improvement of insulin indices after switch from olanzapine to risperidone. Presented at the 15th Congress of the European College of Neuropsychopharmacology, Barcelona, Spain, October 5–9, 2002.

21. Ai D, Roper T, Riley JA. Diabetic ketoacidosis and clozapine. Postgrad Med J 1998; 74:493–494.

22. Colli A, Cocciolo M, Francobandiera F, Rogantin F, Cattalini N. Diabetic ketoacidosis associated with clozapine treatment. Diabetes Care 1999; 22: 176–177.

23. Smith H, Kenney-Herbert J, Knowles L. Clozapine-induced diabetic keto-acidosis. Aust N Z J Psychiatry 1999; 33:120–121.

24. Pierides M. Clozapine monotherapy and ketoacidosis. Brit J Psychiatry 1997; 171:90–91.

25. Peterson GA, Byrd SL. Diabetic ketoacidosis from clozapine and lithium cotreatment. Am J Psychiatry 1996; 153:737–738.

26. Koval MS, Rames LJ, Christie S. Diabetic ketoacidosis associated with clozapine treatment. Am J Psychiatry 1994; 151:1520–1521.

27. Maule S, Giannella R, Lanzio M, Villari V. Diabetic ketoacidosis with clozapine treatment. Diabetes Nutr Metab 1999; 12(2):187–188.

28. Popli AP, Konicki PE, Jurjus GJ, Fuller MA, Jaskiw GE. Clozapine and associated diabetes mellitus. J Clin Psychiatry 1997; 58:108–111.

29. Kamran A, Doraiswamy PM, Jane JL, Hammett EB, Dunn L. Severe hyperglycemia associated with high doses of clozapine. Am J Psychiatry 1994; 151:1395.

30. Koren W, Kreis Y, Duchowiczny K, Prince T, Sancovici S, Sidi Y, Gur H. Lactic acidosis and fatal myocardial failure due to clozapine. Ann Pharmacother 1997; 31:168–170.

31. Kostakoglu AE, Yazici KM, Erbas T, Guvener ET. Ketoacidosis as a side-effect of clozapine: a case report. Acta Psychiatr Scand 1996; 93:217–218.

32. Wirshing DA, Spellberg BJ, Erhart SM, Marder SR. Novel antipsychotics and new onset diabetes. Biol Psychiatry 1998; 44:778–783.

33. Thompson J, Chengappa KN, Good CB, Baker RW, Kiewe RP, Bezner J, Schooler NR. Hepatitis, hyperglycemia, pleural effusion, eosinophilia, hema-turia and proteinuria occurring early in clozapine treatment. Int Clin Psychopharmacol 1998; 13:95–98.

34. Hauptmann B, Kupsch A, Arnold G. Hyperglycemia associated with low-dose clozapine treatment. J Neural Transm 1999; 106:12.

35. Mohan D, Gordon H, Hindley N, Barker A. Schizophrenia and diabetes mellitus. Brit J Psychiatry 1999; 174:180–181.

36. Dickson RA, Hogg L. Pregnancy of a treatment treated with clozapine. Psychiatr Services 1998; 49:1081–1083.

37. Waldman MD, Safferman A. Pregnancy and clozapine. Am J Psychiatry 1993; 150:168–169.

38. Wu G, Dias P, Chun W, Li G, Kumar S, Singh S. Hyperglycemia, hyperlipemia, and periodic paralysis: a case report of new side effects of clozapine. Prog Neuropsychopharmacol Biol Psychiatry 2000; 24:1395–1400.
39. Brugman NJ, Cohen D, de Vries RH. Diabetes mellitus after treatment with clozapine. Ned Tijdschr Geneeskd 2000; 144:437–439.
40. Liebzeit KA, Markowitz JS, Caley CF. New onset diabetes and atypical antipsychotics. Eur Neuropsychopharmacol 2001; 11:25–32.
41. Wirshing DA. Adverse effects of atypical antipsychotics. J Clin Psychiatry 2001; 62:7–10.
42. Mir S, Taylor D. Atypical antipsychotics and hyperglycemia. Int Clin Psychopharmacol 2001; 16:63–73.
43. Jin H, Meyer JM, Jeste DV. Phenomenology of and risk factors for new-onset diabetes mellitus and diabetic ketoacidosis associated with atypical antipsychotics: an analysis of 45 published cases. Ann Clin Psychiatry 2002; 14:59–64.
44. Wehring H, Alexander B, Perry PJ. Diabetes mellitus associated with clozapine therapy. Pharmacotherapy 2000; 20:844–847.
45. Lu HM, Yu HX. Reassessment of the side effect profile of clozapine. Chinese J Clin Psychol Med 1997; 7:298–300.
46. Ramaekers GM, Rambharos R, Matroos G. Diabetes mellitus after treatment with clozapine. Ned Tijdschr Geneeskd 2000; 144:1463–1464.
47. Poersch M, Hufnagel A, Smolenski C. Drug-induced asterixis amplified by relative hypoglycemia. Nervenarzt 1996; 67:323–326.
48. Goldman S. Medical illness in patients with schizophrenia. J Clin Psychiatry 1999; 60:10–15.
49. Lund BC, Perry PJ, Brooks JM, Arndt S. Clozapine and the risk of diabetes, hyperlipidemia, and hypertension: a claims-based approach. Arch Gen Psychiatry 2001; 58:1171–1176.
50. Hagg S, Joelsson L, Mjorndal T, Spigset O, Oja G, Dahlqvist R. Prevalence of diabetes and impaired glucose tolerance in patients treated with clozapine compared with patients treated with conventional depot neuroleptic medications. J Clin Psychiatry 1998; 59:294–299.
51. Henderson DC, Cagliero E, Gray C, Nasrallah RA, Hayden DL, Schoenfeld DA, Goff DC. Clozapine, diabetes mellitus, weight gain, and lipid abnormalities: a five-year naturalistic study. Am J Psychiatry 2000; 157: 975–981.
52. Melkersson KI, Hulting AL, Brismer KE. Different influences of classical antipsychotics and clozapine on glucose-insulin homeostasis in patients with schizophrenia or related psychoses. J Clin Psychiatry 1999; 60:783–791.
53. Yazici KM, Erbas T, Yazici AH. The effect of clozapine on glucose metabolism. Exp Clin Endocrinol Diabetes 1998; 106:475–477.
54. Wang PS, Glynn RJ, Ganz DA, Schneeweiss S, Levin R, Avorn J. Clozapine use and risk of diabetes mellitus. J Clin Psychopharmacol 2002; 22:236–243.
55. Gatta B, Rigalleau V, Gin H. Diabetic ketoacidosis with olanzapine treatment. Diabetes Care 1999; 22:1002–1003.
56. Ober SK, Hudak R, Rusterholz A. Hyperglycemia and olanzapine. Am J Psychiatry 1999; 156:970.

57. Fertig MK, Brooks VG, Shelton PS, English CW. Hyperglycemia associated with olanzapine. J Clin Psychiatry 1998; 59:687–689.

58. Lindenmayer JP, Patel R. Olanzapine-induced ketoacidosis with diabetes mellitus. Am J Psychiatry 1999; 156:1471.

59. Goldstein LE, Sporn J, Brown S, et al. New onset diabetes mellitus and diabetic ketoacidosis associated with olanzapine treatment. Psychosomatics 1999; 40:438–443.

60. Zung A, Blumenson R, Kupchik M, Zadik Z. Are the atypical antipsychotic drugs diabetogenic? Presented at the 38th Annual Meeting of the European Society of Pediatric Endocrinology, Warsaw, Poland, August 29–September 1, 1999.

61. Von Hayek DV, Huttl V, Reiss J, Schweiger HD, Fuessl HS. Hyperglycemia and ketoacidosis associated with olanzapine. Nervenarzt 1999; 70:836–837.

62. Bechara CI, Goldman-Levine JD. Dramatic worsening of type 2 diabetes mellitus due to olanzapine after 3 years of therapy. Pharmacotherapy 2001; 21:1444–1447.

63. Bonanno DG, Davydov L, Botts S. Olanzapine-induced diabetes mellitus. Ann Pharmacother 2001; 35:563–565.

64. Meatherall R, Younes J. Fatality from olanzapine induced hyperglycemia. J Forensic Sci 2002; 47:893–896.

65. Littrell KH, Johnson CG, Peabody CD, Hilligoss N. Antipsychotics during pregnancy. Am J Psychiatry 2000; 157:1342.

66. Muench J, Carey M. Diabetes mellitus associated with atypical antipsychotic medications: new case report and review of the literature. J Am Board Fam Pract 2001; 14:278–282.

67. Bettinger TL, Mendelson SC, Dorson PG, Crismon ML. Olanzapine-induced glucose dysregulation. Ann Pharmacother 2000; 34:865–867.

68. Meyer JM. Novel antipsychotics and severe hyperglycemia. J Clin Psychopharmacol 2001; 21:369–374.

69. Roefaro J, Mukherjee S. Olanzapine-induced hyperglycemic nonketonic coma. Ann Pharmacother 2001; 35:300–302.

70. Kropp S, Emrich HM, Bleich S, Degner D. Olanzapine-related hyperglycemia in a nondiabetic woman. Can J Psychiatry 2001; 46:457.

71. Rigalleau V, Gatta B, Bonnaud S, Masson M, Bourgeois ML, Vergnot V, Gin H. Diabetes as a result of atypical antipsychotic drugs – a case report of three cases. Diabet Med 2000; 17:484–486.

72. Domon SE, Webber JC. Hyperglycemia and hypertriglyceridemia secondary to olanzapine. J Child Adolesc Psychopharmacol 2001; 11:235–238.

73. Paizis M, Cavaleri S, Schwarz M, Levin Z. Acute-onset diabetic ketoacidosis during olanzapine treatment in a patient without pretreatment obesity or treatment-associated weight gain. Primary Psychiatry 1999; 6:37–38.

74. Selva KA, Scott SM. Diabetic ketoacidosis associated with olanzapine in an adolescent patient. J Pediatr 2001; 138:936–938.

75. Rojas P, Arancibia P, Bravo V, Varela S. Diabetes mellitus induced by olanzapine: a case report. Rev Med Chil 2001; 129:1183–1185.

76. Ragucci KR, Wells BJ. Olanzapine-induced diabetic ketoacidosis. Ann Pharmacother 2001; 35:1556–1558.

77. Seaburg HL, McLendon BM, Doraiswamy PM. Olanzapine-associated severe hyperglycemia, ketonuria, and acidosis: case report and review of the literature. Pharmacotherapy 2001; 21:1448–1454.

78. Koller EA, Doraiswamy PM. Olanzapine-associated diabetes mellitus. Pharmacotherapy 2002; 22; 841–852.

79. Melamed Y, Mazeh D, Elizur A. Risperidone treatment for a patient suffering from schizophrenia and IDMM. Can J Psychiatry 1998; 43:956.

80. Brescan DW, Ramirez LF. Risperidone and glucose tolerance. Presented at the 150th Annual Meeting of the American Psychiatric Association, San Diego, CA, May 17–22, 1997.

81. Croarkin PE, Jacobs KM, Bain BK. Diabetic ketoacidosis associated with risperidone treatment. Psychosomatics 2000; 41:369–370.

82. Hardy H, Esch LD, Morse GD. Glucose disorders associated with HIV and its drug therapy. Ann Pharmacother 2001; 35:343–351.

83. Madhusoodanan S, Brenner R, Araujo L, Abazza A. Efficacy of risperidone treatment for psychoses associated with schizophrenia, schizoaffective disorder, bipolar disorder or senile dementia in 11 geriatric patients: a case series. J Clin Psychiatry 1995; 56:514–518.

84. Sajatovic M, Ramirez LF, Vernon L, Brescan D, Simon M, Jurjus G. Outcome of risperidone therapy in elderly patients with chronic psychosis. Int J Psychiatry Med 1996; 26:309–317.

85. Joshi PM, Joshi U. Risperidone in treatment resistant geriatric patients with chronic psychoses and concurrent medical illnesses. Presented 149th Annual Meeting of the American Psychiatric Association, New York, NY, May 4–9, 1996.

86. Sobel M, Jaggers ED, Franz MA. New-onset diabetes mellitus associated with the initiation of quetiapine treatment. J Clin Psychiatry 1999; 60:556–557.

87. Procyshyn RC, Pande S, Tse G. New-onset diabetes mellitus associated with quetiapine. Can J Psychiatry 2000; 45:668–669.

88. Reinstein MJ, Sirotovskaya LA, Jones LE, Mohan SC, Chasanov MA. Effect of clozapine-quetiapine combination therapy on weight and glycemic control: preliminary findings. Clin Drug Invest 1999; 18:99–104.

89. Kingsbury SJ, Fayek M, Trufasiu D, Zada J, Simpson GM. The apparent effects of ziprasidone on plasma lipids and glucose. J Clin Psychiatry 2001; 62:347–349.

90. Lindenmayer JP, Nathan A-M, Smith RC. Hyperglycemia associated with the use of atypical antipsychotics. J Clin Psychiatry 2001; 62:30–38.

91. Uvnas-Moberg K, Ahlenius S, Alster P, Hillegaart V. Effects of selective serotonin and dopamine agonists on plasma levels of glucose, insulin and glucagon in the rat. Peripheral Neuroendocrinol 1996; 63:269–274.

92. Saller CF, Kreamer LD. Glucose concentrations in the brain and blood regulation by dopamine receptor subtypes. Brain Res 1991; 546:235–240.

93. Erle G, Basso M, Federspil G, Sicolo N, Scandellari C. Effect of chlorpromazine on blood glucose and plasma insulin in man. Eur J Clin Pharmacol 1977; 11:15–18.
94. Jori A, Carrara MC. On the mechanism of hyperglycemic effect of chlorpromazine. J Pharm Pharmacol 1966; 18:623–624.
95. Chan JCN, Cockram CS. Drug-induced disturbances of carbohydrate metabolism. Adverse Drug React Toxicol Rev 1991; 10:1–29.
96. Scislowski PW, Tozzo E, Zhang Y, Phaneuf S, Prevelige R, Cincotta AH. Biochemical mechanisms responsible for the attenuation of diabetic and obese conditions in ob/ob mice treated with dopaminergic agonists. Int J Obes Relat Metab Disord 1999; 23:425–431.
97. Bina KG, Cincotta AH. Dopaminergic agonists normalize elevated hypothalamic neuropeptide Y and corticotrophin-releasing hormone, body weight gain, and hyperglycemia in ob/ob mice. Neuroendocrinology 2000; 71:68–71.
98. Jetton TL, Liang Y, Cincotta AH. Systemic treatment with sympatholytic dopamine agonists improves aberrant beta-cell hyperplasia and GLUT2, glucokinase, and insulin immunoreactive levels in ob/ob mice. Metabolism 2001; 50:1377–1384.
99. Pijl H, Ohashi S, Matsuda M, Miyazaki Y, Mahankali A, Kumar V, Pipek R, Iozzo P, Lancaster JL, Cincotta AH, DeFronzo RA. Bromocriptine: a novel approach to the treatment of type 2 diabetes. Diabetes Care 2000; 23:1154–1161.
100. Buijus RM. Vasopressin and oxytocin: their role in neuro-transmission. Pharmacol Ther 1983; 22:127–141.
101. Siaud P, Puech R, Assenmacher L, Alonso G. Microinjection of oxytocin into the dorsal vagal complex decreases pancreatic insulin secretion. Brain Res 1991; 546:190–194.
102. Bagdy G, Kadogeras T. Stimulation of $5\text{-}HT_{1A}$ and $5\text{-}HT_2/5\text{-}HT_{1C}$ receptors induce oxytocin release in the male rat. Brain Res 1993; 611:330–332.
103. Chaouloff F, Baudrie V. Effects of the $5\text{-}HT_{1C}$ / $5\text{-}HT_2$ receptor agonists DOI and alpha-methyl-5-HT on plasma glucose and insulin levels in the rat. Eur J Pharmacol 1990; 187s:435–443.
104. Yamada J, Sugimoto Y, Yoshikawa T, Kimura I, Horisaka K. The involvement of the peripheral 5-HT2A receptor in peripherally administered serotonin-induced hyperglycemia in rats. Life Sci 1995; 57:819–825.
105. Wozniak KM, Linnoila M. Hyperglycemic properties of serotonin receptor antagonists. Life Sci 1991; 49:101–109.
106. Chaouloff F, Baudrie V, Laude D. Evidence that $5\text{-}HT_{1A}$ receptors are involved in the adrenline-releasing effects of 8-OH-DPAT in the conscious rat. Arch Pharmacol 1990; 341:381–384.
107. Chaouloff F, Baudrie V, Laude D. Ganglionic transmission is a prerequisite for the adrenaline-releasing and hyperglycemic effects of 8-OH-DPAT. Eur J Pharmacol 1990; 185:11–18.
108. Chaouloff F, Jeanrenaud B. $5\text{-}HT_{1A}$ and α_2-adrenergic receptors mediate the hyperglycemic and hypoinsulinemic effects of 8-hydroxy-2-(di-n-propylamino) tetralin in the conscious rat. J Pharmacol Exp Ther 1987; 243:1159–1166.

109. Baudrie V, Chaouloff F. Repeated treatment with the 5-HT1A receptor agonist, ipsaperone, does not affect 8-OH-DPAT- and stress-induced increases in plasma adrenaline levels in the rat. Eur J Pharmacol 1991; 198:1129–1135.

110. Foss MC, Paula FJ, Paccola GM, Piccinato CE. Peripheral glucose metabolism in human hyperprolactinemia. Clin Endocrinol 1995; 43:721–726.

111. Sorenson RL, Brelje TC. Adaption of islets of Langerhans to pregnancy: Beta cell growth, enhanced insulin secretion and the role of lactogenic hormones. Horm Metab Res 1997; 29:301–307.

112. Vigas M, Klimes I, Jurcovicova J, Jesova D. Acute elevation of endogenous prolactin does not influence glucose homeostasis in healthy men. Physiol Res 1993; 42:341–345.

113. Skouby SO, Kuhl C, Hornnes PJ, Andersen AN. Prolactin and glucose tolerance in normal and gestational diabetic pregnancy. Obst Gynaecology 1986; 67:17–20.

114. Dwyer DS, Bradley RJ, Kablinger AS, Freeman AM. Glucose metabolism in relation to schizophrenia and antipsychotic treatment. Ann Clin Psychiatry 2001; 13:103–113.

115. Dwyer DS, Pinkofsky HB, Liu Y, Bradley RJ. Antipsychotic drugs affect glucose uptake and the expression of glucose transporters in PC12 cells. Prog Neuropsychopharmacol Biol Psychiatry 1999; 23:69–80.

116. Ardizzone TD, Bradley RJ, Freeman AM, Dwyer DS. Inhibition of glucose transport in PC12 cells by the atypical antipsychotic drugs risperidone and clozapine, and the structural analogs of clozapine. Brain Res 2001; 923:82–90.

117. Tollefson G, Lesar T. Nonketotic hyperglycemia associated with loxapine and amoxapine: case report. J Clin Psychiatry 1983; 44:347–348.

118. Frankenburg FR, Kando J. Eosinophilia, clozapine and pancreatitis. Lancet 1992; 340:251.

119. Martin A. Acute pancreatitis associated with clozapine use. Am J Psychiatry 1992; 149:714.

120. Jubert P, Fernandez R, Ruiz A. Clozapine-related pancreatitis. Intern Med 1995; 122:397.

121. Berent I, Carabeth J, Cordero MM, Cordero R, Sugerman B, Robinson D. Pancreatitis associated with risperidone treatment. Am J Psychiatry 1997; 154:130–131.

122. Zyprexa Product Monograph, Eli Lilly Canada Inc., October 23, 1996.

123. Kellner M, Wiedemann K, Krieg JC, Berg PA. Toxic hepatitis by clozapine treatment. Am J Psychiatry 1993; 150:985–986.

124. Baptista T. Body weight gain induced by antipsychotic drugs: mechanisms and management. Acta Psychiatr Scand 1999: 100:3–16.

125. Green AI, Patel JK, Goisman RM, Allison DB, Blackburn G. Weight gain from novel antipsychotic drugs: need for action. Gen Hosp Psychiatry 2000; 22:224–235.

126. Russell JM, Mackell JA. Bodyweight gain associated with atypical antipsychotics: epidemiology and therapeutic implications. CNS Drugs 2001; 15:537–551.

127. Blin O, Micallef J. Antipsychotic-associated weight gain and clinical outcome parameters. J Clin Psychiatry 2001; 62:11–21.

128. Allison DB, Mentore JL, Heo M, Chandler LP, Cappelleri JC, Infante MC, Weiden PJ. Antipsychotic-induced weight gain: a comprehensive research synthesis. Am J Psychiatry 1999; 156:1686–1696.

129. Wirshing DA, Wirshing WC, Kysar L, Berisford MA, Goldstein D, Pashdag J, Mintz J, Marder SR. Novel antipsychotics: comparison of weight gain liabilities. J Clin Psychiatry 1999; 60: 358–363.

130. Sussman N. Review of atypical antipsychotics and weight gain. J Clin Psychiatry 2001; 62:5–12.

131. Wetterling T. Bodyweight gain with atypical antipsychotics: a comparative review. Drug Saf 2001; 24: 59–73.

132. Wetterling T, Müßigbrodt HE. Weight gain: side effect of atypical neuroleptics? J Clin Psychopharmacol 1999; 19: 316–321.

133. Taylor DM, McAskill R. Atypical antipsychotics and weight gain – a systematic review. Acta Psychiatr Scand 2000; 101:416–432.

134. Jones B, Basson BR, Walker DJ, Crawford AM, Kinon BJ. Weight change and atypical antipsychotic treatment in patients with schizophrenia. J Clin Psychiatry 2001; 62:41–44.

135. Basile VS, Masellis M, McIntyre RS, Meltzer H, Lieberman JA, Kennedy JL. Genetic dissection of atypical antipsychotic-induced weight gain: novel preliminary data on the pharmacogenetic puzzle. J Clin Psychiatry 2001; 62:45–66.

136. Baskin DG, Figlewicz Lattemann D, Seeley RJ, Woods SC, Porte D Jr, Schwartz MW. Insulin and leptin: dual adiposity signals to the brain for the regulation of food intake and body weight. Brain Res 1999; 848:114–123.

137. Bromel T, Blum WF, Ziegler A, Schulz E, Bender M, Fleischhaker C, Remschmidt H, Krieg JC, Hebebrand J. Serum leptin levels increase rapidly after initiation of clozapine therapy. Mol Psychiatry 1998; 3:76–80.

138. Kraus T, Haack M, Schuld A, Hinze-Selch D, Kuhn M, Uhr M, Pollmacher T. Body weight and plasma leptin levels during treatment with antipsychotic drugs. Am J Psychiatry 1999; 156:312–314.

139. Melkersson KI, Hulting AL. Insulin and leptin levels in patients with schizophrenia or related psychoses: a comparison between different antipsychotic agents. Psychopharmacology 2001; 154:205–212.

140. Melkersson KI, Hulting AL, Brismer KE. Elevated levels of insulin, leptin, and blood lipids in olanzapine-treated patients with schizophrenia or related psychoses. J Clin Psychiatry 2000; 61:742–749.

141. Herrán A, Garcia-Unzueta MT, Amado JA, de La Maza MT, Alvarez C, Vasquez-Barquero JL. Effects of long-term treatment with antipsychotics on leptin serum levels. Brit J Psychiatry 2001; 179:59–62.

142. Obuchowicz E, Turchan J. Clozapine decreases neuropeptide Y-like immunoreactivity and neuropeptide Y mRNA levels in rat nucleus accumbens. Eur Neuropsychopharmacol 1999; 9:329–335.

143. Gruber SH, Mathe AA. Effects of typical and atypical antipsychotics on neuropeptide Y in rat brain tissue and microdialysates from ventral striatum. J Neurosci Res 2000; 61:458–463.

144. Tecott LH, Sun LM, Akana SF, Strack AM, Lowenstein DH, Dallman MF, Julius D. Eating disorder and epilepsy in mice lacking 5-HT2C receptors. Nature 1995; 374:542–546.

145. Schuld A, Kraus T, Haack M, Hinze-Selch D, Kuhn M, Pollmacher T. Plasma levels of cytokines and soluble cytokine receptor levels during treatment with olanzapine. Schizophr Res 2000; 43:164–166.

146. Pollmacher T, Hinze-Selch D, Mullington J. Effects of clozapine on plasma cytokine and soluble cytokine receptor levels. J Clin Psychopharmacol 1996; 16:403–409.

147. Hinze-Selch D, Deuschle M, Weber B, Heuser I, Pollmacher T. Effect of coadministration of clozapine and fluvoxamine versus clozapine monotherapy on blood cell counts, plasma levels of cytokines and body weight. Psychopharmacology 2000; 149:163–169.

148. Hagg S, Soderberg S, Ahren B, Olsson T, Mjorndal T. Leptin concentrations are increased in subjects treated with clozapine or conventional antipsychotics. J Clin Psychiatry 2001; 62:843–848.

149. Hinze-Selch D, Schuld A, Kraus T, Kuhn M, Uhr M, Haack M, Pollmacher T. Effects of antidepressants on weight and on the plasma levels of leptin, TNF-alpha and soluble TNF receptors: a longitudinal study in patients treated with amitriptyline or paroxetine. Neuropsychopharmacology 2000; 23:13–19.

150. Bealer SL, Crowley WR. Neurotransmitter interaction in release of intranuclear oxytocin in magnocellular nuclei of the hypothalamus. Ann N Y Acad Sci 1999; 897:182–191.

151. Richelson E. Receptor pharmacology of neuroleptics: relation to clinical effects. J Clin Psychiatry 1999; 60: 5–14.

152. Virkkunen M, Wahlbeck K, Rissanen A, Naukkarinen H, Franssila-Kallunki A. Decrease of energy expenditure causes weight increase in olanzapine treatment – a case study. Pharmacopsychiatry 2002; 35:124–126.

153. Werneke U, Taylor D, Sanders TA. Options for pharmacological management of obesity in patients treated with atypical antipsychotics. Int Clin Psychopharmacol 2002; 17:145–160.

154. Kretschmer E. Body Structure and Character. Berlin: J Springer, 1921.

155. Kraus T, Zimmermann U, Schuid A, Haack M, Hinze-Selch D, Pollmacher T. The physiopathology of weight regulation during treatment with psychotropic drugs. Fortschr Neurol Psychiatr 2001; 69:116–137.

156. Cincotta AH, Meier AH. Bromocriptine (Ergoset) reduces body weight and improves glucose tolerance in obese subjects. Diabetes Care 1996; 19:667–670.

157. Baptista T, Lopez ME, Teneud L, Contreras Q, Alastre T, de Quijada M, Araujo de Baptista E, Alternus M, Weiss SR, Musseo E, Paez X, Hernandez L. Amantadine in the treatment of neuroleptic-induced obesity in rats: behavioural, endocrine and neurochemical correlates. Pharmacopsychiatry 1997; 30:43–54.

158. Kaur G, Kulkarni SK. Studies on modulation of feeding behaviour by atypical antipsychotics in female mice. Prog Neuropsychopharmacol Biol Psychiatry 2002; 26:277–285.
159. Floris M, Lejeune J, Deberdt W. Effect of amantadine on weight gain during olanzapine treatment. Eur Neuropsychopharmacol 2001; 11:181–182.
160. Frankenburg RF, Zanarini MC, Kando J, Centorrino F. Clozapine and body mass change. Biol Psychiatry 1998; 43:520–524.
161. Landau MA, Leeens P, Ulizio K, Cicchetti D, Scahill L, Leckman JF. Risperidone-associated weight gain in children and adolescents: a retrospective chart review. J Child Adolesc Psychopharmacol 2000; 10:259–268.
162. Krishnamoorthy J, King BH. Open-label olanzapine treatment in five pre-adolescent children. J Child Adolesc Psychopharmacol 1998; 8:107–113.
163. Kelly DL, Conley RR, Love RC, Horn DS, Ushchak CM. Weight gain in adolescents treated with risperidone and conventional antipsychotics over 6 months. J Child Adolesc Psychopharmacol 1998; 8:151–159.
164. Ghaeli P, Dufresne RL. Serum triglyceride levels in patients treated with clozapine. Am J Health Syst Pharm 1996; 53:2079–2081.
165. Gaulin BD, Markowitz JS, Caley CF, et al. Clozapine-associated elevation in serum triglycerides. Am J Psychiatry 1999; 156:1270–1272.
166. Su T-P, Elman I, Malhotra AK, Adler CM, Pickar D, Breier AF. Comparison of weight gain during risperidone and clozapine treatment in chronic schizophrenia. Presented at the 149th Annual Meeting of the American Psychiatric Association, New York, USA, May 4–9, 1996.
167. Bouchard RH, Demers MF, Simoneau I, Almeras N, Villeneuve J, Mottard JP, Cadrin C, Lemieux I, Despres JP. Atypical antipsychotics and cardio-vascular risk in schizophrenic patients. J Clin Psychopharmacol 2001; 21:110–111.
168. Sheitman BB, Bird PM, Binz W, Akinli L, Sanchez C. Olanzapine-induced elevation of plasma triglyceride levels. Am J Psychiatry 1999; 156:1471–1472.
169. Osser DN, Najarian DM, Dufresne RL. Olanzapine increases weight and serum triglycerides. J Clin Psychiatry 1999; 60:767–770.
170. Procyshyn RC, Kennedy NB, Marriage S, Wasan KM. Plasma protein and lipoprotein distribution of clozapine. Am J Psychiatry 2001; 158:949–951.
171. Hamner MB, Arana GW. Hyperprolactinemia in antipsychotic-treated patients. CNS Drugs 1998; 10:209–222.
172. Melkersson KI, Hulting AL, Rane AJ. Dose requirement and prolactin elevation of antipsychotics in male and female patients with schizophrenia or related psychoses. Brit J Clin Pharmacol 2001; 51:317–324.
173. Kim K-S, Pae C-U, Chae J-H, Bahk W-M, Jun T-Y, Kim D-J, Dickson RA. Effects of olanzapine on prolactin levels of female patients with schizophrenia treated with risperidone. J Clin Psychiatry 2002; 63:408–413.
174. Turrone P, Kapur S, Seeman MV, Flint AJ. Elevation of prolactin levels by antipsychotics. Am J Psychiatry 2002; 159:1608–1609.

175. Kleinberg DL, Davis JM, de Coster R, Van Baelen B, Brecher M. Prolactin levels and adverse events in patients treated with risperidone. J Clin Psychopharmacol 1999; 19:57–61.
176. Smith SM, O'Keane V, Murray R. Sexual dysfunction in patients taking conventional antipsychotic medication. Brit J Psychiatry 2002; 181:49–55.
177. Compton MT, Miller AH. Priapism associated with conventional and atypical antipsychotics: a review. J Clin Psychiatry 2001; 62:362–366.
178. Lewis R, Bagnall A, Leitner M. Sertindole for schizophrenia. Cochrane Database Syst Rev 2000; 2:CD001715.
179. Seger A, Lamberti JS. Priapism associated with polypharmacy. J Clin Psychiatry 2001; 62:128.
180. Aizenberg D, Modai I, Landa A, Gil-Ad I, Weizman A. Comparison of sexual dysfunction in male schizophrenic patients maintained on treatment with classical antipsychotics versus clozapine. J Clin Psychiatry 2001; 62:541–544.
181. Hummer M, Kemmler K, Kurz M, Kurzthaler I, Oberhauer H, Fleischhacker WW. Sexual disturbances during treatment with clozapine and haloperidol treatment for schizophrenia. Am J Psychiatry 1999; 156:631–633.
182. Feret BM, Caley CF. Possible hypothyroidism associated with quetiapine. Ann Pharmacother 2000; 34:483–486.
183. Meltzer HY. Putting metabolic side effects in perspective: risks versus benefits of atypical antipsychotics. J Clin Psychiatry 2001; 62:35–39.
184. Stanniland C, Taylor D. Tolerability of atypical antipsychotics. Drug Saf 2000; 22:195–214.
185. Fontaine KR, Heo M, Harrigan EP, Shear CL, Lakshminarayanan M, Casey DE, Allison DB. Estimating the consequences of anti-psychotic induced weight gain on health and mortality rate. Psychiatry Res 2001; 101:277–288.
186. Curkendall SM, Mo J-P, Jones JK, Glasser D. Increased cardiovascular disease in patients with schizophrenia. Presented at the 154th Annual Meeting of the American Psychiatric Association, New Orleans, LA, May 5–10, 2001.
187. Kapur S, Remington G. Atypical antipsychotics: new directions and new challenges in the treatment of schizophrenia. Annu Rev Med 2001; 52: 503–517.

6

The Nosology of the Psychotic Disorders

Rhoshel Lenroot and John Lauriello

*University of New Mexico,
Albuquerque, New Mexico, U.S.A.*

I. INTRODUCTION

Nosology refers to the classification of pathological phenomena. While descriptions of individuals exhibiting symptoms of mental disturbance can be found throughout recorded history, the terms used to describe them have varied widely. The language of psychopathology has evolved along with the theories used to explain abnormalities of thought, mood, and behavior. These have ranged from the earliest accounts of "demonic possession" in Vedic and biblical accounts (1), to the theories based upon the imbalances of the humors (2) or "wandering uterus" of Greek and Roman times (3), to the hypotheses of dysfunctional cortical networks now being explored with the growingly sophisticated tools of cognitive neuroscience (4). This introductory chapter will provide a brief overview of the current nosology of the psychotic disorders, including some background in the history of the terms we use today. It should be noted that in this short summary we have not been able to include many of the individuals who have made important contributions to the development of the conceptualization and classification of psychotic disorders, and would refer the reader to other more comprehensive works such as those by Wallace (5) or Berrios (6).

II. ORIGIN OF THE TERM "PSYCHOSIS"

Modern nosology began in the 17th century with Sydenham's definition of the concept of disease (7): "Nature, in the production of diseases, is uniform and consistent; so much so that for the same disease in different persons the symptoms are for the most part the same; and the self-same phenomena that you could observe in the sickness of a Socrates you would observe in the sickness of a simpleton."

Sydenham's definition arose within a historical context in which the classification of natural phenomena was advancing rapidly. Carl Linnaeus created his great botanical classification system during the first part of the 18th century, based upon the principles that species exist which are finite, stable, and discontinuous, and which may be discovered upon application of the correct criteria. Sydenham's definition of disease as a consistent entity independent of the individual in which it occurred opened the way for those who wished to apply the same principles of classification to medicine (8). The earliest figures in this endeavor in the field of psychopathology were Boissier de Sauvages (1768) and William Cullen (1790). While de Sauvages attempted to apply Linnaeus' method directly and ended up with an unwieldy compendium of over 2400 diseases, Cullen followed his predecessor in Edinburgh, Robert Whytt, in attempting to classify diseases according to etiology. He introduced the term "neurosis" in the mid-18th century to refer to all disturbances of general functions of the nervous system, in the absence of fever or specific local lesions (9): "I propose to comprehend, under the title neuroses, all those preternatural affections of sense and motion, which are without pyrexia as part of the primary disease; and all those which do not depend upon a topical affection of the nervous system ... [but] on a more general affection of the nervous system" (10).

The neuroses contained a broad range of disorders, ranging from tetany to melancholia, and were divided into categories by the function affected, including the comata, adynamiae, spasmi, and vesaniae, the last one containing most of what would come to be considered psychotic illnesses (8). During this period the nature of the relationship between the mind and the body and consequent implications for the understanding of behavioral disturbances were being intensely debated. In 19th century Germany, where these debates had been most developed, the primary theoretical positions were held by two opposing groups, the "Somaticists" and the "Mentalists" (11). The Somaticists viewed the mind as separate from the body and incorruptible, and thus "mental disturbances" were caused by diseases of internal organs. The Mentalists also saw the mind as being independent of physical influences, but stated instead that mental illness was due to spiritual factors, i.e., the adverse effects of excessive passion or sins such as envy or greed. While this could eventually have an adverse effect on the body, the source was in the mind.

The term "psychosis" was first used by Ernst Feuchtersleben in 1845 (12). Feuchtersleben was an Austrian physician who recognized that not all nervous system pathology resulted in mental symptoms. He proposed that mind and body reciprocally affected each other, and that mental illnesses arose from both interacting together, rather than stemming primarily from one or the other as argued by the Somaticists and Mentalists. He used the term psychosis to describe the diseases of "personality," defined as the sum of the physical and mental aspects of a given individual, and whose symptoms could include the whole range of mental disturbances. He also coined the term "psychopathy" which he used synonymously with psychosis. He accepted Cullen's classifications, and considered his psychoses to be a subgroup of the neuroses (12): "Every psychosis is at the same time a neurosis, because without the nerves as an intermediary, no psychological change can come to expression, but every neurosis is not a psychosis."

Psychosis proved to be a popular term, although with a different meaning than given by Feuchtersleben. The debate between Somaticists and Mentalists had been replaced by a materialist viewpoint which saw all mental illnesses as being based in pathology of the nervous system. This differed from the earlier Somaticists in that they had emphasized extra-cerebral pathology, while the materialists emphasized intra-cerebral pathology. Rather than Feuchtersleben's concept of a reciprocal interaction between psychological and physical factors, psychoses were taken as the psychological results of organic lesions in the nervous system, with the same organic basis as other types of neurosis (9).

As the term evolved, psychoses came to be classified as "organic," ascribed to specific cerebral changes, and "functional," in which cerebral changes were thought to be present but not yet proven. Bonhoeffer divided the organically based psychoses into the "exogeneous" psychoses, which were conditions such as delirium in which similar symptoms could be produced by different types of external factors, and "endogeneous" psychoses, such as manic-depression and paranoia, which were considered primarily due to the brain disease stemming from the individual's innate disposition (13,14). Wimmer on the other hand separated psychogenic psychoses, which were related to stressful or traumatic life events, from endogeneous psychoses. The concept of endogeneous psychosis was heavily influenced by Benedict Morel's theory of degeneration, which postulated that mental disorders were not only hereditary but became increasingly severe as they were passed from one generation to the next. This theory had the unfortunate consequence of adding to the stigma associated with mental illness (15), as well as the tragic results of being used to help justify the sterilization or extermination of mentally ill individuals by the German Third Reich beginning in the 1930s (16,11). The chronic psychoses came to be seen as rooted in organic pathology of the central nervous system, similar to the later-onset dementias being identified by Alzheimer during this period.

The concept of neurosis was also changing during this period. The study of psychotic illnesses had been based in the asylums where many of the affected individuals resided, and thus came from the tradition of the early psychiatrists who worked in these settings, then called "alienists," as they specialized in patients who were "alienated" from society. The neuroses had traditionally been the province of the neurologists, and as it was much less stigmatizing to have a "neurosis" or "nervous disorder" than be associated with the conditions treated by the alienists, those who were able brought their mental and behavioral complaints to the outpatient office of the neurologist or general physician (16). Researchers in the field of neurology were meanwhile gradually identifying lesions of the nervous system associated with many of the neuroses, and reclassifying these conditions into categories based on these lesions. Those disorders that remained had no identifiable organic pathology, and were theorized by individuals such as Freud to be due to more general disturbances of the nervous system, or "nervous energy" (2,17). The finding that the mental disturbances of shell-shocked World War I veterans could be helped by psychotherapy lent credence to the notion that these disorders could be due to the impact of stressful circumstances on previously healthy individuals, and effectively treated through interactions with a skillful therapist. The combination of these factors led to neuroses being considered "psychological" conditions in which consideration of physical pathology of the nervous system was largely irrelevant. Thus, by the end of World War I, the concept of neuroses and psychoses had come to have nearly opposite meanings from a hundred years previously (3,16).

A. The Evolving Classification of the Psychotic Disorders

Emil Kraepelin (1856–1926), Eugene Bleuler (1857–1939), and Kurt Schneider (1887–1967) were three individuals who were highly influential in creating the modern formulation of the paradigmatic functional psychosis, schizophrenia (18). The lack of success in identifying an anatomic basis for the functional psychoses led Kraepelin to characterize them based instead on detailed clinical observation of the course and outcome of individual cases. This evolved into his now classic division of the functional psychoses into three groups. One was dementia praecox, the first formulation of the syndrome now called schizophrenia. It typically came on early in life and in most cases had a chronic course with a poor outcome (Kraepelin acknowledged that some individuals with dementia praecox experienced remission or recovery, but this did not appear to alter his fundamental conception of the illness). Manic-depressive illness had a later onset, cyclic presentation, and did not show the same chronic deteriorating course. In the third type, paranoia, patients suffered from complex non-bizarre delusions in the absence of significant thought disorder. Kraepelin actually classified paranoia as a type of personality disorder, as he had observed many of these cases to have had premorbid personality abnormalities, and these patients did not display the profound functional impairment or deteriorating course more characteristic of dementia praecox or manic-depressive illness (19–21).

Bleuler took the concept of dementia praecox and attempted to determine its most important features based on signs and symptoms, with more emphasis on the attempt to identify psychological mechanisms of the disorder and less on the clinical course. He objected to the term "dementia praecox" because not all cases began in adolescence or had a poor outcome, and introduced the term schizophrenia as a means of denoting what he saw as a group of related but heterogeneous disorders. The term itself was chosen to reflect the splitting between thought, emotion, and behavior that he felt was the essential characteristic of this group of disorders.

Bleuler made two different divisions in the symptoms of the schizophrenias. One distinction was a clinical one between *basic* and *accessory* symptoms. The basic symptoms were those arising from the unique, characteristic, and generally permanent alterations in fundamental psychic functions which were thought to be at the root of this illness. They included the "four A's": loosening of associations, disturbances of affect, ambivalence, and autism, as well as disturbances of the subjective experience of self and of volition and behavior. In contrast, the accessory symptoms included phenomena such as hallucinations, delusions, mood alterations, and somatic symptoms which were not universally present, could be intermittent in nature, and were found in other types of psychotic illness. The second distinction was between *primary* and *secondary* symptoms. This distinction had a more theoretical basis arising from his views of how the symptoms were produced. Bleuler was influenced by the psychological theories of Freud and Jung, and speculated that the presence of specific kinds of secondary symptoms was created by the interaction of affect-laden psychic complexes with the underlying "latent psychosis" or primary symptoms (18). The primary symptoms were considered those directly related to the basic disease process, such as loosening of associations and the tendency to hallucinate, while the secondary symptoms were a psychologically understandable reaction to the primary symptoms, such as disturbances of affect or autistic withdrawal (22). Both divisions reflected his belief that these illnesses arose from a common underlying process unique to this group that then gave rise to a variety of other less specific symptoms, and thus they overlapped to some degree. Bleuler's emphasis on cross-sectional signs and symptoms made the patient's subjective experience a more important factor in diagnosis than had been the case in Kraepelin's course-based formulation. However, the vagueness of the primary symptoms made diagnosis difficult, and the idea that schizophrenia could be present in a "latent" form without active psychotic symptoms led to the broad application of the term "schizophrenic" to many individuals with non-specific symptoms.

Schneider also sought a cross-sectional description of schizophrenia, but one independent of any particular theoretical stance towards the etiology of the disease or the relationship of symptoms to specific disease processes. He instead chose to place his emphasis on a pragmatic determination of which symptoms could most reliably be used for differential diagnosis. This was intended to both increase reliability of diagnosis and to narrow the range of presentations called "schizophrenic" from Bleuler's broader formulation. He arrived at a set of "first rank criteria," symptoms that he considered to be pathognomic of schizophrenia when present in the absence of organic causes of psychosis. These first rank criteria consisted of delusions and hallucinations such as thought insertion, thought withdrawal, externally controlled behavior, auditory hallucinations of voices in discussion or commenting on the patient's actions, and hallucinations with tightly linked associated delusions. These symptoms are notable for their bizarre nature and the frequent theme of feeling that one's thoughts, bodily sensations, or activities are being controlled by some external agency. Other types of hallucinations and delusions were considered less specific, and could be present in other psychotic disorders such as manic-depressive illness as well as schizophrenia (22).

Schneider was successful at identifying a set of symptoms which could be relatively easily identified and which lent themselves to a categorical approach that could be operationalized into diagnostic criteria for clinical and research purposes. As such they took on a prominent role in the differentiation of schizophrenia from other illnesses in many diagnostic systems, including the International Classification of Diseases (ICD), the Research and Diagnostic Criteria (RDC), and the DSM-III (22). However, over time it has become clear that they are not as pathognomic of schizophrenia as once thought. Schneider himself had been careful to stipulate that these symptoms could be present in cases of organic psychosis, and studies have reported first rank symptoms as being associated with subcortical and limbic lesions as well as some metabolic or toxic encephalopathies (23). In addition, a number of careful studies beginning in the 1970s found that first rank symptoms occurred within a significant proportion of psychoses associated with affective disorders (24–27). Studies have not found that cases of schizophrenia with prominent first rank symptoms ("nuclear" schizophrenia) have a different course or outcome. The high variability in reported base rates of first rank symptoms in schizophrenia populations, ranging from 28 to 72% at different centers, raised questions regarding how reliably they could be identified. These considerations led to a decreased emphasis on the presence of first rank symptoms in the most recent Diagnostic and Statistical Manual (DSM) definition of schizophrenia (28). Instead there was an effort to incorporate recognition of multiple aspects of this syndrome in the criteria, including the chronic course first emphasized by Kraepelin, and the presence of negative symptoms, recognized by both Kraepelin and Bleuler as an essential feature.

While Kraepelin's basic nosological structure has remained the basis for psychiatric classification of the functional psychoses, it has also been long recognized that there were functional psychotic disorders that did not fit into either dementia praecox or manic-depressive illness. These have evolved into the modern concepts of delusional disorder, schizoaffective disorder, and brief psychotic disorder.

As mentioned above, Kraepelin actually divided the functional psychoses into three groups. The third, paranoia, was troublesome for him and has continued to be a source of controversy. The term "paranoia" was originally an ancient Greek word that was a colloquial word for insanity. It was resurrected by Heinroth in the first part of the 19th century to describe mental disorders that primarily affected cognition rather than perception. Schifferdecker and Peters in their review of the origin of the concept of paranoia (21) describe the evolution in France and Germany of the idea of a partial mental disorder, eventually called "monomania" by Esquirol, in which abnormal fixation or agitation regarding only one or a few subjects was present in the absence of significant thought disorder. Kraepelin's concept of paranoia as a disorder distinct from dementia praecox was first defined in the sixth edition of his textbook (this was also the first edition in which he used the term dementia praecox) (29, p. 316): "Paranoia is a chronic, progressive psychosis ... characterized by the gradual development of a stable progressive system of delusions, without marked mental deterioration, clouding of consciousness or involvement of the coherence of thought."

The relationship of paranoia to dementia praecox changed throughout the successive versions of Kraepelin's textbook, and continued to be debated elsewhere in the field. Kraepelin's last edition of his textbook placed the paranoid psychotic disorders that were accompanied by marked deterioration within the category of dementia praecox, and divided the non-deteriorating paranoid disorders into classic paranoia, which was characterized by non-bizarre delusions, and paraphrenia, in which delusions could be bizarre and hallucinations were frequently present. Bleuler considered most paranoias to actually fall within the schizophrenias, while others in the Scandinavian and British schools considered them to be psychogenic reactions arising from stressful circumstances in certain kinds of personalities (19). Schneider considered them to be a subtype of schizophrenia. DSM-III retained the concept of classic paranoia as Paranoid Disorder, which was renamed Delusional Disorder in DSM-III-R and continued in DSM-IV.

Another problematic area was the significant number of cases which would not fit within either schizophrenia or manic-depressive illness, but seemed to have elements of both. Kraepelin had recognized the "disturbingly frequent" number of cases which could not be easily classified and represented an area of overlap between the two categories (30). Jacob Kasanin coined the term "schizo-affective psychosis" in 1933 to describe a group of psychoses with acute onset, short duration, and a combination of delusions, hallucinations, and affective symptoms. He felt that these were usually triggered by stressors, and most of the cases he described would now be considered to fall within the Scandinavian concept of a reactive psychosis or an affective disorder (31). Nonetheless, the term served useful to describe those cases characterized by a combination of schizophrenia-like and affective symptoms, and has remained in use, although with varying definitions of the exact nature and course of the symptoms involved (32).

While in the United States a broad definition of schizophrenia based on Bleuler's criteria had subsumed most functional psychotic disorders, the more restrictive Kraepelinian definition prevalent in Europe during the first part of the century had prompted interest in a new classification for a "third psychosis" to encompass those cases with less severe symptoms and a non-chronic course (33). Gabriel Langfeldt introduced the term schizophreniform disorder in 1939 as way of differentiating two different syndromes that at the time were usually both called schizophrenia but which he saw as having very different potential responses to treatment and outcomes. The first he considered the "genuine type" of schizophrenia, which included factors he felt indicative of poor prognosis and likely progression into a chronic illness, such as poor premorbid personality functioning, insidious onset without precipitating factors, symptoms characteristic of Kraepelin's description of dementia praecox, and an unfavorable environment. The second, which he termed the schizophreniform disorders, were a heterogeneous group characterized by acute onset with identifiable precipitating factors, good premorbid function, the presence of affective symptoms or confusion rather than affective blunting, and favorable surroundings. This group was more likely to return to premorbid functioning (22). Schizophreniform disorder gradually evolved to have the same symptomatic criteria as schizophrenia but with a time course of less than six months. It has thus come to include three different syndromes, including a first psychotic episode which has not yet met the duration criterion for schizophrenia; a first psychotic episode which did not meet duration or intensity criteria for schizophrenia before remission, but is occurring in an individual who will have further psychotic breaks and eventually meet diagnostic criteria for schizophrenia; and the group Langfeldt originally envisioned, in which the affected individual does experience complete remission without relapse (31).

This "third psychosis" was conceptualized slightly differently by Karl Jaspers as a brief reactive psychosis. He stressed the relationship of a precipitating factor to the onset of psychotic symptoms, including stipulations that the stressor must be of adequate severity to precipitate such a severe reaction, that there should be a meaningful connection between the contents of the stressor and of the reaction, and that the psychotic reaction should end when the precipitating factor is removed (33). This diagnosis was eventually subsumed in the most recent version of the DSM under the category Brief Psychotic Disorders, which was defined primarily on the basis of having symptoms of less than a month. The presence of a stressor was also changed from a requirement to a qualifier, as it was felt defining what would be an adequate stressor to precipitate such a reaction was too difficult to be done accurately. Brief Psychotic Disorder thus came to include many of the culturally bound brief psychotic disorders such as koro and amok.

B. Current Classifications of Psychotic Disorders

Difficulties arising from the use of multiple versions of diagnostic criteria in different settings and locations led to the creation of consensus-based classification systems, i.e., diagnostic formulations agreed upon by a body of experts in the field. The American Psychiatric Association developed the Diagnostic and Statistical Manual, whose first version was published in 1952. The World Health Organization also changed to a consensus-based classification system with the publication of the International Classification of Disease (ICD-9) in 1977.

The conceptions of the psychotic disorders have evolved through the different versions of each of these classification systems. In DSM-I and DSM-II, as well as ICD-9, psychotic disorders were seen as illnesses that involved difficulties with reality testing in combination with disruptions of intellect and social function severe enough to markedly impact functioning. They were disorders of the whole person, in contrast to paranoia and the neuroses in which only part of the personality was involved. With DSM-III and the switch to operationalized criteria and a multi-axial system the previous dichotomies of psychotic versus neurotic were dropped. Psychotic became a term used either as an adjective for a patient, or to describe several different disorders which at some point caused all those afflicted to have difficulties with reality testing and abnormalities of thought and/or perception, but which had no other inherent relation. Psychosis continued as a term in common usage as a convenient way to indicate problems with reality testing in conjunction with impaired function, but was no longer a formally defined nosological entity.

Both the DSM and the ICD were designed with the goal of emphasizing reliable and clinically useful descriptions of mental disorders, based on observable phenomena, and relying on as few overt theoretical claims as possible. The ICD-10 is the most commonly used classification system outside the United States, while the DSM has become the standard vocabulary for mental health professionals within the United States. Its descriptions have for the most part become so well accepted that they run the risk of being taken as a more definitive statement of the nature of mental illnesses than was ever intended by its authors. Nevertheless, many criticisms of this classification system remain.

One criticism of the DSM is that validity may have been sacrificed for the goal of reliability, i.e., it is not a true nosology, in which pathological phenomena are sorted into natural categories based on their key features. Part of this is due to the nature of the phenomena of psychopathology, which unlike those of the "harder" sciences such as physics or chemistry does not show the invariant features and highly ordered relationships that lend themselves to the establishment of a natural classification (for example, the periodic table) (34). In the field of medicine, when an etiological framework is available, such as in infectious disease, it is possible to use it to create a natural classification system. This moves a taxonomy from being descriptive to one in which the classification of a phenomenon is itself informative, predicting other likely although yet unobserved attributes and allowing the assignment of relationships between different categories (for example, that pulmonary tuberculosis and miliary tuberculosis are related to a common infectious agent and may respond to similar treatment). But when an etiological framework is not yet available, as in the case of most psychiatric disorders, classification systems must fall back on descriptive measures whose emphasis is chosen to some extent arbitrarily depending on the purposes of the classification system being designed.

The systems arrived at by the three figures above, Kraepelin, Bleuler, and Schneider, are an example of this. Kraepelin emphasized the longitudinal course of the psychoses in order to show how these categories corresponded to what he thought were natural disease entities that had a predictable evolution and prognosis. Bleuler instead focused on clinical features in the attempt both to better diagnose an individual in the absence of extensive longitudinal information, and to describe what he thought were the essential psychological deficits. Thus he gave close descriptions of clinical phenomena, with attempts to create a structure of relationships between them such as "primary" and "secondary" based on his theories of the underlying psychological dynamics. Schneider designed his system to enhance inter-rater reliability and reduce the number of indeterminate cases being diagnosed as schizophrenia, and so he highlighted symptoms such as bizarre hallucinations and delusions which were easily recognizable as being outside of the range of normal functioning and unlike what was usually seen in affective disorders.

The fact that mental disorders are still classified in multiple ways depending on the purposes and contexts involved has led some, such as Foucault in his *Madness and Civilization* or Thomas Szasz and the antipsychiatry movement, to charge that psychiatric disorders are completely arbitrary constructs based on societal values. Such concerns helped motivate cross-cultural studies such as those undertaken by the World Health Organization (WHO) beginning in the 1960s (35–37). While Kraepelin had traveled to the Far East to explore whether illnesses similar to dementia praecox existed in non-European cultures, and others had documented the presence of psychotic illnesses in various Asian and African countries, these earlier investigations had significant methodological limitations. These included problems such as the lack of standardized instruments, biases in case selection, and reliance on cross-sectional or retrospective data. The WHO studies were designed to examine psychotic disorders in a controlled and systematic fashion in multiple countries with different cultures and varying levels of industrial development.

The subjects of the first study, the International Pilot Study of Schizophrenia (IPSS) (36), were patients with psychotic disorders who had been admitted to psychiatric facilities. The IPSS was followed by the Determinants of Outcome Study (DOS) (35), which instead identified subjects when they first presented for help with a possible psychotic disorder to a variety of community agencies, including both medical facilities and traditional healers. This approach was chosen to allow a closer estimation of the actual incidence of the disorder than in the first study. Both studies were able to obtain follow up information for over 75% of the subjects, after 5 years in the IPSS study and after 2 years in the DOS study. The studies found similar incidences of schizophrenia-like illnesses across the different centers, and that patients tended to present with very similar symptoms, including persecutory delusions, beliefs that their mind or body had been invaded by alien forces, and auditory and visual hallucinations. These were seen as abnormal and distressing to patients and their families. Some differences were seen between the different sites, particularly in the better long-term outcomes in developing countries that were found by both studies. However, the overall homogeneity in rates of incidence and presentation of psychotic illnesses across different settings helped support the notion that a fundamental pathologic process was at work rather than a purely sociologic phenomenon.

Evidence from studies such as those of the WHO described above, as well as the experience of countless clinicians, helped to show that while psychiatry was not yet able to lay down a definitive naturalistic classification system, or "carve nature at the joints," at least some psychiatric phenomena could be considered diseases in Sydenham's sense.

Jaspers proposed dividing psychiatric disorders into three groups, which he felt each required a different approach to classification due to their varying approximations to status as disease entities. He included in his Group I those mental disorders which could be ascribed to definite physical causes, such as local lesions such as trauma or tumor, systemic diseases with symptomatic psychoses such as infections or endocrine disorders, and mental disorders due to substances such as street drugs, carbon monoxides, or other toxins. These would generally fall within our modern categories of mental disorders due to a general medical condition, delirium, and mental disorders associated with substance use. Jaspers felt the illnesses of this first group could be definitively considered diseases and could be classified according to etiologies. Group II consisted of schizophrenia, manic-depressive disorder, and epilepsy, and Group III included isolated abnormal reactions not due to the processes found in Group I or Group II; neuroses; and personality disorders. This group was different from the second in that these disorders could conceivably be seen as gradations of normal functioning, and in addition were even more difficult to separate from each other than members of Group II.

Jaspers stated that where the etiological knowledge of Group I was absent, the alternative was a typological classification system. In contrast to a naturalistic classification system as described above, a typological classification is an example of a nominalistic system, in which a structure is arbitrarily imposed upon phenomena by choosing particular aspects to attend according to the purpose at hand (for example, grouping cows and lizards together if one is interested in animals that have four legs). This allows the creation of categories that can serve as a starting point for further investigations or to meet practical needs without being bound to a particular etiological theory unsupported by available knowledge. He saw Group III as requiring a strictly typological framework. The group containing schizophrenia and manic-depressive illness, however, he proposed as reflecting an intermediate stage. In these conditions the ignorance regarding etiology still necessitated a typological classification system, but the similarity of symptoms and course between different individuals, severity of functional impairment, and the presence of positive neuropathological findings showed them as clearly different from normal functioning in a way indicative of a disease process. Therefore their classification could be seen as a typological system guided by a disease concept, and he expected that with the accrual of further information these illnesses would be moved from Group II to Group I, as occurred in the case of epilepsy.

Keeping these differing levels of classification in mind can help to make sense of modern diagnostic compendia such as the DSM-IV, which contains descriptions of mental disorders which would fall within each of these levels (7) (Table 1). As mentioned above, categories such as substance-induced psychotic disorder would belong in Jasper's Group I, while schizophrenia and the major affective disorders would be examples of Group II. Many disorders would be considered to fall within Group III. Ongoing current debates regarding matters such as relative merits of dimensional versus categorical approaches to the personality disorders, or the differences between Social Phobia and Avoidant Personality Disorder, can be seen as attempts to define different typological descriptions of a group of symptoms whose inherent relationships are yet unclear.

Other occasionally problematic aspects to the modern classifications can be seen as intrinsic to the kind of typology used. For example, the DSM-IV uses a prototypal structure rather than a classical model of categorization. As Millon reviewed in his summary of classification of psychopathology (34), in the classical model, disorders are seen as discrete entities clearly delineated by the presence or absence of defining features, such as squares and triangles being separated by their number of sides. This tends not to work as well with many natural phenomena, where such clear divisions may not exist. A prototypal structure instead specifies the most common features of a proposed group, thus describing a "typical" member that others may match in varying degrees. Each member contains at least some of these features, although no one feature is absolute. The classical categories encourage stereotyping of patients and ignoring of aspects that do not fit. The greater flexibility of a prototypal structure is less likely to lead to these pitfalls, but at the expense of allowing heterogeneous presentations to receive the same diagnosis. In addition, while members that match many of the criteria are relatively easy to classify, those that meet

Table 1 Key Features of Psychotic Disorders in the DSM-IV

Disorder	Symptoms	Impairment	Duration	Types
Schizophrenia	Two or more symptoms such as delusions, hallucinations, disorganized speech or behavior, negative symptoms; only one required if delusions bizarre or hallucinations are of voice with running commentary on person, or two or more voices conversing	Major impairment in one or more areas of function	Continuous signs of disturbance for at least 6 months, with at least 1 month of active symptoms	Paranoid Disorganized Catatonic Undifferentiated Residual
Schizophreniforzm disorder	Same as schizophrenia	Same as schizophrenia	Episode lasting at least 1 month but less than 6 months	With or without good prognostic features, i.e., rapid onset, confusion at height of psychotic episode, good premorbid functioning, absence of blunted or flat affect
Brief Psychotic Disorder	Presence of delusions, hallucinations, disorganized speech or disorganized behavior, not consistent with cultural norms	—	At least 1 day but less than 1 month, with return to premorbid functioning	With marked stressors Without marked stressors Postpartum onset

Delusional disorder	Non-bizarre delusions	Functioning not significantly impaired outside of impact of the delusions	At least 1 month	Erotomanic Grandiose Jealous Persecutory Somatic Mixed Unspecified
Shared single psychotic disorder	Delusion developing in individual in context of close relationship with another person(s) who has an already established delusion; delusion is similar to the other person's	—	—	—
Psychotic disorder due to a general medical condition	Prominent hallucinations or delusions; with evidence from history or physical findings that they are the direct physiological consequence of a general medical condition; not occurring exclusively during delirium	—	—	With delusions With hallucinations

(Continued)

Table 1. Continued

Disorder	Symptoms	Impairment	Duration	Types
Substance-induced psychotic disorder	Prominent hallucinations or delusions without insight in context of substance intoxication or withdrawal, or with evidence that medication use is etiologically related to the disturbance; not occurring exclusively during delirium	—	—	Onset during intoxication Onset during withdrawal
Mood disorder with psychotic features	Presence of either delusions or hallucinations in context of major depressive episode or manic episode	—	—	Mood congruent (most common) such as guilt associated with depression or grandiosity with mania Mood incongruent: no relationship between content of hallucinations or delusions to depressive or manic themes; associated with poorer prognosis

Delirium	Disturbance of consciousness with attentional impairments, change in cognition or development of perceptual disturbance such as hallucinations, with evidence that it is a direct physiological consequence of a general medical condition	—	Develops over a short period of time and tends to fluctuate during the course of a day	—
Dementia	Development of multiple cognitive deficits; presentation depends on type of dementia	Significant functional decline	Suddenness of onset varies by type of dementia; usually chronic	Delusions can be a prominent feature, hallucinations also not infrequently present

only a few can form a fuzzy borderline area that is hard to assign to one category or another.

III. CONCLUSION

Sydenham's formulation of disease allowed modern medical classification to begin. Symptoms could be conceptualized apart from the individual affected, their characteristics described and grouped in ways that could help to show common processes and mechanisms. In much of medicine enough has been learned about these underlying etiologies that they can be the basis for classification, making the act of diagnosis not only one of assigning a convenient name, but potentially a source of information regarding other aspects of a particular disease that may be occurring in an individual patient. Most of the subject matter of psychiatry is still far from this point, however, and so psychiatric nosological systems must still be designed on a more arbitrary basis, depending on the amount of information available and the purposes intended. The classification systems for psychotic illnesses have undergone many changes, from Feuchtersleben's early formulation of psychosis as an illness that affected both the mind and the nervous system, to Morel's theory that psychosis represented an inherited deficiency in the nervous system that inevitably worsened from generation to generation, to the most recent operationalized criterion of the DSM-IV and ICD-10 in which "psychosis" as a particular disease entity has become a less useful concept than "psychotic," an adjective describing individuals having particular types of observable behaviors and subjective experiences.

Such a transition has both pros and cons. The presence of individual symptoms such as hallucinations or delusions is not unusual, and may not always be considered as indicative of a psychotic disorder. For example, hallucinations may be directly associated with pathology of systems associated with sensory processing, both in the peripheral and central nervous systems. In some cases these are easy to differentiate from a primary psychotic disorder, such as the visual hallucinations termed "phantom vision." This is a condition experienced by up to a half of individuals who have undergone surgical removal of an eye, in which spontaneous visual phenomena are experienced while insight into the falsity of the visual phenomena is preserved (38). In other cases, such as the transient auditory hallucinations sometimes associated with temporal lobe seizure activity, the presence of a neural lesion may be less clear, and the distinction from a primary psychotic disorder much harder to make.

Cultural considerations can also affect whether a given symptom or belief is interpreted as representing a psychotic disorder. In some cultures (e.g., Hispanic), hallucinations of recently deceased loved ones are felt to be an acceptable form of grief, and not a harbinger of severe mental illness. In the case of delusions, the relationship of a given belief of an individual to his or her cultural context is explicitly taken into account in determining whether the belief is to be considered delusional or not. Given the ever-changing nature of what can be considered an unremarkable belief, even within one cultural stream (for example, the belief that individuals could be regularly consorting with the biblical Lucifer was taken quite seriously in the United States during the Salem witch trials), such an approach is currently necessary to avoid over-pathologizing unfamiliar beliefs. Yet it can be far from easy to apply – besides the difficulty of knowing what beliefs may be a current part of a given culture, the bizarre and sometimes dangerous practices of some cults can raise questions about when a mass belief should be given the sanction of being a cultural phenomenon. Some investigators are attempting to bypass this difficulty by developing ways of directly assessing the cognitive processes by which individuals adopt and hold beliefs, independent of content and thus of cultural considerations (39), but such efforts are still in their very early stages.

On the other hand, much as separating out the mechanism of the inflammatory process from the insults that trigger it allowed better understanding of both, attempting to understand the mechanism of non-specific symptoms such as delusions and hallucinations apart from a particular disease construct such as "psychosis" may open the way to more satisfactory formulations than presently available. Kraepelin himself recognized that the division of dementia praecox, paranoia, and manic-depressive illness failed to adequately classify many cases, although he held that if more complete information were available these problems would diminish. Current classification systems such as the DSM-IV are also acknowledged to have many problems (40), such as how to make sense of the heterogeneity of possible presentations within the common diagnosis of "schizophrenia" or how to meaningfully classify individuals who have both prominent affective and psychotic symptoms. Many different approaches to these questions are currently being debated, including division of schizo-phrenia into subtypes (41), concentrating on a more dimensional approach to symptoms (42,43), or a return to the idea of a unitary psychosis which stretches across many of the current diagnostic categories (44).

While such debates are not new, the tools currently being developed in neuroimaging are making possible new kinds of observation of the physiologic processes accompanying particular symptoms and experiences, and thus may have the potential to add the additional information needed to improve nosological categories that Kraepelin sought. As the chapters in this volume attest, the reliability afforded by current diagnostic classification systems coupled with new investigative tools are making possible enormous progress in the treatment of psychotic disorders.

REFERENCES

1. Mack AH, Forman L, Brown R, Frances A. A brief history of psychiatric classification. From the ancients to DSM-IV. Psychiatr Clin North Am 1994; 17(3):515–523.
2. Hare E. The history of 'nervous disorders' from 1600 to 1840, and a comparison with modern views. Brit J Psychiatry 1991; 159:37–45.
3. Knoff WF. Four thousand years of hysteria. Compr Psychiatry 1971; 12(2):156–164.
4. Friston KJ. Schizophrenia and the disconnection hypothesis. Acta Psychiatr Scand Suppl 1999; 395:68–79.
5. Wallace ERI. Psychiatry and its nosology: a historico-philosophical overview, In: Sadler JZ, Wiggins OP, Schwartz MA, eds, Philosophical Perspectives on Psychiatric Diagnostic Classification. Baltimore, Maryland, John Hopkins University Press, 1994:16–88.
6. Berrios GE. The History of Mental Symptoms: Descriptive Psychopathology Since the Nineteenth Century. Cambridge: Cambridge University Press, 1996.
7. Wiggins OP, Schwartz MA. The limits of psychiatric knowledge and the problem of classification. In: Sadler JZ, Wiggins OP, Schwartz MA, eds. Philosophical Perspectives on Psychiatric Diagnostic Classification. Baltimore: Johns Hopkins University Press, 1994:89–103.
8. Pichot P. Nosological models in psychiatry. Brit J Psychiatry 1994; 164(2):232–240.
9. Beer MD. The dichotomies: psychosis/neurosis and functional/organic: a historical perspective. Hist Psychiatry 1996; 7(26 Pt 2):231–255.
10. Cullen W. First Lines in the Practice of Physic. Vol 3. Edinburgh: Elliott and Cadell, 1784:121–122.
11. Beer MD. Psychosis: a history of the concept. Compr Psychiatry 1996; 37(4):273–291.
12. Beer MD. Psychosis: from mental disorder to disease concept. Hist Psychiatry 1995; 6(22 Pt 2):177–200.
13. Ban TA. Diagnostic criteria in psychoses. Dialogues Clin Neurosc 2001; 3(4):257–263.
14. Beer MD. The endogenous psychoses: a conceptual history. Hist Psychiatry 1996; 7(25):1–29.
15. Shorter E. A History of Psychiatry: From The Era of the Asylum to the Age of Prozac. New York: John Wiley & Sons, Inc. 1997.
16. Colp R. Psychiatry, past and future. In: Sadock BJ, Sadock VA, eds. Kaplan & Sadock's Comprehensive Textbook of Psychiatry. Vol 2. Philadelphia: Williams & Wilkins, 2000:3320–3333.

17. Knoff WF. A history of the concept of neurosis, with a memoir of William Cullen. Am J Psychiatry 1970; 127(1):80–84.
18. Hoenig J. The concept of Schizophrenia. Kraepelin-Bleuler-Schneider. Brit J Psychiatry 1983; 142:547–556.
19. Kendler KS, Tsuang MT. Nosology of paranoid schizophrenia and other paranoid psychoses. Schizophr Bull 1981; 7(4):594–610.
20. Kendler KS. Kraepelin and the diagnostic concept of paranoia. Compr Psychiatry 1988; 29(1):4–11.
21. Schifferdecker M, Peters UH. The origin of the concept of paranoia. Psychiatr Clin North Am 1995; 18(2):231–249.
22. Berner P, Katschnig H, Kieffer W, Koehler K, Lenz G, Nutzinger D, Schanda H, Simhandl C. Diagnostic Criteria for Functional Psychoses. Cambridge, Cambridge University Press, 1992.
23. Cummings JL. Organic delusions: phenomenology, anatomical correlations, and review. Brit J Psychiatry 1985; 146:184–197.
24. Carpenter WT Jr, Strauss JS. Cross-cultural evaluation of Schneider's first-rank symptoms of schizophrenia: a report from the International Pilot Study of Schizophrenia. Am J Psychiatry 1974; 131(6):682–687.
25. Taylor MA. Schneiderian first-rank symptoms and clinical prognostic features in schizophrenia. Arch Gen Psychiatry 1972; 26(1):64–67.
26. Taylor MA, Abrams R. The phenomenology of mania. A new look at some old patients. Arch Gen Psychiatry 1973; 29(4):520–522.
27. O'Grady JC. The prevalence and diagnostic significance of Schneiderian first-rank symptoms in a random sample of acute psychiatric in-patients. Brit J Psychiatry 1990; 156:496–500.
28. Andreasen NC, Flaum M. Characteristic symptoms of schizophrenia. In: DSM-IV Sourcebook. Vol 1. Washington, DC: American Psychiatric Press, 1994; 351–380.
29. Kraepelin E. Clinical Psychiatry: A Textbook for Students and Physicians. New York: Macmillan, 1904.
30. Angst J. Historical aspects of the dichotomy between manic-depressive disorders and schizophrenia. Schizophr Res 2002; 57(1):5–13.
31. Lauriello J, Erickson BR, Keith SJ. Schizoaffective disorder, schizophreniform disorder, and brief psychotic disorder. In: Sadock BJ, Sadock VA, eds. Kaplan & Sadock's Comprehensive Textbook of Psychiatry. Vol 1. Philadelphia: Williams & Wilkins, 2000:1232–1243.
32. Bertelsen A, Gottesman II. Schizoaffective psychoses: genetical clues to classification. Am J Med Genet 1995; 60(1):7–11.
33. Jauch DA, Carpenter WT Jr. Reactive psychosis. I. Does the pre-DSM-III concept define a third psychosis? J Nerv Ment Dis 1988; 176(2): 72–81.
34. Millon T. Classification in psychopathology: rationale, alternatives, and standards. J Abnorm Psychol 1991; 100(3):245–261.
35. Jablensky A, Sartorius N, Ernberg G, Anker M, Korten A, Cooper JE, Day R, Bertelsen A. Schizophrenia: manifestations, incidence and course in different

cultures. a World Health Organization ten-country study. Psychol Med Monogr Suppl 1992; 20:1–97.

36. Leff J, Sartorius N, Jablensky A, Korten A, Ernberg G. The International Pilot Study of Schizophrenia: five-year follow-up findings. Psychol Med 1992; 22(1):131–145.

37. World Health Organization. Schizophrenia: An International Follow-up Study. Chichester: John Wiley and Sons, 1979.

38. Benson DF, Gorman DG. In: Fogel BS, Schiffer RB, eds. Neuropsychiatry. Baltimore: Williams & Wilkins, 1996:307–324.

39. Mujica-Parodi LR, Sackeim HA. Cultural invariance and the diagnosis of delusions: information processing as a neurobiologically preferable criterion. J Neuropsychiatry Clin Neurosci 2001; 13(3):403–410.

40. Frances AJ, First MB, Widiger TA, Miele GM, Tilly SM, Davis WW, Pincus HA. An A to Z guide to DSM-IV conundrums. J Abnorm Psychol 1991; 100(3):407–412.

41. Andreasen NC, Carpenter WT Jr. Diagnosis and classification of schizophrenia. Schizophr Bull 1993; 19(2):199–214.

42. Andreasen NC, Arndt S, Alliger R, Miller D, Flaum M. Symptoms of schizophrenia. Methods, meanings, and mechanisms. Arch Gen Psychiatry 1995; 52(5):341–351.

43. Maziade M, Roy MA, Martinez M, Cliche D, Fournier JP, Garneau Y, Nicole L, Montgrain N, Dion C, Ponton AM. Negative, psychoticism, and disorganized dimensions in patients with familial schizophrenia or bipolar disorder: continuity and discontinuity between the major psychoses. Am J Psychiatry 1995; 152(10):1458–1463.

44. Crow TJ. From Kraepelin to Kretschmer leavened by Schneider: the transition from categories of psychosis to dimensions of variation intrinsic to homo sapiens. Arch Gen Psychiatry 1998; 55(6):502–504.

7

Acute Efficacy of Atypical Antipsychotic Drugs

Joseph M. Pierre and Stephen R. Marder
*David Geffen School of Medicine at UCLA, and
VA Greater Los Angeles Healthcare System,
Los Angeles, California, U.S.A.*

I. INTRODUCTION

The availability of the atypical (also referred to as "novel" or "second-generation") antipsychotic medications for the treatment of schizophrenia and other psychotic disorders in the United States began in 1988 with the publication of the pivotal trial supporting the effectiveness of clozapine in patients with treatment-resistant schizophrenia and the consequent release of clozapine in 1990. Since that time, five additional atypical antipsychotic medications (risperidone, olanzapine, quetiapine, ziprasidone, aripiprazole) have come to market. The use of atypical antipsychotics in clinical practice is therefore a relatively recent phenomenon with both clinical and clinical research experience with these medications confined to just the past 10 or 15 years (or less for the more recently released drugs).

Clinical research in psychiatry was born in part out of efforts to prove, in the face of early skepticism, that the first generation of antipsychotic medications (now called "conventional" or "typical" antipsychotics) were indeed effective. In order to reduce the bias inherent in clinical observations, various research methods were established for clinical drug trials, including randomization (ensuring random assignment to treatments being compared), prospective data collection, use of validated clinical rating scales, and double-blind clinical assessments (in which neither the research subject nor the rater are aware of the treatment being received). Before a new medication is approved by the U.S. Food and Drug Administration (FDA) and released to market, it must show favorable results in three investigative phases of clinical trials – phase I (small-scale studies examining safety and dosing issues in healthy volunteers), phase II (larger studies evaluating efficacy and appropriate dosing of a new drug compared to placebo or a standard treatment), and phase III (studies including thousands of patients in order to firmly establish both efficacy and safety). Phase IV studies are trials performed after the release of a new drug that aim to answer questions beyond that of efficacy. The cumulative results of these clinical research studies provide essential information about the optimal use of antipsychotic medications from which to guide rational "evidence-based" clinical practice.

While clinical psychiatric research is designed to provide objective and reliable information about the efficacy and safety of various therapies, evidence-based medicine has its limits. One stems from the phenomenon of "publication bias" in which studies with positive findings (those showing that a particular treatment is effective) are more likely to be published. Therefore, clinicians may be unaware of data from negative studies (those showing no efficacy for a particular treatment). Another limitation is that clinical trials usually include a relatively "pure" study sample, meaning that certain patients are inevitably excluded. These patients typically include those younger than 18 or older than 65, patients with serious medical illness, patients with active comorbid substance abuse ("dual diagnosis" patients), or pregnant women. As a result, clinicians have limited or in some cases no data upon which to base clinical decisions for these unstudied but commonly encountered patient populations.

II. BASIC CONCEPTS

A. Defining an Adequate Trial

Studies investigating the efficacy of atypical antipsychotic medications typically involve comparison to treatment with either placebo or conventional antipsychotic medications such as chlorpromazine or haloperidol. Acute efficacy studies generally last 4 to 8 weeks and include patients in the acute stage of schizophrenia. The acute stage is characterized by active psychotic symptoms that would usually require immediate clinical attention. These symptoms may represent a first psychotic episode or, more commonly, a relapse in an individual who has experienced multiple episodes. Treatment during this phase focuses on alleviating the most prominent psychotic symptoms such as hallucinations and delusions.

In clinical practice and investigative studies, an "adequate trial" of an antipsychotic medication is necessary in order to judge its efficacy in an individual. The concept of an adequate trial includes both adequate dose and adequate duration of treatment. Early studies by Van Putten and colleagues showed that a patient's subjective response to a medication within hours of their first dose of medication was a powerful predictor of treatment adherence and response (1). The early subjective response of a patient to an antipsychotic is almost always determined by the medication's side effects rather than its therapeutic effect. Therefore, patients should usually be started on a low initial antipsychotic dose before titrating up to the effective dose range in order to maximize tolerability. In the past, loading dose techniques were sometimes employed with conventional antipsychotic agents as a means of "rapid tranquilization." Double-blind studies have consistently shown no benefit and an increase in side effects from such strategies, as compared to initiating and treating with more standard antipsychotic doses (2). Although the atypical antipsychotic drugs generally are better tolerated than conventional agents, when one considers the high rate of treatment nonadherence in schizophrenia, it is still prudent to initiate treatment with doses that will decrease the risk of side effects and subjective intolerability.

Likewise, patients should generally be treated with the lowest effective dose of an antipsychotic medication for an adequate duration in order to judge a therapeutic effect. To determine this ideal dose, dose increases must proceed slowly. Once a patient has achieved a steady state drug level at a potentially therapeutic dose, it is usually best to avoid the temptation to increase the antipsychotic dose further within the first few weeks, even if the patient is not improving. A full 4 to 6 weeks of treatment may be necessary to determine whether an antipsychotic trial is effective. The lowest effective dose can therefore be surpassed if the antipsychotic dose is increased too quickly within this time period, resulting in a patient being treated with a higher than required antipsychotic dose and unnecessary side effects. When a patient does improve in the setting of aggressive dose escalation, it can be difficult to know whether the observed response was a result of increasing the dose or simply from additional days of treatment. In addition, some patients will demonstrate evidence of immediate improvement (becoming quieter, calmer, or less agitated), but this may be a consequence of the sedating and tranquilizing properties of antipsychotic medications rather than a true antipsychotic effect. The goal of pharmacotherapy during acute treatment is to begin an adequate dose of antipsychotic, monitor the patient for side effects, ensure their comfort and safety, and wait until the patient begins to show a response. While various pressures such as psychotic agitation or length of hospital stay can make the additional time required to achieve an effective dose of medication problematic, the "start low, go slow" strategy will likely contribute to better long-term results.

B. Defining Acute Efficacy

Once a patient has received an adequate trial of an antipsychotic medication, the clinician must then decide whether the patient has responded to that trial. In the treatment of schizophrenia, where the goal of treatment is symptomatic improvement rather than cure, this can be one of the most difficult questions to answer. That is, what degree of improvement is satisfactory? In clinical research, various scales have been devised to quantify psychopathology and measure its change. Ideally, these scales are administered by individuals who have received sufficient training to attain a suitable degree of inter-rater reliability (a measure of how much raters agree with one another or with a "gold standard" rater). In clinical trials involving schizophrenia, the most commonly used rating scales include the Brief Psychiatric Rating Scale (BPRS) and the Positive and Negative Syndrome Scale (PANSS) (3,4). These scales include items measuring positive and negative symptoms associated with schizophrenia, as well as other general symptoms such as anxiety, depression, and hostility. Negative symptoms in schizophrenia are typically quantified using the negative symptom subscale of the PANSS or with another scale devised to specifically measure negative symptoms in schizophrenia, the Schedule for the Assessment of Negative Symptoms (SANS) (5). Improvement is then analyzed by examining the difference between the mean group score on one of these rating scales at baseline and the mean score at endpoint, either at the end of the study (as in a completers analysis) or at the time of study drop-out (as with an "intent to treat" or "last observation carried forward" (LOCF) analysis). In addition, an *a priori* definition of treatment response is sometimes examined, such as a 20% improvement on the total BPRS or PANSS score. In other cases, treatment response is examined in a post-hoc fashion, by examining various definitions of improvement such as a 30%, 40%, or 50% improvement. Using these various measures of treatment response, studies then use statistical methods to determine whether an observed numerical difference is significant – whether it is a "real" difference and not simply due to chance.

Of note, the degree of improvement quantified by these research methods may or may not be significant or satisfactory for an individual patient in the clinical setting where specific improvements such as functional status or quality of life may be more important than overall symptomatic improvement. Some studies are now including scales to measure these types of outcomes as well.

III. EFFICACY OF ATYPICAL ANTIPSYCHOTIC MEDICATIONS: ACUTE TRIALS

A. Clozapine

Clozapine, the first atypical antipsychotic, was synthesized more than 40 years ago. Early trials performed in Germany during the late 1960s and early 1970s provided evidence that it was effective in the treatment of schizophrenia, but this was regarded with skepticism since it violated the time honored observation that antipsychotic efficacy was inextricable from extrapyramidal side effects (EPS) (6). Clozapine was released in Europe in 1972, but was withdrawn 2 years later after eight patients taking clozapine died from complications of agranulocytosis. It was not until clozapine was shown to be effective in patients with schizophrenia who had failed previous trials of conventional antipsychotic medications and that the reversibility of agranulocytosis was established that it was approved by the FDA and released in the United States in 1990. The development and release of all subsequent atypical agents have been, to a large extent, attempts to replicate the success of clozapine as an antipsychotic with better efficacy than the conventional agents and negligible EPS, but without the risk of agranulocytosis.

The landmark clinical trial that led to the release of clozapine in the United States was a multicenter study involving patients with schizophrenia who had severe psychosis despite at least three previous adequate trials of conventional antipsychotic medications (7). The study included 268 patients randomized to either treatment with clozapine or chlorpromazine (plus benztropine) for 6 weeks. On the basis of an *a priori* definition of treatment response (20% improvement total BPRS score), 30% of patients treated with clozapine improved compared to only 4% of those treated with chlorpromazine. While this degree of improvement (30% of patients improving by 20%) may seem modest, it needs to be considered in the context that the patients included in the study were highly symptomatic and had never benefited from any previous antipsychotic treatment. In addition, clozapine demonstrated efficacy for a broad range of psychopathology including positive and negative symptoms, anxiety, and depression without causing EPS. This breadth of improvement suggested that clozapine was not only more effective than conventional antipsychotics, but qualitatively different. A recent meta-analysis of 30 randomized and mostly double-blind trials, involving patients with both refractory and non-refractory schizophrenia, confirmed that clozapine is convincingly more effective than conventional antipsychotic medications in the acute treatment of schizophrenia (8). Expert consensus also supports the notion that clozapine can be more effective than conventional antipsychotic therapy and is currently the most effective antipsychotic medication available for treatment-refractory schizophrenia (9).

In addition to providing information regarding efficacy, clinical trials have also yielded important information about how to optimally prescribe clozapine. For example, the therapeutic dose range for clozapine is between 200 mg and 800 mg per day. The mean daily dose of clozapine in European studies is lower than in the United States, for reasons that are not altogether clear (10). Owing to its considerable sedative and hypotensive effects, clozapine should be initiated at 25 mg per day in divided doses and increased by 25 or 50 mg increments every 2 days as tolerated to the target dose. The length of time required for titration to a therapeutic dose means that an adequate trial of clozapine will likely require more than 6 weeks of treatment. There is also evidence that plasma levels may be of use in judging whether a patient has had an adequate trial of clozapine. Trough plasma levels of clozapine above a threshold of 350 ng/ml have been shown to be predictive of treatment response (11,12). This suggests that if trough levels do not exceed this threshold, further dose increases are likely to be of benefit. Conversely, dose increases once this threshold has been attained may not be helpful. Plasma levels are however notoriously inconsistent and it is probably best to use an average level based on several tests on different days at a steady state dose.

B. Risperidone

Risperidone was first introduced in the United States in 1994 or about 4 years after the approval of clozapine. The agranulocytosis associated with clozapine and the required blood monitoring limited its use in clinical practice and put clozapine in a class by itself. As such, risperidone was the first of a new class of "first line" atypical antipsychotic medications sharing the more favorable EPS profile of clozapine without its myelotoxicity.

The efficacy of risperidone has been established in a number of important clinical trials. The pivotal studies were both 8 week comparisons of four different fixed doses of risperidone (2, 6, 12, and 16 mg) to haloperidol 20 mg per day and placebo (13,14). Improvements were measured using the PANSS. The results of these two studies, carried out in Canada and the U.S. and including acutely ill patients with schizophrenia, were strikingly similar. In the larger US trial (14), risperidone at doses above 2 mg and haloperidol 20 mg were consistently more effective (as measured by mean improvement in total PANSS and its positive symptom subscale) than placebo. The most effective dose of risperidone was 6 mg per day – at this dose, risperidone was significantly more effective than haloperidol and the rate of EPS was comparable to placebo. The Canadian study (13) also concluded that 6 mg was the optimal dose of risperidone based on improvements in positive and negative symptoms and a low incidence of EPS. Unlike the U.S. study, risperidone at 2 mg per day was found to be more effective than placebo for overall PANSS improvement.

The largest clinical trial involving risperidone was an 8-week multinational study involving 1362 subjects randomized to five different daily doses of risperidone (1, 4, 8, 12, and 16 mg) or haloperidol 10 mg per day (15). Consistent with the North American trials, 4 and 8 mg per day were found to be the optimal doses of risperidone based on efficacy and side effects. Interestingly, while risperidone 1 mg was found to be less effective than higher doses of risperidone for improvements in total PANSS score, this dose was as effective as haloperidol 10 mg. In addition, more than 50% of subjects treated with 1 mg met criteria for treatment response (20% reduction in PANSS score). This suggests, along with the Canadian data, that doses of risperidone as low as 1–2 mg may be effective for some patients. The choice of only 10 mg of haloperidol as a comparison dose in this study is important given criticisms that 20 mg of haloperidol may have been too high (thereby biasing the results against haloperidol due to EPS) in the North American studies. However, risperidone was still found to have a lower incidence of EPS compared to this lower dose of haloperidol 10 mg per day.

These clinical trials suggest an optimal therapeutic dose of risperidone of 4 to 6 mg per day. The package insert for risperidone, on the other hand, recommends increasing to 6 mg per day by the third day of treatment. There is now an emerging consensus that this may be too aggressive – the average dose of risperidone for the treatment of schizophrenia in both Europe and the United States is now about 4 mg per day. Some patients will require higher doses, but this dose represents a reasonable target for the initial titration of risperidone during the first six weeks of acute treatment.

C. Olanzapine

Olanzapine was introduced in the United States, Canada, and most of Europe in 1996. Its chemical structure is remarkably similar to clozapine, yet it has a significantly improved side effect profile with regard to subjective tolerability and myelotoxicity. It is also much easier to initiate, being one of the only available atypical antipsychotics (along with aripiprazole) for which dosing recommendations suggest starting at a single effective daily dose of 10 mg.

The pivotal study of olanzapine was an international multicenter trial involving 1996 subjects with schizophrenia, schizoaffective disorder, and schizophreniform disorder (16). Olanzapine and haloperidol were dosed flexibly between 5 and 20 mg per day over 6 weeks – the mean doses at endpoint were 13.2 mg for olanzapine and 11.8 mg for haloperidol. The results of this study showed that olanzapine was significantly better than haloperidol at improving total PANSS scores, PANSS negative symptom subscale scores, and depressive symptoms. An earlier study comparing three dose ranges of olanzapine (2.5–7.5, 7.5–12.5, and 12.5–17.5 mg per day), to haloperidol (10–20 mg per day) or placebo showed that the medium and high dose ranges of olanzapine were most effective (17). The high dose range was superior to both placebo and haloperidol for negative symptom improvement. This study therefore indicates that the higher daily dose range of 12.5 to 17.5 mg is probably the most appropriate for treating acute psychosis in schizophrenia. This is consistent with clinical experience in the United State, where the average daily dose of olanzapine for acute schizophrenia is in the range of 15 to 20 mg.

D. Quetiapine

Quetiapine distinguishes itself from risperidone and olanzapine by having a lower affinity for dopamine D_2 receptors and a short half-life of about 7 hours. A number of studies have demonstrated that quetiapine is an effective antipsychotic medication. One such study compared a low dose of quetiapine (no more than 250 mg per day) and a higher dose (no more than 750 mg per day) to placebo for 6 weeks (18). The efficacy of the higher dose range was significantly greater than either the lower dose or placebo, based on BPRS ratings as well as measures of negative symptom improvement. However, the mean doses in the high and low groups were not actually that different and were both in the medium range of recommended dosing for quetiapine (360 mg per day and 209 mg per day respectively). Another 6-week trial compared five different daily doses of quetiapine (75, 150, 300, 600, and 750 mg) to haloperidol 12 mg per day and placebo (19). This study showed that quetiapine was significantly more effective than placebo at doses of 150 mg and above. Subsequent clinical experience, on the other hand, suggests that higher daily doses of quetiapine in the 400 to 800 mg range are often most effective.

While the short half-life of quetiapine implies that it should be taken in divided doses as frequently as three times a day, this does not seem to be necessary (20). Although D_2 occupancy is minimal (0–27%) 12 hours after the last dose of quetiapine during fixed dose treatment, the transient 58–64% occupancy of D_2 receptors that occurs up to 3 hours after a single dose of quetiapine appears to be sufficient for an antipsychotic effect (21). Such findings have given rise to the notion that this "fast dissociation" from D_2 receptors is what confers "atypicality" to atypical antipsychotic medications and results in their low liability for EPS (22).

E. Ziprasidone

Ziprasidone, released in 2001, is one of the newest of the available antipsychotic medications. It has some unique receptor affinities compared to other antipsychotic medications, including a higher ratio of affinity to 5-HT_{2A} to D_2 receptors than any of the other atypical agents, 5-HT_{1A} agonism, and serotonin and norepinephrine reuptake inhibition (23). These additional receptor affinities raise the possibility that ziprasidone could be particularly effective at reducing anxious or depressive symptoms as are medications such as buspirone (a 5-HT_{1A} agonist) and venlafaxine (a serotonin and norepinephrine reuptake inhibitor), though this has not yet been clearly demonstrated in clinical trials.

Clinical trials with ziprasidone have established its efficacy and optimal dosing in the treatment of schizophrenia. A preliminary dose finding study of only 4 weeks duration compared several doses of ziprasidone (4, 10, 40, and 160 mg per day) to haloperidol 15 mg per day. Ziprasidone 160 mg per day was found to be as effective as haloperidol, with a decreased rate of EPS (24). Ziprasidone at 40 mg or lower did not appear as effective at reducing psychopathology measures. Another 4 week study compared ziprasidone 40 mg and 120 mg per day to placebo and found that 120 mg was superior to placebo for BPRS improvement as well depressive symptom improvement (25). The 40 mg daily dose failed to distinguish itself from placebo treatment. A third, larger, 6-week multicenter study compared ziprasidone 80 mg and 160 mg per day to placebo (26). This trial found that both of these doses were superior to placebo. Taken together, these studies indicate an effective dose range for ziprasidone between 80 and 160 mg per day. Because the half-life of ziprasidone is less than 7 hours, current recommendations are for twice a day divided dosing.

F. Aripiprazole

Aripiprazole was approved by the FDA in November 2002. Although it shares many of the receptor affinities of the other atypical antipsychotic medications, its activity at the dopamine D_2 receptor is unique among antipsychotic drugs. At this receptor, it acts as a partial agonist/antagonist, which in theory would tend to normalize either hyper- or hypo-dopaminergic transmission. This could result in the ability to impact both positive and negative symptoms, without causing substantial EPS. The first published study on the efficacy of aripiprazole in schizophrenia was a 4-week study comparing two doses (15 and 30 mg per day) of aripiprazole to haloperidol and placebo (27). Both doses of aripiprazole were found to be superior to placebo and as effective as haloperidol 10 mg per day as measured by mean improvement in PANSS scores. A recent review of shortterm phase II and III studies reported on the side effect profile and safety of aripiprazole (28). It found that aripiprazole was comparable to placebo with a very low rate of EPS, minimal weight gain, little sedation, and trivial effects on lipids or glucose.

IV. EFFICACY OF ATYPICAL ANTIPSYCHOTIC MEDICATIONS: META-ANALYSES

The clinical trials described above include comparisons of the various atypical antipsychotic drugs to either haloperidol or placebo. In the case of a placebo controlled study, the intent is to assess for superiority for the atypical drug, whereas with a haloperidol controlled trial, the intent is to assess for either superiority or equivalency, since haloperidol is a medication with established efficacy in schizophrenia. While it is widely believed that the atypical antipsychotics are more effective than their conventional anti-psychotic counterparts, the studies reviewed here suggest that this has only been shown for clozapine, risperidone and olanzapine. However, the studies concluding an advantage for risperidone and olanzapine involved a control dose of haloperidol 20 mg per day, whereas the trials with quetiapine, aripiprazole and ziprasidone used 10–15 mg haloperidol doses. The optimal comparison dose of haloperidol has not been established however. Because one of the clearest advantages of the atypical antipsychotics compared to conventional agents is their decreased rate of EPS, it has been argued that haloperidol 20 mg is too high a dose to use as a comparator, since this could bias the results in favor of the atypical drug. This is potentially true not only with respect to EPS, but for psychopathology measures as well. For example, EPS could result in higher ratings of depressive and negative symptoms due to bradykinesia or anxiety and tension due to akathisia.

A series of recent meta-analyses have examined the consistency and degree of atypical antipsychotic superiority compared to placebo or conventional drugs. The meta-analysis of nine placebo controlled studies involving risperidone, olanzapine, and quetiapine found that the placebo response rates, based on different *a priori* definitions of response, varied from 8% to 58% with an average rate across studies of 35% (29). The response rate for different therapeutic doses of the atypical antipsychotics ranged from 24% to 100% with an average response rate of 57%. Superiority of the atypical agents over placebo was established in 67% of studies when defined response outcomes were compared, whereas 87% of studies showed superiority for the atypicals when mean symptomatic improvement outcomes (as measured by changes in a standardized rating scale) were compared. These findings indicate that treatment with atypical antipsychotic medications is consistently more effective than with placebo, although the placebo response rate is not trivial in acute trials involving schizophrenia.

Two recent meta-analyses have examined whether, and to what degree, the atypical antipsychotic medications are superior to conventional antipsychotics. The first examined 19 trials comparing risperidone, olanzapine, or quetiapine to haloperidol (30). It found that these atypical antipsychotic medications as well as haloperidol were consistently superior to placebo treatment as noted above. It also confirmed that both risperidone and olanzapine were significantly more effective than treatment with haloperidol. However, the effect size or magnitude of this difference was small and only statistically significant because the studies had very large sample sizes. On the other hand, the magnitude of difference with regard to producing EPS (as measured by the use of anti-parkinson medications) was large and favored the atypical agents. The second meta-analysis was more elaborate, examining 52 trials (five of which were long term studies) involving a variety of first and atypical antipsychotic medications including clozapine, risperidone, olanzapine, and quetiapine (31). It reported that patients were more likely to have greater symptomatic improvement with clozapine, risperidone, and olanzapine compared to conventional antipsychotic medications, though again the effect size was modest. Importantly, the study also found that when lower doses of conventional antipsychotic medications (e.g., haloperidol 12 mg per day or less) were used for comparison, there were no significant differences between conventional and atypical agents with regard to efficacy or study dropout, though a small advantage for the atypical antipsychotics remained with respect to EPS. This study, which was carried out in the United Kingdom, therefore argued that when cost is taken into account, conventional antipsychotic medications should still be used as first line therapy.

From these meta-analyses, it can be concluded that while the atypical antipsychotic medications are at least as effective or slightly more effective than haloperidol, their major advantage lies within their reduced liability for EPS. This is consistent with recently published expert consensus conclusions that while superior efficacy of the atypical antipsychotic medications has not been firmly established, their clearest advantage relative to first-generation drugs lies within their superior safety profile (9). This distinction should not be discounted because EPS can cause substantial discomfort, stigmatization, functional impairment, and treatment nonadherence for patients. From this perspective, the atypical antipsychotic medications are preferable to their conventional counterparts.

V. EFFICACY OF ATYPICAL ANTIPSYCHOTICS: HEAD TO HEAD TRIALS

Since most comparative trials involving the atypical antipsychotic medications involve a fairly standard study design – 4 to 8 weeks of double-blind comparison to a standard treatment (usually haloperidol) or placebo, it is possible, to some extent, to compare the efficacy and safety of new medications from one study to another. However, a more accurate way of examining the differential efficacy of the atypical antipsychotic drugs is to specifically compare two or more drugs in a "head to head" trial. Such studies are not required for a drug to be released and are therefore typically reserved for post-marketing phase IV studies. Since many of the atypical antipsychotic medications have only recently been released, head to head comparisons are at this time limited in number.

One of the first double-blind head to head studies involving atypical antipsychotic drugs compared clozapine 400 mg per day to risperidone 4 mg or 8 mg per day in hospitalized patients over 4 weeks (32). Using BPRS improvement as the major outcome measure, both doses of risperidone were found to be as effective as clozapine, although risperidone was better tolerated. This German study is interesting in that it provides information about the efficacy of clozapine in non-refractory schizophrenia (in the United States, clozapine is only approved for treatment of refractory schizophrenia).

Another double-blind study by Conley et al. (33) was an 8-week multicenter comparison of 377 patients randomized to treatment with risperidone 2 to 6 mg (mean modal dose 4.8 mg per day at endpoint) to olanzapine 5 to 20 mg (mean modal dose 12.4 mg per day at endpoint). On most measures, including treatment response as defined by a 20% or 30% reduction in PANSS score, risperidone and olanzapine were found to be equally effective. A significant difference did emerge however when 40% PANSS improvement was examined, as well as when looking at change in PANSS score for subjects in the completers analysis, with an advantage for risperidone. In addition, significantly greater weight gain was noted with olanzapine treatment. While a discussion of long-term studies is reserved for the next chapter, a similar, but longer-term study warrants side by side comparison. This double-blind trial by Tran et al. (34) was a 28-week study involving risperidone 4 to 12 mg (mean modal dose 7.2 mg per day at endpoint) and olanzapine 10 to 20 mg (mean modal dose 17.2 mg per day at endpoint). In contrast to the Conley et al. study, it found several advantages for olanzapine over risperidone, with respect to both efficacy and solicited side effects. Overall, both studies suggest that risperidone and olanzapine were effective treatments and dosing differences probably accounted for their disparate conclusions. For example, in the Tran et al. study, risperidone was rapidly titrated to 6 mg with a mean modal dose of 7.2 mg per day (34). As noted previously, while such dosing is consistent with the package insert instructions, this dose of risperidone exceeds what is now thought to be the optimal acute dose range of 4 to 6 mg. The higher dose may have therefore contributed to the increased rate of EPS and lesser degree of negative symptom improvement found in the study. Likewise, in the Conley et al. study, the mean dose of olanzapine 12.4 mg could be considered on the low side of efficacy compared to risperidone 4.8 mg (33). Another important consideration is the distinction between statistical versus clinical significance. Although statistically significant, the advantages for olanzapine with respect to negative symptoms (1.4 SANS points) in the Tran et al. study and for risperidone for positive symptoms (0.8 PANSS points) in the Conley et al. study were very small, with limited clinical relevance (33,34). Finally, it should be noted that both of these studies were funded by pharmaceutical companies – Conley et al. was funded by Janssen (makers of risperidone) while Tran et al. was funded by Eli Lilly (makers of olanzapine) – and therefore subject to potential biases of both study design and interpretation of the results.

An additional head to head trial comparing olanzapine to ziprasidone has been presented but has not yet been published (35). This 6-week study found that olanzapine (mean dose 11 mg per day) and ziprasidone (mean dose 130 mg per day) were equally effective in terms of mean BPRS improvement and responder rates.

On the basis of these limited data from head to head comparisons of atypical antipsychotic medications, there do not yet appear to be large between-drug differences when one looks at overall treatment response or improvements in positive and negative symptoms across groups of patients. It is however possible that an individual patient might do better in terms of efficacy on one medication than another. Additional studies will be needed in order to clarify whether certain patients might respond preferably to a particular antipsychotic medication or whether there are predictors of individual drug response. In addition, there may be some subtle differences between antipsychotics in terms of negative or cognitive symptom improvement that could be clinically important.

VI. SPECTRUM OF EFFICACY

Research in schizophrenia now supports the notion of distinct spheres of impairment in schizophrenia – positive or psychotic symptoms, negative symptoms, and cognitive symptoms (36,37). Antipsychotic drugs are most effective in treating the positive symptom dimension of schizophrenia. This is especially true of the conventional agents since rigidity or bradykinesia from extrapyramidal side effects can worsen negative symptoms and the adjunctive anticholinergic medications that are necessary to treat these same side effects can impair cognition. Historically, clinicians were therefore usually satisfied when an antipsychotic medication reduced psychotic symptoms. These expectations have changed since the release of clozapine and the other atypical antipsychotic medications, which seem to have an impact on negative and cognitive symptoms in addition to positive symptoms. This impact is believed to be highly significant from a clinical standpoint, given that negative and cognitive symptoms are, more so than positive symptoms, associated with substantial impairments in social and vocational functioning for patients with schizophrenia (38,39).

A. Negative Symptoms

The term "negative symptom" was originally coined to describe the loss of normal neurological function and was added to the diagnostic criteria for schizophrenia in 1994 with the publication of the fourth edition of the *Diagnostic and Statistical Manual for Mental Disorders* (DSM-IV) (40). In schizophrenia, negative symptoms include impoverishment of thinking and speech (alogia), flattening of affect, loss of motivation and energy (avolition and apathy), and diminished interest in recreational and social activities (anhedonia and asociality) (41). Therefore, despite adequate positive symptom control, persistent negative symptoms can leave the patient with schizophrenia in a state of inactivity and social isolation.

The distinction between primary and secondary negative symptoms is vital with regard to intervention. Secondary negative symptoms are those that may be due to some other condition, such as EPS, depression, positive symptoms, medical illness, or environmental factors. EPS due to conventional antipsychotic therapy are a common cause of secondary negative symptoms particularly when patients are experiencing akinesia, a side effect that can be manifest in decreased speech, decreased motivation, and decreased spontaneous gestures. Comorbid depression, medical illnesses such as hypothyroidism or anemia, or the effects of various drugs such as beta-blockers, benzodiazepines, alcohol, or marijuana can also resemble negative symptomatology. Patients may also develop negative symptoms due to functionally impairing positive symptoms – a common example is the patient who is isolative or uncommunicative due to paranoia. Finally, negative symptoms might be the result of life in an unstimulating institutional setting with low expectations and a low threshold of tolerance for psychotic behavior. The management of secondary negative symptoms involves treatment of the underlying cause. For example, EPS should be managed with a reduction in antipsychotic dose, with adjunctive anti-parkinson medications, or a change to another antipsychotic medication with a decreased risk of EPS. Depression, medical illness, and substance abuse should be identified and treated accordingly. Environmental causes are best addressed through a change in setting, social skills training, and other forms of rehabilitation such as a day treatment program.

In contrast to secondary negative symptoms, primary negative symptoms in schizophrenia are those attributable to the core disease process, and are therefore a diagnosis of exclusion (42). The concept of the "deficit state" was developed to characterize a subtype of schizophrenia characterized by enduring primary negative symptoms and a distinct pathophysiology, course, and treatment response (43). Diagnosis of the deficit state is based on the longitudinal assessment of enduring primary negative symptoms that are present both during and between episodes of positive symptom exacerbation. The Schedule for the Deficit Syndrome (SDS) was developed as a standardized diagnostic tool for the deficit state (44).

While conventional antipsychotic medications do seem to have some impact on negative symptoms (45), clinical experience suggests that the atypical antipsychotic agents may improve negative symptoms to a greater degree. A number of clinical studies have been performed in order to determine whether, or to what extent, this is true. In the landmark study of clozapine in treatment-resistant schizophrenia, clozapine was found to be more effective at reducing negative symptoms than chlorpromazine, which was ineffective (7). Negative symptom improvement was measured using items extracted from the BPRS, but no attempt was made to differentiate between primary or secondary negative symptoms. Patients treated with clozapine did however experience significantly greater positive symptom improvement and fewer EPS than chlorpromazine treated patients. There-fore it could be argued that clozapine's advantage was due to its impact on secondary negative symptoms due to positive symptoms and EPS rather than primary negative symptoms. In support of this argument, a 10-week double-blind comparison of clozapine to haloperidol showed that improve-ment in negative symptoms was significantly greater with clozapine treatment, but that neither clozapine nor haloperidol improved negative symptoms in patients with the deficit syndrome as diagnosed by the SDS (46). In the case of risperidone, the U.S. study found that while risperidone 6 mg and 16 mg per day were more effective than placebo in reducing negative symptoms, no dose was significantly more effective than haloperidol (14). The Canadian study revealed a negative symptom advantage for risperidone over placebo (but not haloperidol) only at 6 mg per day (13). More recently, the U.S. and Canadian data were combined and reanalyzed using factor analysis to examine the impact of risperidone on five symptomatic dimensions including negative symptoms (47). This study concluded that a significant and sizeable advantage for risperidone over haloperidol did emerge for negative symptom improvement. Furthermore, this differential efficacy was found to be unrelated to EPS. On the other hand, another multicenter study pitting several different doses of risperidone against a lower dose of haloperidol 10 mg per day (a dose that would be expected to cause fewer secondary negative symptoms due to EPS) found no advantage with risperidone for negative symptoms (15). With olanzapine, the pivotal trial found a significant benefit with olanzapine compared to haloperidol for negative symptom improvement (16). However, this overpowered study allowed the detection of small differences (in this case a 1.3 point difference on the PANSS negative symptom subscale) that while statistically significant, are of questionable clinical pertinence. Also, a subsequent open-label trial examining the effect of olanzapine on patients with the deficit syndrome found no benefit (48).

In summary, there is evidence that the atypical antipsychotic medications (clozapine, risperidone, and olanzapine) are indeed more effective than conventional antipsychotic medications at treating negative symptoms. Antipsychotic pharmacotherapy does not seem to improve primary negative symptoms associated with the deficit syndrome however, suggesting that the differential efficacy in favor of atypical antipsychotics is largely related to their impact on secondary negative symptoms due to EPS and depressive symptoms. Even if this is the case, this represents a considerable benefit of the atypical antipsychotic medications over conventional antipsychotics in the overall symptomatic control of schizophrenia. Further research is needed to specifically address and clarify the potential benefits of all of the atypical agents, as well as adjunctive therapies, on both primary and secondary negative symptoms.

B. Cognitive Symptoms

Cognitive impairments in schizophrenia were recognized as far back as the late 1800s when the illness was described as "dementia praecox". As with negative symptoms, they have received renewed attention due to the apparent newfound ability to remediate them pharmacologically. Neuro-cognitive deficits in schizophrenia affect memory, attention, and executive functioning, but are not always obvious on routine examination and typically require neuropsychological testing to detect and quantify. However, as noted in a review by Green (39), such impairments are highly relevant since they have been found to have a substantial negative impact on functional outcome, particularly in the areas of social problem solving, social skill acquisition, and social and occupational functioning. The specific domains of neurocognition found to be most consistently related to functional outcome in schizophrenia include verbal working memory, secondary verbal memory, executive functioning, and vigilance (49). These domains are important for basic tasks such as recalling written information (secondary memory), memorizing a telephone number (verbal working memory), planning and adapting to change (executive function), and sustaining attention (vigilance). Impairments in these domains can interfere with normal functioning in educational, vocational, or social settings.

The conventional antipsychotic medications generally have little impact on neurocognition or acutely worsen certain cognitive measures (50). These effects may be due to the sedative and anticholinergic properties of the low potency conventional antipsychotics, to EPS, or to the use of adjunctive anticholingeric medications. In any case, while many of the studies examining the effects of antipsychotic therapy on neurocognition suffer from methodological problems, there is now evidence that the atypical antipsychotic medications may be able to improve neurocognitive deficits to a greater degree than was possible in the conventional antipsychotic era (51). For example, risperidone has been found to be associated with greater improvements in secondary memory and verbal working memory compared to haloperidol (49,52). Olanzapine has been associated with improvements in verbal learning and memory and verbal fluency, while clozapine studies have demonstrated a favorable impact on verbal fluency and attention (53).

The available data support the consensus opinion that the atypical antipsychotic medications are more effective than conventional antipsychotics at improving cognitive deficits in schizophrenia. This advantage appears to be independent of any effect on positive symptoms, though the effect of EPS or anticholinergic medications remains controversial. In addition, it appears that different atypical agents have a differential impact on specific neurocognitive impairments. Cognitive improvements in schizophrenia may continue beyond the usual time frame of acute trials. Longer-term studies have recently been published that add to the characterization of differences between cognitive improvements in patients treated with atypical antipsychotic medications (54,55).

VII. TREATMENT-REFRACTORY SCHIZOPHRENIA

Treatment-refractory or treatment-resistant schizophrenia are terms used to describe patients who have not responded to previous antipsychotic therapy. Approximately 20 to 30% of patients with schizophrenia do not improve significantly despite an adequate trial of an antipsychotic medication (56). When approaching the patient with treatment-resistant schizophrenia, it is first important to determine whether the patient has improved at all. Improvements sometimes occur gradually and are only apparent after the antipsychotic medication is withdrawn and the patient worsens. Partial responders may need several weeks or even months of treatment in order to achieve a full response and switching to another antipsychotic should therefore be considered only after an adequate trial of an antipsychotic medication has failed to produce any detectable improvement.

Sometimes symptoms do not improve with antipsychotic therapy because of underlying factors that will continue to be problematic despite switching to another medication. Therefore, when a patient has not responded despite an adequate trial, several considerations should be made before changing medications. First, it is important to ensure that the patient is actually taking the medication. Treatment nonadherence is common in schizophrenia and can have various causes including lack of insight, delusional beliefs, intolerance of side effects, and cognitive impairments. These factors must be addressed accordingly through education, skills training, dosing adjustments or adjunctive medications, and fostering of the therapeutic alliance which is itself a powerful predictor of adherence (57). Oftentimes the clinician is inclined to consider a long-acting depot medication for nonadherent patients, but this option does not guarantee treatment adherence since patients must still show up for injection appointments and consent to treatment. Other important considerations for nonresponsive patients relate to diagnosis – first, whether the patient actually has schizophrenia or another psychotic disorder and second, whether there are other comorbid conditions such as medical illness, substance abuse, mood disorders, or environmental factors that are exacerbating the psychosis. The patient who does not actually have psychotic symptoms is best treated without antipsychotic therapy, while those with comorbidities might require specific treatments in addition to antipsychotic therapy.

Treatment options for patients who have not responded to previous antipsychotic trials are by definition limited. Prior to the release of the atypical antipsychotic medications, standard treatment strategies for refractory patients included changing to another antipsychotic drug from a different chemical class (e.g., from a phenothiazine to a butyrophenone or vice versa) or increasing the antipsychotic dose beyond the usual therapeutic range. Both of these strategies have been subsequently found to be ineffective (58). As noted previously, the first atypical antipsychotic clozapine was released despite problems with agranulocytosis because of its demonstrated ability to help patients with refractory schizophrenia – patients who had previously not responded despite years of antipsychotic therapy. With the release of each subsequent atypical agent comes the possibility that it might also be effective for refractory patients.

Several studies have now addressed the question of whether patients who have not responded to previous antipsychotic trials will respond to atypical antipsychotic medications. These studies usually take one of two forms – comparison of an atypical agent to clozapine, where the goal is to establish equivalency or noninferiority, or comparison to a conventional antipsychotic medication where the goal is to assess superiority. Only patients with treatment-refractory schizophrenia are included in these studies, though the definition of treatment refractory can vary from trial to trial. The landmark study involving clozapine used stringent criteria to define treatment resistance, including nonresponse to three previous adequate trials of conventional antipsychotic medications from different chemical classes (7). In addition, patients had to have had no period of good functioning over the previous 5 years and severe baseline levels of psychopathology based on the BPRS and another rating scale. Finally, all patients who improved during a prospective 6-week trial of haloperidol were subsequently excluded from the study. On the basis on of these stringent criteria for treatment resistance, 30% of these patients were found to be responders compared to only 4% for patients treated with chlorpromazine. The low rate of response to chlorpromazine was expected since the study sample included patients refractory to conventional antipsychotic therapy.

The results of subsequent studies involving the other atypical antipsychotic medications have varied along with different criteria to define treatment resistance. For example, two studies have used loosely defined criteria for treatment resistance and included patients who were either nonresponders or were intolerant of previous antipsychotic trials. One found equivalent rates of response for clozapine (65%) and risperidone (67%) while another found that the response rate for olanzapine (47%) was significantly better than with haloperidol (35%) (59,60). These relatively high response rates indicate that the patients were less refractory than those in the original Kane et al. study (7). In contrast, another study including only nonresponders (as opposed to patients with drug intolerance) and stringent criteria for treatment resistance found equivalently low rates of response with either olanzapine (7%) and chlorpromazine (0%) (61). Likewise, a comparison of risperidone to haloperidol using stringent criteria for treatment resistance showed an advantage for risperidone after 4 weeks, but not at 8-week endpoint (62). These findings indicate that risperidone and olanzapine may be effective for some patients who have only responded partially to conventional antipsychotic medications. Quetiapine has also been shown to be more effective than haloperidol in partial responders (63). On the other hand, the atypical antipsychotic medications seem to be less effective for the most severely ill treatment-refractory patients in which only clozapine has established efficacy and superiority over conventional antipsychotic agents.

It should be noted that the design of stringent treatment-refractory studies comparing an atypical to a conventional agent are biased against the conventional drug since patients are defined as refractory based on previous conventional drug nonresponse. Also, the information provided by these studies regarding the likelihood of treatment response to an atypical antipsychotic after conventional antipsychotic failure is of limited clinical pertinence since most patients in the United States are now primarily treated with atypical agents. Therefore, what the clinician now needs to know is whether patients will respond to one atypical antipsychotic medication after failure of another atypical drug. Unfortunately, few data are available to address this question. In a single open-label study, Conley et al. found that 41% of treatment-refractory patients who had previously had a poor response to olanzapine did respond to clozapine (64). This is again consistent with the idea that clozapine remains the most unambiguously effective atypical antipsychotic medication for patients with refractory schizophrenia.

On the basis of these results, when a patient has not responded to two or more antipsychotic medication trials, a trial of clozapine should be strongly considered. Current expert consensus suggests that a trial of one atypical antipsychotic medication following conventional antipsychotic failure is reasonable prior to clozapine, but that the likelihood of success with further trials remains unclear (9). Owing to concerns about clozapine's potential toxicities and the difficulties associated with its use (i.e., blood draws, frequency of visits), clinicians may be inclined to continue successive trials of atypical antipsychotic drugs before resorting to clozapine. This strategy must be weighed against the potential costs (in terms of prolonged suffering and actual economic cost) of delaying a clozapine treatment in favor of trials of potentially less effective medications.

Some patients will prove to be refractory despite previous adequate trials of conventional antipsychotic medications as well as all of the available atypical medications including clozapine. There are currently no empiric data to guide the treatment of this group of refractory patients. Strategies that are becoming increasingly common in clinical practice for refractory schizophrenia include combination antipsychotic treatment and high dose atypical antipsychotic therapy. The most rational approach to combination antipsychotic treatment involves using two medications with the most disparate modes of action such as clozapine along with a low dose of a high potency conventional agent. There is some evidence to support the use of high potency conventional drugs and risperidone for clozapine augmentation (65). High dose atypical antipsychotic therapy is also gaining popularity, and a wealth of anecdotal and some controlled evidence is accumulating regarding the potential benefits of olanzapine (up to 40 mg per day or more) and quetiapine (beyond 800 mg per day) in treatment-refractory patients (66). These strategies should be thought of as desperation measures to be reserved for patients who have thoroughly failed mono-therapy with all of the atypical agents including clozapine and at least one conventional agent.

VIII. SIDE EFFECTS

A. Extrapyramidal Side Effects

All of the antipsychotic drugs, both first and atypical, act on many of the same receptors and therefore share many of the same potential side effects. For example, since they all antagonize alpha-1, histamine-1, and muscarinic-1 receptors, each has the propensity to cause orthostasis and reflex tachycardia, sedation, and anticholinergic symptoms such as tachycardia and constipation. However, each drug has varying affinities at these receptors, such that each causes these and other side effects to varying degrees. Patients can acclimatize to some of these side effects, so that education, careful monitoring, and gradual dose titration will usually minimize difficulties arising from them.

As noted throughout this chapter, the greatest difference between the conventional and atypical drug side effects is the decreased risk of EPS with the atypical antipsychotic medications. EPS include a spectrum of different conditions, including akathisia (the subjective feeling and objective manifestation of motoric restlessness), dystonia (the sustained and often painful muscular contraction), drug-induced parkinsonism (rigidity, tremor, bradykinesia), and tardive dyskinesia (TD; involuntary choreiform movements usually arising from chronic antipsychotic exposure). Among the atypical antipsychotic medications, the greatest risk of encountering the neuroleptic threshold (the dose at which EPS occur) at therapeutic doses is with risperidone. The risk of EPS with risperidone is dose related and typically occurs once a daily dose of 8 to 10 mg has been achieved. When EPS occurs with risperidone therapy, this is generally a clue to the clinician that the ideal dose has been surpassed and that addition efficacy is unlikely to be attained with further dose increases. Instead, a trial of dose reduction, rather than use of adjunctive anticholinergic medications, should be instituted. Acute EPS are relatively infrequent with the other atypical antipsychotic medications with routine dosing. Akathisia seems to be the most likely form of EPS to emerge with atypical antipsychotic therapy and is best treated with a reduction in antipsychotic dose or a trial of propranolol.

Because the risk of tardive dyskinesia increases with cumulative antipsychotic exposure, the long-term rate of tardive dyskinesia with the atypical antipsychotic medications in unclear. Based on the observation that acute EPS are a risk factor for TD, it is expected that the atypical antipsychotic medications will cause much less TD than the conventional agents, even in the long run. Studies involving risperidone and olanzapine have supported a much lower yearly incidence of TD than with conventional antipsychotic medications (67,68). In addition, patients switched from conventional agents to atypical agents often experience a reduction in TD – therefore, if a patient on conventional antipsychotic therapy has moderate to severe TD, a trial of an atypical antipsychotic medication is warranted.

B. Weight Gain and Metabolic Effects

Atypical antipsychotic induced obesity and its associated metabolic effects are currently an area of intense interest and investigation. Because of the association between many of the atypical antipsychotic medications and clinically pertinent weight gain, this side effect is being called the "EPS of the new millennium." Increases in weight are associated with a heightened risk of coronary artery disease and hypertension and therefore increased morbidity and mortality due to cardiac disease. In addition, weight gain can lead to problems such as low self-esteem, osteoarthritis, and obstructive sleep apnea, all of which have been reported with novel antipsychotic drug treatment. Even in acute studies, the atypical antipsychotic medications have been associated with substantial weight gain. Allison et al. performed an extensive meta-analysis in order to estimate the weight gain associated with various antipsychotic medications at 10 weeks (69). They found that clozapine (9.8 lbs) and olanzapine (9.1 lbs) were associated with the most weight gain, with risperidone (4.6 lbs) causing half as much weight gain, and ziprasidone (0.1 lbs) being relatively weight neutral. Wirshing et al. found a similar pattern of liability from a retrospective analysis of longer-term studies, with maximum adjusted weight gain as follows: clozapine (15.2 lbs), olanzapine (15.0 lbs), and risperidone (5.0 lbs) (70). Early experience with quetiapine suggests a similar liability to risperidone, while aripiprazole seems to be more weight neutral like ziprasidone.

In addition to weight gain, reports of diabetes associated with antipsychotic therapy are becoming increasingly frequent. Weight gain and in particular the development of abdominal or omental adiposity are known risk factors for the development of diabetes. Accordingly, the number of reports of new onset diabetes associated with the atypical antipsychotic medications has been proportional to the weight gain liability of each drug. Clozapine and olanzapine have been associated with the most reports of diabetes, with a few reports involving quetiapine and risperidone as well (71). There have not yet been any reports of diabetes associated with ziprasidone or aripiprazole. Although weight gain and obesity are believed to underlie most cases of antipsychotic induced diabetes, some cases of new onset diabetes have occurred in patients taking antipsychotic medications who developed diabetic ketoacidosis in the absence of weight gain.

Much still needs to be learned about the risks of obesity and diabetes and the now emerging association between dyslipidemia and atypical antipsychotic therapy. In the meantime, these reported side effects suggest that clinicians need to monitor weight changes, glucose levels, and lipids in patients treated with the atypical antipsychotic medications.

C. Prolactin Elevation and Sexual Side Effects

Hyperprolactinemia is a well-known liability of the conventional antipsychotic medications and is clinically important because it can result in galactorrhea, gynecomastia, amenorrhea, anovulation, impaired spermatogenesis, decreased libido and sexual arousal, impotence, and anorgasmia. The loss of the protective effects of estrogen may also increase the risk of cardiac morbidity and osteoporosis in women (72). Among the atypical antipsychotic medications, risperidone carries the greatest risk of hyperprolactinemia while the other available novel antipsychotic medications do not appear to cause significant or sustained prolactin elevation (71). Aripiprazole is associated with a decrease in mean prolactin (28). When hyperprolactinemia is detected in the context of related morbidity, switching to an atypical antipsychotic medication with neutral effects on prolactin can be both diagnostic and therapeutic. However, switching medications could result in loss of antipsychotic effectiveness as well as increased fertility and risk of pregnancy.

Sexual side effects are often neglected in clinical research and practice, but current data suggest that conventional antipsychotic medications, clozapine, and risperidone are all associated with sexual side effects (71,73). These side effects warrant monitoring in routine clinical practice, as well as continued study of the relative toxicities of the atypical antipsychotic medications and appropriate interventions, due to their presumed negative impact on treatment adherence and quality of life.

D. QTc Prolongation

The propensity of antipsychotic medications to prolong cardiac conduction (as measured by the QTc interval) has received renewed attention with the release of ziprasidone. However, this side effect is not limited to ziprasidone and is shared by tricyclic antidepressants, some of the low potency conventional antipsychotics, pimozide, and all of the atypical antipsychotic medications to some degree. Several medications, including the atypical antipsychotic sertindole, have been removed from or were never released to the market due to concerns about QTc prolongation. This concern stems from the fact that QTc prolongation can lead to the development of the potentially fatal ventricular arrhythmia, *torsade de pointes*. In response to FDA concerns about ziprasidone, investigators at Pfizer performed an open-label prospective study of QTc changes in patients treated with atypical and some conventional antipsychotic medications (74). They found that the greatest degree of mean QTc prolongation occurred with thioridazine (35.6 msec) followed by ziprasidone (20.3 msec), quetiapine (14.5 msec), risperidone (11.6 msec), olanzapine (6.8 msec), and haloperidol (4.7 msec). No subjects developed increases in QTc to above 500 msec (a threshold for increased risk of *torsade de pointes*). Although concerns about QTc delayed the release of ziprasidone, data from this study enabled Pfizer to eventually release it without recommendations for a baseline electro-cardiogram (EKG). In addition, thioridazine and its relative mesoridazine were given black box warnings for QTc prolongation with new instructions to limit their use only to patients with refractory schizophrenia. In order to err on the side of caution and as a matter of routine primary care, screening EKGs should probably be performed on any patient starting antipsychotic therapy and especially those with known cardiac disease or who are taking other medications with the potential to cause QTc prolongation.

E. Clozapine

Owing to the troubling and serious side effects associated with clozapine, its prescription is often deferred in favor of another trial with an atypical antipsychotic despite robust evidence for its efficacy in treatment-refractory schizophrenia. Commonly encountered side effects including sedation, orthostasis, tachycardia, sialorrhea, and constipation require gradual and careful titration during dose escalation and sometimes specific intervention. For example, addition of a beta-blocker might be necessary for tachycardia, an aggressive bowel regimen might be needed in order to prevent bowel obstruction, and patients might need to sleep with a towel in order to cope with excessive salivation. Clozapine can also cause seizures in a dose-related fashion. Patients who develop clozapine induced seizures can usually be managed with a reduction in dose or addition of an anticonvulsant such as valproic acid without leukopenic side effects (carbamazepine should not be prescribed).

The most concerning side effect of clozapine is agranulocytosis, since it is potentially lethal. The mechanism of action is unknown and the side effect does not seem to be dose-related. Defined as an absolute neutrophil count (ANC) below 500/mm^3, clozapine induced agranulocytosis usually occurs within the first 3 months of therapy and is usually reversible if detected early, taking about 2 to 3 weeks for blood counts to normalize after discontinuation. As a result, in the United States, complete blood counts (CBC) must be monitored on a weekly basis until 6 months of therapy, at which time they can be checked every 2 weeks. If either the white blood count (WBC) falls below 3000 or ANC falls below 1500/mm^3, clozapine must be discontinued at least until these values normalize. No one developing WBC below 2000/mm^3 or ANC below 1000/mm^3 should be rechallenged with clozapine. Since the implementation of the National Clozapine Registry and mandatory CBC monitoring, the incidence of agranulocytosis has decreased from 1–2% to 0.38% with a death rate of only 0.012% (75). Despite these data supporting clozapine's safety, many clinicians remain reluctant to prescribe and patients often refuse it due to this risk and the requirement of frequent blood monitoring.

IX. SUMMARY OF MAIN POINTS

1. An adequate trial of antipsychotic medication consists of at least 4 to 6 weeks of sustained treatment at a potentially therapeutic dose.
2. All of the available atypical antipsychotic medications have been demonstrated to be effective for the treatment of acute schizophrenia. It is not yet clear whether there are important between drug differences with regard to efficacy of the atypical antipsychotic medications, with the exception of clozapine which appears to be the most effective medication for treatment-refractory schizophrenia.

3. Antipsychotic therapy is most effective at reducing positive symptoms. The atypical antipsychotic medications seem to also be effective at improving secondary negative symptoms and neurocognitive deficits in schizophrenia.
4. The clearest benefit of atypical antipsychotic medications compared to first-generation medications is the reduced risk of EPS. However, atypical antipsychotic medications have important and potentially serious side effects such as weight gain, glucose intolerance and diabetes, sexual side effects, and the potential for QTc prolongation. There appear to be important between-drug differences with regard to these side effects.

X. GUIDELINES FOR CLINICIANS

1. Patients requiring treatment with an antipsychotic medication should be treated with the lowest effective dose for at least 4 to 6 weeks in order to gauge the efficacy of antipsychotic therapy. Partial responders may require a longer duration of treatment in order to achieve the full benefits of an antipsychotic trial.
2. Patients who have not responded to an adequate trial of two or more antipsychotic medications, at least one of which is an atypical agent, should be considered for a trial of clozapine for refractory positive symptoms. Combination and high dose antipsychotic therapy should be reserved for patients who have not responded to or are ineligible for clozapine therapy.
3. Patients with refractory positive or negative symptoms should be assessed carefully for treatment nonadherence and secondary causes of negative symptoms prior to switching antipsychotic medications.
4. Judicious monitoring for side effects (weight gain, glucose intolerance, lipid abnormalities, sexual and prolactin-related changes) associated with atypical antipsychotic medications should be performed on a regular basis in order to reduce morbidity and enhance treatment adherence and overall antipsychotic effectiveness.

REFERENCES

1. Van Putten T, May PR, Marder SR. Response to antipsychotic medication: The doctor's and the consumer's view. Am J Psychiatry 1984; 141:16–19.

2. Baldessarini RJ, Cohen BM, Teicher MH. Significance of neuroleptic dosing and plasma level in the pharmacological treatment of psychoses. Arch Gen Psychiatry 1988; 45:79–91.

3. Overall JE, Gorman DR. The brief psychiatric rating scale. Psychol Rep 1962; 10:799–812.

4. Kay SR, Opler LA, Lindenmayer JP. Reliability and validity of the positive and negative syndrome scale for schizophrenics. Psychiatry Res 1998; 23:99–110.

5. Andreasen NC. Scale for the assessment of negative symptoms (SANS). Brit J Psychiatry 1989; 155(suppl 7):53–58.

6. Hippius H. A historical perspective of clozapine. J Clin Psychiatry 1999; 60 (suppl 12):22–23.

7. Kane JM, Honigfeld G, Singer J, Meltzer H, and the Clozaril Collaborative Study Group. Clozapine for the treatment-resistant schizophrenic: a double-blind comparison versus chlorpromazine. Arch Gen Psychiatry 1988; 45:789–796.

8. Wahlbeck K, Cheine M, Essali A, Adams C. Evidence of clozapine's effectiveness in schizophrenia: a systematic review and meta-analysis of randomized trials. Am J Psychiatry 1999; 156:990–999.

9. Marder SR, Essock SM, Miller AL, Buchanan RW, Davis JM, Kane JM, Lieberman J, Schooler NR. The Mount Sinai Conference on the pharmacotherapy of schizophrenia. Schizophr Bull 2002; 28:5–16.

10. Fleischhacker WW, Hummer M, Kurz M, Kurzthaler I, Lieberman JA, Pollack S, Safferman AZ, Kane JM. Clozapine dose in the United States and Europe: implications for therapeutic and adverse effects. J Clin Psychiatry 1994; 55(9, suppl B):78–81.

11. Miller DD, Fleming F, Holman TL, Perry PJ. Plasma clozapine concentrations as a predictor of clinical response: a follow-up study. J Clin Psychiatry 1994; 55(9, suppl B):117–121.

12. Kronig MH, Munne RA, Szymanski S, Safferman AZ, Pollack S, Cooper T, Kane JM, Lieberman JA. Plasma clozapine levels and clinical response for treatment-refractory schizophrenic patients. Am J Psychiatry 1995; 152:179–182.

13. Chouinard G, Jones B, Remington G, Bloom D, Addington D, MacEwan GW, Labelle A, Beauclair L, Arnott W. A Canadian multicenter placebo-controlled study of fixed doses of risperidone and haloperidol in the treatment of chronic schizophrenic patients. J Clin Psychopharmacol 1993; 13:25–40.

14. Marder SR, Meibach RC. Risperidone in the treatment of schizophrenia. Am J Psychiatry 1994; 151:825–835.

15. Peuskens, J. Risperidone in the treatment of patients with chronic schizophrenia: a multi-national, multi-centre, double-blind, parallel-group study versus haloperidol. Brit J Psychiatry 1995; 166:712–726.

16. Tollefson GD, Beasley CM Jr, Tran PV, et al. Olanzapine versus haloperidol in the treatment of schizophrenia and schizoaffective and schizophreniform disorders: results of an international collaborative trial. Am J Psychiatry 1997; 154:457–465.

17. Beasley CM, Tollefson G, Tran P, Satterlee W, Sanger T, Hamilton S, and the Olanzapine HGAD Study Group. Olanzapine versus placebo and

haloperidol: acute phase results of the North American double-blind olanzapine trial. Neuropsychopharmacology 1996; 14:111–123.

18. Small JG, Hirsch SR, Arvantis LA, Miller BG, Link CGG, and the Seroquel Study Group. Quetiapine in patients with schizophrenia: A high- and low-dose double-blind comparison with placebo. Arch Gen Psychiatry 1997; 54:549–557.

19. Arvanitis LA, Miller BG, and the Seroquel Trial 13 Study Group. Multiple fixed doses of "Seroquel" (quetiapine) in patients with acute exacerbation of schizophrenia: a comparison with haloperidol and placebo. Biol Psychiatry 1997; 42: 233–246.

20. King DJ, Link CG, Kowalcyk B. A comparison of bid and tid dose regimens of quetiapine (Seroquel) in the treatment of schizophrenia. Psychopharmacology 1998; 137:139–146.

21. Kapur S, Zipursky R, Jones C, Shammi CS, Remington G, Seeman, P. A positron emission tomography study of quetiapine in schizophrenia: a preliminary finding of an antipsychotic effect with only transiently high dopamine D2 receptor occupancy. Arch Gen Psychiatry 2000; 57: 553–559.

22. Kapur S, Seeman P. Does fast dissociation from the dopamine D_2 receptor explain the action of atypical antipsychotics? A new hypothesis. Am J Psychiatry 2001; 158:360–369.

23. Seeger TF, Seymour PA, Schmidt AW, Zorn SH, Schulz DW, Lebel LA, McLean S, Guanowsky V, Howard HR, Lowe JA 3rd, Heym J. Ziprasidone (CP-88,059): a new antipsychotic with combined dopamine and serotonin receptor antagonist activity. J Pharmacol Exp Ther 1995; 275:101–113.

24. Goff DC, Posever T, Herz L, Simmons J, Kleti N, Lapierre K, Wilner KD, Law CG, Ko GN. An exploratory haloperidol-controlled dose-finding study of ziprasidone in hospitalized patients with schizophrenia or schizoaffective disorder. J Clin Psychopharmacol 1998; 18:296–304.

25. Keck P Jr, Buffenstein A, Ferguson J, Feighner J, Jaffe W, Harrigan EP, Morrissey MR. Ziprasidone 40 and 120 mg/day in the acute exacerbation of schizophrenia and schizoaffective disorder: a 4-week placebo-controlled trial. Psychopharmacology 1998; 140:173–184.

26. Daniel DG, Zimbroff DL, Potkin SG, Reeves KR, Harrigan EP, Lakshminarayanan M, and the Ziprasidone Study Group. Ziprasidone 80 mg/day and 160 mg/day in the acute exacerbation of schizophrenia and schizoaffective disorder: a 6-week placebo-controlled trial. Neuropsychopharmacology 1999; 20:491–505.

27. Kane JM, Carson WH, Saha AR, McQuade RD, Ingenito GG, Zimbold DL, Ali MW. Efficacy and safety of aripiprazole and haloperidol versus placebo in patients with schizophrenia and schizoaffective disorder. J Clin Psychiatry 2002; 63:763–771.

28. Marder SR, McQuade RD, Stock E, Kaplita S, Marcus R, Safferman AZ, Saha A, Ali M, Iwamoto T. Aripiprazole in the treatment of schizophrenia: safety and tolerability in short-term, placebo-controlled trials. Schizophrenia Res 2003; 61:123–126.

29. Woods SW, Stolar M, Sernyak MJ, Charney DS. Consistency of atypical antipsychotic superiority to placebo in recent clinical trials. Biol Psychiatry 2001; 49:64–70.

30. Leucht S, Pitschel-Walz G, Abraham D, Kissling W. Efficacy and extrapyramidal side-effects of the new antipsychotics olanzapine, quetiapine, risperidone, and sertindole compared to conventional antipsychotics and placebo. A meta-analysis of randomized controlled trials. Schizophrenia Res 1999; 35:51–68.

31. Geddes J, Freemantle N, Harrison P, Bebbington P for the National Schizophrenia Guideline Development Group. Atypical antipsychotics in the treatment of schizophrenia: systematic overview and meta-regression analysis. Brit Med J 2000; 321:1371–1376.

32. Kleiser E, Lehmann E, Kinzler E, Wurthmann C, Heinrich K. Randomized, double-blind, controlled trial of risperidone versus clozapine in patients with chronic schizophrenia. J Clin Psychopharmacol 1995; 15(suppl 1):45S–51S.

33. Conley RR, Mahmoud R. A randomized double-blind study of risperidone and olanzapine in the treatment of schizophrenia or schizoaffective disorder. Am J Psychiatry 2001; 158:765–774.

34. Tran PV, Hamilton SH, Kuntz AJ, Potvin JH, Andersen SW, Beasley C, Tollefson GD. Double-blind comparison of olanzapine versus risperidone in the treatment of schizophrenia and other psychotic disorders. J Clin Psychopharm 1997; 117:407–418.

35. Simpson G, Weiden P, Pigott T, Romano SJ. Ziprasidone vs olanzapine in schizophrenia: results of a double-blind trial. 155th Annual Meeting of the American Psychiatric Association, Philadelphia, PA, May 18–23, 2002.

36. Buchanan RW, Carpenter WT. Domains of psychopathology: an approach to the reduction in heterogeneity in schizophrenia. J Nerv Ment Dis 1994; 182:193–204.

37. Andreason NC, Arndt S, Alliger R, Miller D, Flaum M. Symptoms of schizophrenia: methods, meanings, and mechanisms. Arch Gen Psychiatry 1995; 52:341–351.

38. Tamminga CA, Buchanan RW, Gold JM. The role of negative symptoms and cognitive dysfunction in schizophrenia outcome. Int Clin Psychopharmacol 1998; 13(suppl 3):S21–S26.

39. Green MF. What are the functional consequences of neurocognitive deficits in schizophrenia? Am J Psychiatry 1996; 153:321–330.

40. American Psychiatric Association. Diagnostic and Statistical Manual for Mental Disorders. 4th ed. Washington DC: American Psychiatric Association, 1994.

41. Andreasen NC. Negative symptoms in schizophrenia. Arch Gen Psychiatry 1982; 39:784–788.

42. Carpenter WT, Heinrichs DW, Wagman AMI. Deficit and nondeficit forms of schizophrenia: the concept. Am J Psychiatry 1999; 145:578–583.

43. Kirkpatrick B, Buchanan RW, Ross DE, Carpenter WT. A separate disease within the syndrome of schizophrenia. Arch Gen Psychiatry 2001; 58:165–171.

44. Kirkpatrick B, Buchanan RW, McKenney PD, Aphs LD, Carpenter WT Jr. The schedule for the deficit syndrome: an instrument for research in schizophrenia. Psychiatry Res 1989; 30:119–124.

45. Goldberg SC. Negative and deficit symptoms in schizophrenia do respond to neuroleptics. Schizophr Bull 1985; 11:453–456.

46. Breier A, Buchanan RW, Kirkpatrick B, Davis OR, Irish D, Summerfelt A, Carpenter WT Jr. Effects of clozapine on positive and negative symptoms in outpatients with schizophrenia. Am J Psychiatry 1994; 151:20–26.

47. Marder SR, Davis JM, Chouinard G. The effects of risperidone on the five dimensions of schizophrenia derived by factor analysis: combined results of the North American trials. J Clin Psychiatry 1997; 58:538–546.

48. Kopelowicz A, Zarate R, Tripodis K, Gonzalez V, Mintz J. Differential efficacy of olanzapine for deficit and nondeficit negative symptoms in schizophrenia. Am J Psychiatry 2000; 157:987–993.

49. Green MF, Marshall BD Jr, Wirshing WC, Ames D, Marder SR, McGurk S, Kern RS, Mintz J. Does risperidone improve verbal working memory in treatment-resistant schizophrenia? Am J Psychiatry 1997; 154:799–804.

50. Sharma T, Mockler D. The cognitive efficacy of atypical antipsychotics in schizophrenia. J Clin Psychopharmacol 1998; 18(suppl 1):12S–19S.

51. Keefe RSE, Silva SG, Perkins DO, Lieberman JA. The effects of atypical antipsychotic drugs on neurocognitive impairment in schizophrenia: a review and meta-analysis. Schizophr Bull 1999; 25:201–222.

52. Kern RS, Green MF, Marshall BD Jr, Wirshing WC, Wirshing DA, McGurk S, Marder SR, Mintz J. Risperidone versus haloperidol on secondary memory: Can newer medications aid learning? Schizophr Bull 1999; 25: 223–232.

53. Meltzer HY, McGurk SR. The effects of clozapine, risperidone, and olanzapine on cognitive function in schizophrenia. Schizophr Bull 1999; 25:233–255.

54. Purdon SE, Jones BD, Stip E, Labelle A, Addington D, David SR, Breier A, Tollefson GD for the Canadian Collaborative Group for Research on Cognition in Schizophrenia. Neuropsychological change in early phase schizophrenia during 12 months of treatment with olanzapine, risperidone, or haloperidol. Arch Gen Psychiatry 2000; 57:249–258.

55. Bilder RM, Goldman RS, Volavka J, Czobor P, Hoptman M, Sheitman B, Lindenmayer JP, Citrome L, McEvoy J, Kunz M, Chakos M, Cooper TB, Horowitz TL, Lieberman JA. Neurocognitive effects of clozapine, olanzapine, risperidone, and haloperidol in patients with chronic schizophrenia or schizoaffective disorder. Am J Psychiatry 2002; 159:1018–1028.

56. Conley RR, Buchanan RW. Evaluation of treatment-resistant schizophrenia. Schizophr Bull 1997; 23:663–674.

57. Fenton WS, Blyler CR, Heinssen RK. Determinants of medication compliance in schizophrenia: empirical and clinical findings. Schizophr Bull 1997; 23: 637–651.

58. Marder SR. An approach to treatment resistance in schizophrenia. Brit J Psychiatry 1999; 174(suppl 37):19–22.

59. Bondolfi G, Dufour H, Patris M, et al. Risperidone versus clozapine in treatment-resistant chronic schizophrenia: a randomized double-blind study. Am J Psychiatry 1998;155:499–504.
60. Breier A, Hamilton SH. Comparative efficacy of olanzapine and haloperidol for patients with treatment-resistant schizophrenia. Biol Psychiatry 1999;45:403–411.
61. Conley RR, Tamminga CA, Bartko JJ, Richardson C, Peszke M, Lingle J, Hegerty J, Love R, Counaris C, Zaremba S. Olanzapine compared to chlorpromazine in treatment-resistant schizophrenia. Am J Psychiatry 1998; 155:914–920.
62. Wirshing DA, Marshall BD, Green MF, Mintz J, Marder SR, Wirshing WC. Risperidone in treatment-refractory schizophrenia. Am J Psychiatry 1999; 156:1374–1379.
63. Emsley RA, Raniwalla J, Bailey PJ, Jones AM on behalf of the PRIZE study group. A comparison of the effects of quetiapine ('Seroquel') and haloperidol in schizophrenia patients with a history of and a demonstrated, partial response to conventional antipsychotic treatment. Int Clin Psychopharmacol 2000; 15:121–131.
64. Conley RR, Tamminga CA, Kelly DL, Richardson CM. Treatment-resistant schizophrenic patients respond to clozapine after olanzapine non-response. Biol Psychiatry 1999; 46:73–77.
65. Buckley P, Miller A, Olsen J, Garver D, Miller DD, Csernansky J. When symptoms persist: Clozapine augmentation strategies. Schizophr Bull 2001; 27:615–628.
66. Citrome L, Volavka J. Optimal dosing of atypical antipsychotics in adults: a review of the current evidence. Harvard Rev Psychiatry 2002; 10:280–291.
67. Beasley CM, Delleva MA, Tamura RN, Morgenstern H, Glazer WM, Ferguson K, Tollefson GD. Randomized double-blind comparison of the incidence of tardive dyskinesia in patients with schizoprehnia during long-term treatment with olanzapine or haloperidol. Brit J Psychiatry 1999; 174:23–30.
68. Jeste DV, Lacro JP, Bailey A, Rockwell E, Harris MJ, Caligiuri MP. Lower incidence of tardive dyskinesia with risperidone compared to haloperidol in older patients. J Am Geriatr Soc 1999; 47:716–719.
69. Allison DB, Mentore JL, Heo M, Chandler LP, Cappelleri JC, Infante MC, Weiden PJ. Antipsychotic-induced weight gain: a comprehensive research synthesis. Am J Psychiatry 1999; 156:1686–1696.
70. Wirshing D, Wirshing W, Kysar L, Berisford MA, Goldstein D, Pashdag J, Mintz J, Marder SR. Novel antipsychotics: comparison of weight gain liabilities. J Clin Psychiatry 1999; 60:358–363.
71. Wirshing DA, Pierre JM, Erhart S, Boyd J. Understanding the new and evolving profile of adverse drug effects in schizophrenia. Psychiatr Clin N Am 2003; 26:165–190.
72. Dickson RA, Glazer WM. Neuroleptic-induced hyperprolactinemia. Schizophrenic Res 1999; 35:S75–S86.
73. Wirshing DA, Pierre JM, Marders SM, Saunders CS, Wirshing WC. Sexual side effects of novel antipsychotic medications. Schizophr Res 2002; 56:25–50.

74. Food and Drug Administration. Center for Drug Evaluation and Research. Briefing information for Psychopharmacologic Drugs Advisory Committee Meeting; 2000: available at http://www.fda.gov/ohrms/dockets/ac/00/backgrd/3619b1.htm.

75. Honigfeld G, Arellano F, Sethi J, Bianchini A, Schein J. Reducing clozapine-related morbidity and mortality: 5 years of experience with the clozapine national registry. J Clin Psychiatry 1998; 59(suppl 3):3–7.

8

Long-Term Efficacy, Effectiveness, and Safety of Atypical Antipsychotic Drugs

Robert R. Conley and Deanna L. Kelly

University of Maryland,
Baltimore, Maryland, U.S.A.

I. INTRODUCTION

Long-term outcomes for people with schizophrenia are usually disappointing. With conventional antipsychotic treatment, two-thirds of those treated have persistent positive symptoms. The same proportion also experiences persistent parkinsonian side effects. Rates of unemployment and rehospitalization are high, quality of life ratings are low, and the lifetime risk of suicide is approximately 10% (1). Atypical antipsychotics represent a significant advance in the treatment of schizophrenia. Treatment with these medications may improve long-term outcomes for people suffering from this devastating illness.

The efficacy and safety of atypical antipsychotics for the acute treatment of psychoses have been widely established. Clozapine, risperidone, olanzapine, quetiapine, ziprasidone, and aripiprazole have all been found to have comparable or superior efficacy to conventional antipsychotics in numerous short-term trials. Treatment with atypical antipsychotics is generally associated with improved safety and tolerability profiles as compared to conventional agents, notably with regards to extrapyramidal symptoms. However, little information is available regarding the impact of atypical antipsychotics on long-term outcomes. This chapter will review the efficacy, effectiveness, and safety of long-term treatment of atypical antipsychotic medications for the treatment of schizophrenia.

II. OUTCOME ASSESSMENT

Psychopathology varies greatly among people with schizophrenia. Additionally, domains of the illness are represented by many characteristics and dimensions of impairment. Those afflicted suffer from positive symptoms (hallucinations and delusions), negative symptoms (affective flattening, alogia, and avolition), disorganization (formal thought disorder and inappropriate affect), and relational dysfunctions (problems with intimacy, closeness, and forming relationships). These dimensions occur relatively independently of each other in terms of severity and recovery (2). Traditionally, short-term reductions in positive symptoms were the primary determinant of medication effectiveness. More recently, however, it has been recognized that other domains such as rehabilitative (work, school, social functioning) and humanitarian (quality of life, treatment satisfaction) are also important for improving outcomes.

Existing randomized controlled trials focus primarily on the reduction of positive symptoms and short-term data are not sufficient to answer many research questions. It is well accepted that the efficacy of a treatment under optimal research conditions overestimates its effectiveness in typical clinical practice, referred to as the efficacy–effectiveness gap (3). While some long-term trials exist with antipsychotics, most long-term treatment of psychosis is now largely empiric. It is currently accepted that people with schizophrenia should be on lifelong medication. In the recent past it was argued that long-term treatment with antipsychotics might not be an option, or even an ethical choice. Now it is argued that any gap in medication treatment may be unethical. As comparative trials are developed in this area, it is important to remember that neither of these positions may represent the best choice. It is critical to perform larger trials over longer periods of time. Yet, to accomplish this, better methods for determining efficacy must be determined (4). Efficacy studies evaluate the intended effect of a drug under ideal conditions in controlled clinical trials, usually with small, homogeneous patient samples that may not be representative of the entire universe of people with schizophrenia or psychosis. Efficacy studies are complemented by studies of the effectiveness of medications, in which an investigation occurs under usual practice setting conditions. Although the majority of people with schizophrenia are maintained in outpatient clinical settings, studies of the effectiveness of medications outside of clinical trials (which are often conducted in inpatient settings) are relatively rare (5). It is largely unknown how the results of clinical trials (efficacy studies) compare with treatment patterns and outcomes (effectiveness) in regular clinical practice settings.

Some advancements have occurred in the last couple of years as many have begun to study efficacy in many domains over longer periods reflecting a move toward effectiveness research. Time to relapse, rehospitalization, and tolerability as well as examining subject satisfaction, quality of life, and neurocognitive effects are included in many longer-term studies.

III. LONG-TERM EFFICACY AND EFFECTIVENESS

A. Clozapine

Clozapine was the first atypical antipsychotic marketed in the United States and has been in clinical use now for over a decade. Much data exist demonstrating both the short- and long-term efficacy and effectiveness of clozapine treatment, however only a few double-blind long-term comparative studies are available. In the early 1990s reports began to emerge that evaluated long-term therapy with clozapine. Lindenmayer et al. (6) found that after 12 weeks of treatment many domains of psychopathology showed significant improvement including positive, negative, cognitive, excitement, and depressive symptoms. These improvements were maintained throughout 26 weeks of treatment. These authors noted that there were no further significant improvements after 12 weeks and that improvement at 12 weeks reliably predicted scores observed at 26 weeks. Brier and colleagues (7) also noted that sustained response was evident at 12 months. In addition to symptomatology, other benefits of clozapine were noted to occur after long-term treatment such as improvements in disruptiveness, aggressiveness, neuropsychological testing, social functioning, and decreasing hospitalization (8–11). A large 12-month double-blind trial was conducted in the late 1990s comparing clozapine and haloperidol in 423 subjects. Fifty-seven percent of subjects on clozapine continued on the medication for the entire year while only 28% continued haloperidol treatment ($p < 0.001$). PANSS assessments for those treated with clozapine were significantly lower than haloperidol-treated subjects at all follow-up evaluations. This important study also found clozapine to be associated with fewer mean days of hospitalization for psychiatric reasons than haloperidol. While drug costs and outpatient services were significantly higher with clozapine, overall treatment costs between haloperidol and clozapine did not significantly differ (12). A second double-blind long-term study comparing clozapine to "usual care" (conventional antipsychotics) found no differences between clozapine and haloperidol on symptom response in chronic inpatients. However, many other benefits were evident (9) such as decreased hospitalization and resource utilization.

Other recent studies have examined efficacy and effectiveness over several treatment years. Essock et al. (13) found that clozapine treatment up to 2 years is more cost-effective than conventional antipsychotics on most measures of effectiveness. Other follow-ups also found sustained and significant improvements in many symptom domains with treatment up to 2 years (14–16).

B. Risperidone

Risperidone is the only atypical antipsychotic with a U.S. Food and Drug Administration (FDA) approved indication for relapse prevention in schizophrenia. There are numerous data to support the long-term efficacy of risperidone. Furthermore, much data suggest long-term benefits superior to conventional antipsychotics.

Recently, a double-blind randomized study comparing haloperidol (mean 11.7 mg) to risperidone (mean 4.7 mg) has been published involving 397 subjects. The risk of a relapse estimated by Kaplan–Meier survivor analysis was 34% for risperidone which was significantly lower than haloperidol's associated relapse risk of 60% at 1 year. Additionally, risperidone had greater reductions in the mean severity of psychotic symptoms and extrapyramidal side effects than haloperidol-treated subjects. More subjects treated with haloperidol discontinued treatment for reasons other than a relapse than those treated with risperidone (17). Another 12-month study in subjects with chronic schizophrenia also found significantly greater improvements in symptom ratings for those treated with risperidone as compared to haloperidol. At 12 months the rate of response for risperidone-treated subjects was 30% while only 15% in haloperidol-treated subjects (18). Malla et al. (19) found that risperidone treatment may be more advantageous over haloperidol in first-episode schizophrenia subjects as well. Six of 19 (32%) haloperidol-treated subjects were rehospitalized during the first year as compared to only 1 of 19 (5%) in the risperidone group. Subjects in the risperidone group showed a statistically significantly lower length of first hospitalization, utilization of inpatient beds during the course of treatment, and the use of anticholinergic medications. Other long-term open-label and retrospective studies support the long-term treatment benefits of risperidone (20–24).

A long-acting injectable formulation of risperidone has recently been approved in the United States for schizophrenia. This drug formulation is gradually released into the body using a microsphere technology which allows for stable blood levels for 2 weeks. The active drug is contained in a saline-based solution rather than oil based, thus only 2% of subjects complain of injection site pain. Long-acting risperidone is an aqueous suspension containing risperidone in a matrix of a glycolic acid–lactate copolymer. A gradual hydrolysis of the copolymer at the site of injection occurs over 2 weeks. Therapeutic plasma levels are usually reached from 3–4 weeks after starting the depot microspheres. Effectiveness studies have reported benefits for up to 1 year (25,26).

C. Olanzapine

The efficacy of olanzapine has been demonstrated in both short- and long-term studies. The data from double-blind maintenance phase therapy of olanzapine following three acute treatment studies were combined to evaluate the long-term maintenance treatment with olanzapine. This analysis included patients who had responded to either olanzapine or haloperidol during acute treatment. In this large sample of 627 patients on olanzapine and 180 patients on haloperidol significantly more patients were found to have relapse on haloperidol in the following 12 months than on olanzapine (28 vs. 20%, $p = 0.034$). The mean doses used in this analysis of pooled studies were 13.6 mg and 13.5 mg for haloperidol and olanzapine, respectively. Nine percent of patients on olanzapine discontinued due to an adverse event as did 11% on haloperidol (27). Glick and Berg (28) performed a review of long-term outcomes with olanzapine treatment as compared to haloperidol and risperidone using large registry data sets. The authors concluded that for evaluating time to discontinuation of anti-psychotic due to adverse events or lack of efficacy, olanzapine showed superiority over haloperidol and no difference compared to risperidone. In real-world effectiveness studies olanzapine has been found to have significant improvements on Brief Psychiatric Rating Scale (BPRS) and Clinical Global Impression (CGI) scales during 6 months of treatment (29).

D. Quetiapine

Several short-term trials have demonstrated the efficacy of quetiapine, however, data on long-term treatment are lacking with this medication. A 4-month randomized open-label study compared quetiapine to risperidone in a flexible-dose design. Subjects enrolled in the study had a wide range of psychotic disorders including schizophrenia, bipolar disorder, dementia, and substance induced. At the end of 4 months both groups improved similarly on the CGI scale and Positive and Negative Symptom Scale (PANSS). At the study endpoint the quetiapine group had significantly lower Hamilton Depressio Scale (HAM-D) scores ($p = 0.028$) than did those treated with risperidone (30). An open-label study also evaluated quetiapine use in a mixed psychotic population in elderly subjects over 52 weeks where significant improvements were noted on the BPRS and CGI, but did not include a control population (31). A small 12-month retrospective study found that quetiapine treatment was associated with sustained clinical improvements and a decreased usage of inpatient services (32). Another recent study of 23 subjects found only five subjects (22%) to complete between 77–96 weeks of the study. In many of these male subjects therapeutic tolerance and rebound psychoses were noted to occur. Those who completed the study, however, had significantly higher doses of quetiapine than those who did not complete (592 vs. 362 mg/day) (33).

E. Ziprasidone

The efficacy of ziprasidone has been evaluated in a few long-term trials demonstrating significant benefits in long-term treatment. A 28-week double-blind study evaluated the efficacy of ziprasidone compared with haloperidol in 301 outpatients with stable chronic schizophrenia. Subjects received flexible-dose ziprasidone 80 to 160 mg/day ($N = 148$) or haloperidol 5 to 15 mg/day ($N = 153$). For study inclusion, subjects had to have a baseline PANSS negative subscale score of 10 and a Global Assessment of Functioning Scale (GAF) score greater than 30. Clinical efficacy was evaluated using several parameters including, PANSS total score, PANSS negative subscale score, BPRS core items score, CGI severity scale and the Mortgomery-Asberg Depressin Rating Scale (MADRS) score. Mean PANSS total scores at the baseline were 72.9 and 74.4 in the ziprasidone and haloperidol recipients and these scores improved by approximately 12% and 11%, respectively. A PANSS negative symptom response (defined as a 20% decrease in the PANSS negative subscale score) was seen in significantly more ziprasidone compared with haloperidol recipients (48 vs. 32%, $p < 0.05$). There was a trend toward greater improvement on the MADRS scale for those treated with ziprasidone as mean scores decreased by approximately 11% and 3.5% in ziprasidone and haloperidol subjects respectively (34).

A second study also evaluated the efficacy of ziprasidone (80 to 160 mg/day) compared to haloperidol (5 to 15 mg/day) in a 40-week randomized double-blind trial in 599 outpatients. In both the last-observation-carried-forward analysis and completer analysis there was a greater improvement noted in the ziprasidone group as compared to those treated with haloperidol with regards to negative symptoms. Superiority of ziprasidone was noted on the GAF but no differences were noted for other symptom domains (35).

One year data are available from a double-blind placebo controlled study involving 278 chronically ill stable inpatients. This ZEUS trial evaluated fixed dosing of 40, 80, or 160 mg/day. Efficacy was assessed by the PANSS and the CGI-S. Relapse was estimated by Kaplan–Meier survival curves. For those who remained in the study at 6 months, the incidence of impending relapses was seven times higher among the placebo group than the ziprasidone recipients (42 vs. 6%, $p = 0.001$). Subjects treated with 160 mg/day had the greatest improvements in negative symptoms with half of the improvements noted as direct effects by path analysis and the remaining improvements related to positive, depressive, and extrapyramidal symptoms (36).

Ziprasidone was compared to olanzapine in a 6-week trial which reported similar efficacy between medications. A 6-month blinded continuation studied followed subjects who had completed the 6-week randomization with a satisfactory clinical response with flexible dosing of ziprasidone (80, 120, and 160 mg/day) and olanzapine (5, 10, and 15 mg/day). Both antipsychotics had similar sustained improvements on all clinical measures that continued to 1 year including total BPRS, CGI-S, PANSS, Calgary Depression Scale for Schizophrenia (CDSS), and positive and negative subscales. Furthermore, the percentage of those maintaining response was greater than 80% in both groups (37).

F. Aripiprazole

Aripiprazole has been shown to be effective in the short-term treatment of schizophrenia as well as maintaining efficacy in long-term treatment. A 28-week study evaluated relapse of aripiprazole (15 mg/day) as compared to a placebo in 310 subjects. The primary efficacy measure was time from randomization to relapse. Relapse was defined as minimally worse on the CGI, 20% increase in total PANSS, or moderately severe on hostility or uncooperativeness on the PANSS on two successive days. The aripiprazole group experienced a significantly lower number of subjects who relapsed and lower number who discontinued due to lack of efficacy as compared to the placebo group. The estimated probability of not experiencing a relapse prior to week 26 was 39% in the placebo group versus 63% in the aripiprazole group (38).

A second double-blind trial compared aripiprazole (30 mg/day) to haloperidol (10 mg/day) in 1294 acutely ill subjects in a 52-week trial. The primary efficacy measure in this study was the time to failure to maintain response. A responder was defined as a 20% decrease in total PANSS score.

The percentage of subjects who discontinued from the study early was significantly higher in the haloperidol group (70%) as compared to aripiprazole (57%). For the subjects who had a response there were no differences between haloperidol and aripiprazole in the time to failure to maintain a response. The percent of subjects on treatment and still characterized as responders was significantly higher at all study time points with aripiprazole. Aripiprazole appeared to have significant improvements over haloperidol in negative and depressive symptoms that continued to improve up to 1 year after initiation (39).

In summary, most of the atypical antipsychotics appear to maintain efficacy and are effective in the longer-time trials. Data for long-term maintenance therapy are most striking for clozapine and risperidone, however these medications have been available for the longest periods. A few reports and clinical experiences have found some therapeutic tolerance developing with some of the newer antipsychotics. However, long-term post marketing studies are needed. Nonetheless, all the new agents appear to at least be equivalent if not superior in efficacy to traditional agents for most subjects during long-term maintenance treatment. In one of the few long-term naturalistic prospective comparative studies, 150 subjects were switched from conventional antipsychotics to either risperidone, olanzapine, or quetiapine and were monitored for 2–6 years. This study found that the majority (85%) of subjects benefited from a switch to novel antipsychotic drugs. Risperidone was significantly better in improving negative symptoms while olanzapine was more effective than conventional agents for anxiety and depressive symptoms (40). As seen with a recent meta-analysis of short-term trials (41), risperidone and olanzapine may offer superior efficacy in symptom domains as compared to traditional agents while the other atypical antipsychotics may provide long-term benefits in other domains of adverse effects and neurocognition. More long-term comparative trials are needed to discern true efficacy differences among the atypical antipsychotic medications.

IV. NONADHERENCE AND RISK FOR RELAPSE

Long-term goals of antipsychotic treatment include preventing the onset of acute episodes of psychosis and to maintain positive symptom treatment at current levels. Negative symptoms and cognitive deficits generally remain after a psychotic episode. Thus, these also become a focus of long-term rehabilitation. Yet, inevitably relapses are common during the course of schizophrenia. Weiden and Olfson (175) estimated that the average relapse rate on conventional antipsychotics was 3.5% per month, thus resulting in a 42% annual relapse rate. Many studies have shown that the most powerful predictor of relapse and rehospitalization is nonadherence with drug treatment (42–45).

People with schizophrenia are often known to be noncompliant with medication. Side effects, lack of insight, and belief that the mediation is ineffective all contribute to nonadherence with therapy. Specific factors have predicted higher rates of nonadherence. Older, grandiose, substance abusing, and deficit subjects have more difficulty with adherence. Adherence is difficult to quantify, measure, and study because adherence is rarely an all-or-none phenomenon, but may include mistakes in dosing, timing, omitting doses, or taking medications that are not prescribed. Estimates of nonadherence on traditional antipsychotics range from approximately 24% to 88% with a mean of approximately 50% of people with schizophrenia who are noncompliant with prescribed therapy (1). Subjects who are noncompliant have approximately a four-fold greater risk of a relapse than those who are compliant. Physicians often overestimate the adherence of their subjects which, in turn, does not allow them to consider nonadherence as a likely explanation for treatment failures.

Between 25% and 66% of subjects who discontinue prescribed antipsychotic therapy cite adverse effects as the primary reason for nonadherence (46) (Table 1). Both self- and physician ratings of side effects are associated with higher rates of nonadherence. Extrapyramidal side effects, most notably akathisia, sexual dysfunction, and weight gain are the adverse effects that lead to the greatest nonadherence (47). Atypical antipsychotic drugs are associated with better rates of adherence most likely attributable to better side effect profiles (40). This leads to lower rates of relapse and rehospitalization, improving subject care and reducing overall costs (48). Yet while pharmacy prescription data have found higher rates of adherence with atypical antipsychotics as compared to rates with

Table 1 Variables Related to Nonadherence

Subject-related factors	1) Greater illness severity or grandiosity
	2) Lack of insight
	3) Substance abuse comorbidity
Medication-related factors	1) Dysphoric medication side effects
	2) Subtherapeutic or excessively high doses
Environmental factors	1) Inadequate support or supervision
	2) Practical barriers, such as lack of money or transportation
Clinician-related factors	1) Poor therapeutic alliance

conventionals, it appears that 45% of subjects may continue to be nonadherent (49). A good relationship between the subject and the physician is important to establish rapport and trust, the groundwork for enhancing the subject's acceptance of the therapy. Subject and family education, including expectations and potential adverse effects, is important. The emergent of adverse events should be taken seriously and treated immediately. While in multiepisode subjects long-term continuous maintenance treatment appears to offer the best benefits, first-episode subjects may benefit from intermittent treatment; however, more studies are needed in this area (50).

V. REHOSPITALIZATION RATES

Avoiding hospital readmission is important for improving the lives of people with schizophrenia. The decision to readmit subjects usually indicates symptomatology or behavior that can no longer be safely managed in the community or is intolerable outside of an institutional setting. Atypical antipsychotics were developed to provide more effective and tolerable treatments for those who suffer from schizophrenia. The benefits of these medications include higher rates of adherence which can improve long-term outcomes by decreasing relapse and rehospitalization.

The estimated annual risk of rehospitalization with the use of atypical antipsychotics in the United States has ranged from 13% to 20%. A 20% relapse rate was reported for olanzapine as compared to 28% for haloperidol at 1 year (51). Previously reported data examining outcomes of risperidone's first year of release found a 17% rehospitalization risk at 1 year following discharge (52). Conley et al. (52) and Essock et al. (9) reported risks of rehospitalization with clozapine of 13% and 18%, respectively. These are all lower than the previously published risks of 28–50% with traditional oral agents (9,51,53). A recent report from Israel examining rehospitalization for 2 years following discharge found the rehospitalization risk with atypical antipsychotics to be significantly lower than those with conventional antipsychotics (31–33% vs. 48%). This separation was evident even in a chronically ill population of subjects that had failed at least two previous antipsychotic trials (54). Other recent work has estimated the annual risk of rehospitalization to be 10%, 12%, and 13% for chronic subjects treated with clozapine, risperidone, and olanzapine, respectively. In contrast those treated with fluphenazine and haloperidol decanoate had estimated risks of 21% and 35%, respectively (55). These studies have demonstrated that the risk of hospital readmission with atypical antipsychotics is clinically and significantly lower than with traditional antipsychotics, most likely due to the increases in medication adherence. Service utilization of outpatient resources has not been shown to be increased in subjects on atypical antipsychotics and, in fact, the atypicals in general are most likely cost-effective as compared to conventional antipsychotics (56).

VI. LONG-TERM SAFETY

The emergence of chlorpromazine and the other conventional antipsychotics sparked a revolution in the treatment of schizophrenia by improving symptoms. These improvements, however came at the price of severe and potentially disabling adverse effects. Extrapyramidal side effects (EPS) commonly occurred with treatment while persistent disfigurement and mannerisms from tardive dyskinesia (TD) were caused by treatment with first-generation antipsychotic (FGA) medications. Atypical antipsychotics have rapidly changed the face of schizophrenia treatment. Great excitement surrounded the new class of medications as rates of EPS were low and very few cases of TD were occurring. Since their introduction, the atypical antipsychotics have moved fairly quickly into first-line treatment while initially one of the only limitations to routine use has been their high drug costs.

Recently, because of expanded use of the atypical antipsychotics, much literature with regards to weight gain and related consequences during treatment has emerged. Newer medications have real advantages in regard to the production of extrapyramidal symptoms, but the overall safety of these drugs is now coming under close scrutiny. The reemergence of debilitating long-term consequences of weight gain has the potential to surpass the problems of EPS and TD if these problems are not studied and addressed. Metabolic disturbances of long-term antipsychotic treatment may lead to morbidities such as cardiovascular disease, cancer, osteo-arthritis, type 2 diabetes, and early death. Other issues may affect long-term adherence and safety such as prolactin-related effects and changes in the QTc interval. All of these adverse effects will be discussed in regards to their known or potential effects during long-term treatment.

A. Weight Gain

In the United States, one-half of adults are currently overweight (body-mass index (BMI) 25 kg/m^2) and a fifth of the population is considered to be obese (BMI 30 kg/m^2). BMI among people with schizophrenia, however, exceeds the general population estimates. Many psychiatric patients, including those with schizophrenia have sedentary lifestyles with little exercise as well as potentially already being predisposed to metabolic effects associated with weight gain. Obesity in general increases the risk for a myriad of medical disorders such as hypertension, stroke, cancer, diabetes, and atherosclerosis. People with schizophrenia exhibit high relative rates of smoking and drug abuse and have several medical disorders that also compound the high rates of morbidity and mortality seen in this population (57).

Many short-term studies describe weight gain among people taking various antipsychotic agents. The most comprehensive report to date is a meta-analysis of over 80 studies. Weight gain is highly variable among antipsychotics, however, two atypical antipsychotics, olanzapine and clozapine, clearly appear to be associated with the highest degree of weight gain (4–4.5 kg over 10 weeks) (58).

Several reports describe the effects of long-term clozapine treatment on body weight. Hummer et al. (59) reported that after 1 year of clozapine treatment 36% of subjects gained more than 10% of their initial body weight with the average being about 3.5 kg. A 5-year naturalistic study examined the records of 83 outpatients with schizophrenia or schizoaffective disorder. Subjects were noted to experience significant weight gain that continued until approximately month 46 from initiation of treatment with clozapine (60). Another study examined 93 treatment-resistant subjects that were weighed monthly for 4 months during clozapine treatment. Subjects gained an average of 2.4 kg in body weight with the subjects with the lowest BMI demonstrating the greatest weight gains (61). Another 1-year open-label study found gains of 5.8 kg over 1 year with clozapine (62). Long-term comparative studies are lacking for clozapine treatment, however. In one study, 96 neuroleptic-resistant chronic schizophrenia subjects were compared on BMI changes during treatment with either clozapine or conventional antipsychotics for an average of 1.8 years. This group concluded that weight gain was similar between drug groups during long-term treatment (63). Significant weight gain also is widely known to occur with olanzapine treatment. Olanzapine weight gains at doses of 12.5–17.5 mg/day have been found to average 12 kg after 1 year of use (64). Kinon et al. (65) reported mean weight gains after 1.05 years of 6.3 kg. This number is most likely conservative as it was reported in an intent to treat design. Weight gain with olanzapine appears to peak after 40 weeks of treatment and may be greater than gains associated with clozapine treatment (66). Weight gain with risperidone appears to plateau early on and remain at about 2–3 kg at 1 year. A long-term flexible-dose comparative study of risperidone and haloperidol reported a mean increase in weight of 2.3 kg in risperidone-treated subjects which was significantly greater than haloperidol over 52 weeks (17). Studies on long-term quetiapine treatment have reported weight gains of approximately 1–2 kg over at least 1 year (67,68). Ziprasidone is associated with no or minimal (1 kg) weight gain in subjects followed for up to 1 year (34,36). Aripiprazole is associated with about 1 kg weight gains in subjects treated for 6–12 months (39). Most data imply that weight gain is generally not dose dependent with the atypical antipsychotics and that subjects with low BMIs may gain the most weight.

B. Glucose Dysregulation

Metabolic disturbances, particularly impaired glucose metabolism were first described in psychotic subjects prior to the introduction of antipsychotic medications. The risk for type 2 diabetes mellitus (DM) is also known to be higher in schizophrenia subjects than in the general population. In addition, antipsychotic medications are associated with impaired glucose metabolism, exacerbation of existing type 1 and 2 diabetes, new-onset type 2 diabetes mellitus, and diabetic ketoacidosis (DKA). Possible consequences of DM include retinopathy, cataracts, infection, neuropathy, kidney failure, and circulatory disorders. Clozapine and olanzapine have been implicated as having the highest likelihood of DM occurring. Abdominal or central adiposity may contribute to glucose dysregulation. However, DM may occur with olanzapine and clozapine independent of weight change. The incidence of DM, glucose dysregulation as well as risk factors in a schizophrenia population on antipsychotics have not been well characterized.

The best description of long-term effects of clozapine on glucose dysregulation and the occurrence of DM perhaps is the 5-year naturalistic study by Henderson et al. (60). During the follow-up, 43 of 82 subjects (52%) experienced elevated fasting blood glucose greater than 140 mg/dl and 25 of 82 subjects (31%) were diagnosed with adult-onset type 2 diabetes mellitus by primary care physicians. Age was found to be a risk factor for developing type 2 diabetes, while family history, dose, and weight change were not found to be risk factors. Olanzapine treatment has also been associated with diabetes. Many studies and case reports exist for olanzapine while none to few case reports exist for risperidone, quetiapine, ziprasidone and aripiprazole (69–75). Furthermore, a recent population-based nested case-control study of approximately 20,000 schizophrenia subjects found those taking olanzapine to have a significantly increased risk of developing diabetes than those taking conventional antipsychotics (odds ratio 4.2). Risperidone treatment was found to have a slightly elevated but nonsignificant risk as compared to conventional antipsychotic treatment (odds ratio 1.6) (76). Koller et al. (77,78) have recently published epidemiological reports detailing both spontaneously reported cases of DM that have been reported to the U.S. FDA's MedWatch Drug Surveillance

System and published case reports through the spring of 2001. For clozapine, 384 reports were identified, most occurring within 6 months of initiation. Eighty cases of DKA were reported for clozapine and 25 deaths occurred during hyperglycemic episodes. Likewise there were 237 cases of DM reported for olanzapine with 80 patients experiencing DKA and death in 15 patients. With both these medications, improvements in glycemic control were evident in most cases once they were discontinued.

C. Hyperlipidemia

Increases in plasma lipid levels have been noted with the phenothiazines but negligible effects on lipids have occurred with the higher potency agents such as haloperidol. Early on, clozapine use was noted to have a profound increase in serum triglycerides as well as small increases in total cholesterol levels (79). Henderson et al. (60) found that over 60 months mean triglyceride levels increased from 175 mg/dl to approximately 400 mg/dl. They also noted a slight but nonsignificant increase in serum cholesterol levels. Studies have also suggested that olanzapine use is associated with the development of hyperlipidemia. A report by Sheitman et al. (80) suggested that olanzapine treatment may result in marked increases in triglyceride levels for some subjects. Another cohort study of 25 inpatients treated with olanzapine for 12 weeks showed a mean increase of 60 mg/dl in fasting triglycerides (81). Others have also reported significant increases in triglycerides during longer-term treatment (75,82). In a recent study using the U.K.-based General Practice Research Database, the prescription of olanzapine was associated with a statistically significant four-fold increase in the odds of developing hyperlipidemias compared to those not prescribed antipsychotics. No significant increase was noted for risperidone in the sample of approximately 20,000 (83). In a recent 1-year study, triglyceride levels significantly increased by 104.8 mg/dl in subjects treated with olanzapine while small increases (31.7 mg/dl) were noted for risperidone (84). A few cases of high triglyceride levels have been reported with quetiapine (82). Aripiprazole appears to have neutral effects on triglycerides and total cholesterol levels, however long-term studies on lipid changes are lacking (85).

D. Prolactin-Related Adverse Effects/Sexual Dysfunction

While there may be many contributing factors leading to sexual dysfunction, the evidence for elevated prolactin levels contributing to sexual dysfunction is convincing (86–90). The atypical antipsychotics as a class vary in their propensity to cause prolactin elevations and very little long-term data are available. Direct correlations between prolactin levels and sexual dysfunction have not been firmly established, however rating instruments have not been systematically used. In addition to sexual disturbances, other potential long-term consequences of elevated prolactin may include osteoporosis and breast cancer, however more research is needed in this area (91–93).

Clozapine has a low propensity to block dopamine in the tuber-infundibular pathway and has a negligible effect on plasma prolactin levels (94). Sexual function during clozapine treatment has been comparatively better than during treatment with conventional antipsychotics (95–98). This relatively low incidence of sexual problems may be due to its prolactin-sparing effects. Case reports of priapism and impotence with clozapine have been reported and are likely related to alpha adrenergic and muscarinic blockade as opposed to being related to hyperprolactinemia (99).

Of all the atypical antipsychotics, risperidone has the highest propensity to elevate plasma prolactin levels and does so in a dose-related fashion (100). Mean prolactin levels at doses at 3 mg are about 27 ng/ml, significantly higher than olanzapine or clozapine (94). Studies, that have actively questioned patients have produced fairly high rates of prolactin-related effects as menstrual changes were reported to occur in 24% of patients treated with risperidone as compared to 20% with olanzapine (101). A recent retrospective chart review reported a significantly higher proportion of sexual dysfunction with risperidone as compared to haloperidol and clozapine (98) and other prospective comparative studies have found higher rates of both sexual dysfunction and reproductive side effects with risperidone as compared to olanzapine, quetiapine, and haloperidol (102). Additionally, several case reports in the literature describe sexual dysfunction during risperidone treatment. For male patients, reports describe gynecomastia (103–105), galactorrhea (104), ejaculatory difficulties (103,106,107), and priapism (108,109) occurring with risperidone treatment. For women, menstrual irregularities are the most commonly reported and have occurred at doses as low as 1 mg/day. Amenorrhea and galactorrhea are also reported to occur with fairly low doses of risperidone (110,111).

Olanzapine causes transient elevations in plasma prolactin levels. During treatment in adults prolactin levels remain slightly elevated in about a third of patients (112). Elevation of prolactin appears to be a dose-related phenomenon (113). Mean prolactin levels during 10–30 mg daily treatment with olanzapine are approximately 17 ng/ml, which is higher than that of normal, drug-free patients and clozapine-treated patients (114). This same study found levels with haloperidol to be about twice the level of olanzapine. Possibly because of olanzapine's lower propensity to elevate prolactin, few case reports have been published with regards to sexual dysfunction and menstrual changes. Rates of sexual dysfunction in studies actively questioning patients have been reported between 30–35% (101,102). At least seven case reports have discussed cases of priapism occurring with olanzapine treatment which may be due to the alpha and muscarinic blockade of this medication (99).

Quetiapine has negligible effects on the elevation of prolactin. In all of the large trials of quetiapine, prolactin levels were reported to decrease from baseline to endpoint during quetiapine treatment and no differences were noted between quetiapine and placebo (115–118). In over 2000 patients treated with quetiapine, menstrual changes occurred in less than 1% of patients treated (119). One case of priapism occurring with a quetiapine overdose has been reported and was postulated to be secondary to alpha1 antagonism (120). Impotence, abnormal ejaculation, and amenorrhea were reported in pivotal trials to occur in less than 0.1% of patients (121). Quetiapine in a recent comparative trial had the lowest risk of sexual dysfunction (18%) as compared to rates of 35–43% in patients on risperidone, olanzapine, and haloperidol. Of these medications, quetiapine may also have the lowest propensity for reproductive side effects (<3%) (102).

Very little data are available pertaining to either plasma prolactin levels or sexual functioning with ziprasidone. It appears that slight elevations may occur with ziprasidone. In a double-blind study prolactin levels were approximately 19 ng/ml and 60 ng/ml for ziprasidone and risperidone treatment respectively at the end of 52 weeks (122). Impotence, abnormal ejaculation, amenorrhea, galactorrhea, and anorgasmia occurred in premarketing studies infrequently (<0.1%). One case of priapism in premarketing trials was reported (121) and only a few case reports have been reported in the literature (123,124).

Serum prolactin levels during treatment trials with aripiprazole have been found to decrease from baseline across all dose ranges. Levels decreased by about 7 ng/ml during short-term trials (125) and are similar to placebo (<15 ng/ml). This remains fairly consistent across longer-term trials. The lack of increased prolactin levels may be explained by aripiprazole's partial agonism at D_2 receptors, in contrast to the D_2 antagonism of other atypical antipsychotics. Sexual dysfunction was infrequently reported in clinical trials as noted in product labeling. More studies are needed to specifically address prolactin and sexual dysfunction with aripiprazole.

E. Tardive Dyskinesia

Tardive dyskinesia (TD) is a syndrome characterized by abnormal chorei-form (rapid, objective, purposeless, irregular, and spontaneous movement) and athetoid (slow and irregular) movements occurring late in onset in relation to initiation of antipsychotic therapy. This adverse effect usually develops over several months and occurs after at least 3 months of conventional antipsychotic treatment. The estimated average prevalence is 20% with a range of 13–36%. The incidence of new cases per treatment year is approximately 5%. TD is reversible in one-third to one-half of cases with the cessation of the antipsychotic. When the antipsychotic is tapered or discontinued, there is usually worsening of abnormal movements initially. Risk factors include older age, duration of antipsychotic treatment, higher rates of EPS, substance abuse, and mood disorders.

The characteristic signs and symptoms usually involve bucco-lingual-masticatory syndrome or orofacial movements. Typically, these are the first detectable signs of TD and can progress to movements severe enough to interfere with chewing, speech, respiration, or swallowing. These include lip smacking, puckering, sucking, pouting, tongue writhing, protrusion, and tremor. Other facial movements include frequent blinking, grimacing, and tics. Trunctal and limb movements usually are seen as TD progresses. This includes twisting, spreading, flexion and extension of the fingers, and toe dorsiflexion. Unusual posture, hyperextension, pelvic thrusting, exaggerated lordosis (bending backward), rocking, and swaying may all occur in the trunctal area. Younger adults report more trunctal movements while older adults experience more orofacial movements (126).

Clozapine treatment has not been shown to cause tardive dyskinesia. In fact, improvements in choreic and athetoid movements are seen with long-term clozapine treatment (126). Cases of discontinuation and dose reduction of clozapine, however, have reported the reemergence of preexisting tardive dyskinesia (127,128). Olanzapine, risperidone, and quetiapine have all been implicated in a few case reports to both treat preexisting tardive dyskinesia and cause this adverse effect (129). The incidence, however, with all of the atypical antipsychotic medications appears to be minimal and much lower than the risk on traditional antipsychotics. Beasley et al. (130) published a double-blind comparison of olanzapine and haloperidol in over 1600 subjects for up to 2.6 years. The relative risk of TD over 1 year was 7.5% with haloperidol and 0.5% with olanzapine. In two long-term studies of risperidone in elderly adults the risk of spontaneous TD was less than 1% (23,131). Long-term studies are not available for quetiapine, ziprasidone, or apripiprazole, however, the risk appears to be low with all the newer antipsychotics.

F. Effects on the QTc Interval

Psychotropic agents can cause a wide variety of effects which impact on the cardiovascular system. Among the most serious cardiac complications that have been associated with psychotropic medication use is the arrhythmia known as Torsades de Pointes (TdP). This potentially fatal polymorphic ventricular arrhythmia may occur in patients who have a lengthening of the QTc interval.

The QT interval is the period extending from the beginning of depolarization (QRS complex) to the end of repolarization (T wave) of the ventricles. The QT interval is shorter with faster heart rates and longer with slower heart rates. Therefore, a correction for rate (the corrected QT or QTc) is applied to make the reporting of the interval more meaningful. QTc intervals are generally considered to be prolonged if they are greater than 450 msec in males or 470 msec in females. In either gender, QTc prolongation greater than 500 msec may place a patient at higher risk for TdP (132,133). Recently, the effects of antipsychotic drugs on the QTc have received great attention. In a large study, Reilly et al. reported that droperidol and thioridazine were the most likely to cause QTc prolongation out of 20 classes of psychotropic medications studied (134). Furthermore, TdP has been reported to occur in patients receiving most of the conventional antipsychotic medications.

Several of the atypical antipsychotics were compared to haloperidol and thioridazine for QTc changes in a study presented to the FDA prior to the approval of ziprasidone (135). The mean change at steady state in the QTc for thioridazine, using Bazett's correction, was the most significant (35.6 msec). Ziprasidone prolonged the interval by an average of 20.3 msec, quetiapine by 14.5 msec, risperidone by 11.6 msec, and olanzapine by 6.8 msec. Those treated with haloperidol had a mean increase of 4.7 msec at steady state. Very little long-term safety data is currently available assessing QTc changes, however the risk of sudden death and TdP is extremely low. One case of sudden death has been reported for risperidone (136) and significant QTc prolongations have been reported rarely for quetiapine, ziprasidone and olanzapine but generally in high- or overdose situations (137–141). Although clozapine has been associated with cardiomyopathy, unique to this antipsychotic, the risk for QTc prolongation is low. A review of the global Novartis databases, which consisted of 2.8 million patient-years, demonstrated that at therapeutic doses clozapine is rarely associated with a prolongation in the QTc interval (142). Of all the atypical antipsychotics, ziprasidone is associated with the greatest prolongation in QTc and it is recommended not to coadminister this medication with other agents, which may prolong the QTc such as quinidine, pimozide, sotolol, thioridazine, moxifloxacin, and sparfloxacin.

Metabolic inhibitors with ziprasidone have not been studied during long-term use. Ketoconazole (400 mg/day), a potent CYP3A4 inhibitor, administered with ziprasidone (40 mg/day) in short-term studies was found to increase the steady state mean plasma concentrations of ziprasidone by 34%. The mean plasma concentration of the M9 metabolite, thought to have both therapeutic activity and an effect on the QTc was increased by 59% (143). This is postulated to be secondary to a shift in metabolism towards aldehyde oxidase, the enzyme responsible for production of the M9 metabolite. While the sample size was small ($N = 14$) and only descriptively reported, there appeared to be more adverse events seen with the combination of ziprasidone and ketoconazole (71%) than with ziprasidone and placebo (30%). Dizziness was reported in 36% of those receiving both drugs versus 8% receiving ziprasidone alone. No data for QTc changes were included other than the mention that no prolongation greater than 500 msec occurred and no treatment-emergent or significant changes in laboratory measures of vital signs were encountered. Erythromycin, another commonly used CYP450 specific inhibitor, has not been systematically studied for concomitant use with ziprasidone. Even when employed alone macrolide antibiotics can prolong QTc intervals by blocking K^+ channels. However, this effect most often occurs with high doses or intravenous administration (144,145). However, cases of TdP have been reported both for erythromycin and clarithromycin when used alone (146). Other considerations for using drugs that may prolong the QTc include metabolic abnormalities (hypokalemia, hypomagnesia, hypothyroidism, hypocalcemia), female gender, hyperglycemia, alcoholism, bradycardia, and cardiac disease (myocarditis, heart failure, myocardial ischemia or infarction, rheumatic fever, or mitral valve prolapse) (147,148). Also, low-energy diets, consumption of a large meal, obesity, Parkinson's disease, liver disease, or renal insufficiency (147,149,150). Patients with diabetes may be at an additional risk as QTc intervals appear to be significantly associated with fasting glucose (148). In fact, even acute hyperglycemia induced in healthy adults can produce significant increases in the QTc (151). Despite the higher propensity to prolong the QTc, ziprasidone has not yet been linked to cases of TdP and has only been rarely reported to be associated with elevations in the QTc interval in excess of 500 msec.

VII. DOSING ISSUES

Although the establishment of appropriate dosage ranges for antipsychotics has important ramifications both for short-term treatment and long-term therapeutic outcomes, difficulties in dosing persist. Since the introduction of chlorpromazine in the 1950s, clinicians and researchers have utilized a variety of methods to determine the appropriate dosage ranges for antipsychotics. These methods have remained somewhat unsatisfactory.

Decades after the introduction of antipsychotics, optimal dosage ranges remain controversial with prescribed doses of these agents varying from 25 to 7000 mg/day chlorpromazine equivalents (152). The subjective nature of psychiatric symptoms, difficulties in diagnosis, and the lack of simple physiologic correlates of response (such as blood pressure or blood glucose levels) further complicate dosing.

Appropriate dosing for the atypical antipsychotics similarly has been difficult to establish (153). There is no clear biochemical model, such as dopamine-D_2-receptor occupancy, to help establish appropriate clinical dosing for these drugs. Also, as these drugs have substantially fewer and less prominent extrapyramidal side effects, with the exception of risperidone (154), there is no longer a natural barrier to the use of excessive doses. Furthermore, therapeutic effects of these agents may be confused with lack of effectiveness. When individuals are switched to these agents from conventional antipsychotics, families, support staff, and even clinicians may interpret increased vocalization, improvements in motivation and socialization, and higher activity levels as agitation, anxiety, or excitement, and consider increasing the dose.

The current dosing recommendations for atypical antipsychotics originate from doses used in initial clinical efficacy trials. These efficacy trials of 6 to 8 weeks tend to focus on a carefully selected group of acutely psychotic individuals with few or limited comorbid disorders. Subjects are often excluded if they require concomitant medications, especially other psychoactive agents. Furthermore, long-term follow-up studies in naturalistic populations are rarely conducted and are generally not available prior to marketing. Efficacy trials may not reflect how people in "real-world" clinical settings will be treated or will respond to treatment. Hence, dosing recommendations based on stringent efficacy trials may not adequately reflect the most effective doses.

Risperidone is a prime example of a drug whose dosage recommendation and initial product labeling conflicted with its use in the real-world. The first multicenter studies of risperidone displayed a dose–efficacy curve that appeared to peak at 6 mg/day (155). This same trial reported an increasing risk of EPS as the dose increased above 6 mg/day. Thus, the manufacturer recommended administering risperidone 1 mg BID on day one, 2 mg BID on the second day and 3 mg BID on the third day. Although the routine dosing titration was recommended to 6 mg/day, product labeling listed the maximum dosage as 16 mg/day, supported by the observation of a few responders at higher levels. However, these pivotal studies examined only a few widely spaced dosage levels, 2 mg, 6 mg, 10 mg, and 16 mg daily.

In the years since risperidone's introduction, many clinicians have recognized that routine titration to 6 mg/day in 3 days is not appropriate for most people. A European multicenter study of 1362 subjects reported risperidone to have a bell-shaped dose–response curve peaking at about 4 mg/day for its therapeutic effects (156). The greater effectiveness of lower dosing has been since demonstrated in numerous observational studies and clinical trials (101,157–160) and mean maintenance dosing in the United States is currently around 4–5 mg/day.

The clinical benefits of olanzapine have been demonstrated at doses generally between 10 and 20 mg/day. In the pivotal trials doses of 10 and 15 mg/day were significantly more effective than placebo while the 15 mg/day also appeared to be numerically superior to the lower doses (161). These results combined with other fixed dose studies have shown that there is a significant linear trend between increasing olanzapine dose and greater clinical improvement (162). Plasma concentrations have not been routinely found to predict response, however one recent report found olanzapine plasma concentrations in excess of 23.2 ng/ml to predict therapeutic response (163). Males require a higher olanzapine dose to reach this threshold concentration than do females (163,164). Although olanzapine is commonly used in doses exceeding 20 mg/day, the efficacy and safety have not been extensively studied in clinical trials. In a recent 14-week double-blind trial approximately 40 subjects were assigned to receive 20 mg/day of olanzapine. After the initial 8 weeks subjects then received a variable dose of the antipsychotic. The mean dose after the period of fixed dosing was 30 mg/day and some subjects were noted to improve at doses of 30–40 mg/day (66). While olanzapine dosing is gravitating upwards and a few studies have reported greater benefits of this drug at higher dosing, results of treatment-resistant studies have not confirmed the superiority of higher doses and side effects may be more prominent (165,166).

Appropriate clozapine dosing is associated with therapeutic response. The manufacturer's recommended target dose is 300–450 mg/day. The initial dose is much lower and is increased gradually over several days to minimize adverse effects. Plasma levels greater than 350 ng/ml have been found to be associated with the greatest likelihood of response (167). This plasma concentration usually corresponds to doses of 300–500 mg/day. Maintenance treatment has been achieved with once-daily doses for long-term treatment. If dosing is interrupted, retitration is necessary.

Optimal dosing for quetiapine, ziprasidone, and aripiprazole is not well established. In the registration trial for quetiapine maximal effects were demonstrated at 300 mg day (168). It appears, however, that doses of at least 300 mg are associated with the greatest efficacy as a mean dose of 209 mg in another study was not superior to placebo (169). In subjects with chronic schizophrenia, a greater response was noted for efficacy at doses of 600 mg/day as compared to haloperidol (170). While plasma concentrations have not been useful for response, higher doses (>300 mg/day) may be needed to maximize response. Ziprasidone also, may be useful in higher doses as registration trials have shown greatest benefits at doses greater than 120 mg/day (171,172). Doses greater than 200 mg/day, however, have not been systematically evaluated. Ziprasidone should be given with meals to maximize drug absorption. Aripiprazole dosing is recommended in a range of 10–30 mg/day while doses of greater than 15 mg may have the greatest efficacy (125).

Long-term use and dosing in real-world settings also provide clues to the optimal doses that clinicians are using for actual treatment. In the New York State Mental Health system, dosing above package labeling has continued to drop for clozapine and risperidone while dosing is being escalated for olanzapine and quetiapine (152). More studies are needed to determine the most appropriate dosing for long-term treatment.

VIII. SUGGESTED GUIDELINES FOR CLINICIANS

Owing to the severity and chronicity of schizophrenia, people will most likely be on lifelong treatment with antipsychotic medications. While outcomes for treatment are better with atypical antipsychotics as compared to traditional agents, many considerations will surround both acute and maintenance treatment of these medications. Little is currently available in the literature to assist clinicians in long-term treatment, however some recent suggested guidelines are available (107,108,174).

1. Atypical antipsychotics, other than clozapine should be selected before conventional antipsychotics for people experiencing first-episode schizophrenia or for subjects whose history of response to antipsychotics is not available.
2. An adequate trial for atypical antipsychotics is 4 weeks. If patients demonstrate a partial response to atypical antipsychotics at 4 weeks, a trial of 12 weeks may be beneficial.
3. Clozapine is the most effective antipsychotic for treatment-refractory people. Clinicians should assess a person's response to at least one other atypical antipsychotic before beginning clozapine.
4. For subjects who are nonadherent, depot or atypical antipsychotics should be considered first-line treatment.
5. Subjects who demonstrate continued aggressive behavior should be considered for clozapine treatment.
6. Monitoring for metabolic adverse effects is recommended as shown in Table 2.

Table 2 Suggested Monitoring of Atypical Antipsychotics for Metabolic Side Effects

	BP/pulse	Weight	Fasting blood glucose	Cholesterol/triglycerides	EPS
Clozapine	Every visit until stable	Every visit for 6M; then q 3M	BL; 3M, 6M[a]; if weight gain >7% then q 1 yr	BL; 3M[a]; if weight gain >7% then q 1 yr	BL; q 1 yr
Olanzapine	BL; q 1 yr	Same as above	Same as above	Same as above	BL, every visit as long as a problem; then q 1 yr
Risperidone	BL; q 1 yr	Same as above	Same as above	Same as above	same as above
Quetiapine	Every visit until stable then q 1 yr	Same as above	Same as above	Same as above	BL; q 1 yr
Ziprasidone	BL; q 1 yr	BL; 3M, q 1 yr	Same as above	Same as above	BL, every visit as long as a problem; then q 1 yr

BL = baseline, **BP** = blood pressure, M = months, q = repetition interval, yr = year.
[a]3M and 6M glucose added as new literature provides evidence of glucose dysregulation and hyperlipidemia independent of weight gain.
Source: Adapted from Ref. 173.

7. Monitoring for tardive dyskinesia should occur at baseline and annually with atypical antipsychotics.
8. Baseline and follow-up EKGs are indicated when there is a suspicion of cardiac conditions or concomitant medications that could be prolonging the QTc, particularly in the case of ziprasidone.

IX. SUMMARY

While long-term prognosis for schizophrenia remains poor, significant benefits may occur with the treatment of atypical antipsychotics. The incidence of side effects and relapse rates are notably lower with this newer class of medications. Adherence to therapy may be increased and these benefits may provide for better overall subject satisfaction and outcomes. This class of antipsychotics differs significantly among agents most prominently with regards to the side effect profiles and potential long-term health outcomes associated with use. Thus, careful attention should be paid to selection and monitoring of these medications, which will most likely be utilized for the long term.

REFERENCES

1. Weiden P, Aquila R. Standard J: Atypical antipsychotic drugs and long-term outcome in schizophrenia. J Clin Psychiatry 1996; 57:53–60.
2. Lehman AF. Evaluating outcomes of treatments for persons with psychotic disorders. J Clin Psychiatry 1996; 57(suppl 11):61–67.
3. Zito JM. Pharmacoeconomics of the new antipsychotics for the treatment of schizophrenia. Psychiatric Clin North Amer 1998; 21(1):181–202.
4. Conley RR. Evaluating clinical trial data: outcome measures. J Clin Psychiatry 2001; 62 (suppl 9):23–26.
5. Dixon LB, Lehman AF, Levine J. Conventional antipsychotic medications for schizophrenia. Schizophrenia Bull 1995; 2(4): 567–577.
6. Lindenmayer JP, Grochowski S, Mabugat L. Clozapine effects on positive and negative symptoms: a six-month trial in treatment-refractory schizophrenics. J Clin Psychopharmacol 1994; 14:201–204.
7. Brier A, Buchanan RW, Irish D, Carpenter WT Jr. Clozapine treatment of outpatients with schizophrenia: outcome and long-term response patterns. Hosp Community Psychiatry 1993; 44:1145–1149.
8. Pollack S, Woerner MG, Howard A, Fireworker RB, Kane JM. Clozapine reduces hospitalization among schizophrenia patients. Psychopharmacol Bull 1998; 34:89–92.

9. Essock SM, Hargreaves WA, Covell NH, Goethe J. Clozapine's effectiveness for patients in state hospitals: results from a randomized trial. Psychopharmacol Bull 1996; 32:683–697.

10. Buchanan RW, Holstein C, Brier A. The comparative efficacy and long-term effect of clozapine treatment on neuropsychological test performance. Biol Psychiatry 1994; 36:717–725.

11. Joffe G, Vanalainen E, Tupala J, Hiltunen O, Wahlbeck K, Gadeke R, Rimon R. The effect of clozapine on the course of illness in chronic schizophrenia: focus on treatment outcomes in out-patients. Int Clin Psychopharmacol 1996; 11:265–272.

12. Rosenheck R, Cramer J, Xu W, Thomas J, Henderson W, Frisman L, Fye C, Charney D. A comparison of clozapine and haloperidol in hospitalized patients with refractory schizophrenia. Department of Veterans Affairs Cooperative Study Group on Clozapine in Refractory Schizophrenia. N Engl J Med 1997; 337:809–815.

13. Essock SM, Frisman LK, Covell NH, Hargreaves WA. Cost-effectiveness of clozapine compared with conventional antipsychotic medication for patients in state hospitals. Arch Gen Psychiatry 2000; 57:987–994.

14. Conley RR, Carpenter WT Jr, Tamminga CA. Time to clozapine response in a standardized trial. Am J Psychiatry 1997; 154:1243–1247.

15. Ciapparelli A, Dell'Osso L, Pini S, Chiavacci MC, Fenzi M, Cassano GB. Clozapine for treatment-refractory schizophrenia, schizoaffective disorder, and psychotic bipolar disorder: a 24-month naturalistic study. J Clin Psychiatry 2000; 61:329–334.

16. Mattes JA. Clozapine for refractory schizophrenia: an open study of 14 patients treated up to 2 years. J Clin Psychiatry 1989; 50:389–391.

17. Csernansky JG, Mahmoud R, Brenner R, the risperidone USA-79 study group. A comparison of risperidone and haloperidol for the prevention of relapse in patients with schizophrenia. N Engl J Med 2002; 346:16–22.

18. Bouchard RH, Merette C, Pourcher E, Demers MF, Villeneuve J, Roy-Gagnon MH, Gauthier Y, Cliche D, Labelle A, Filteau MJ, Roy MA, Maziade M. J Clin Psychopharmacol 2000; 20:295–304.

19. Malla AK, Norman RM, Scholten DJ, Zirul S, Kotteda V. A comparison of long-term outcome in first-episode schizophrenia following treatment with risperidone or a typical antipsychotic. J Clin Psychiatry 2001; 62:179–184.

20. Moller HJ, Gagiano CA, Addington DE, Von Knorring L, Torres-Plank JF, Gaussares C. Long-term treatment of chronic schizophrenia with risperidone: an open-label, multicenter study of 286 patients. Int Clin Psychopharmacol 1998; 13:99–106.

21. Gutierrez Fraile M, Segarra Echevarria R, Gonzalez-Pinto Arrillaga A, Martinez Junquera G. Risperidone in the early treatment of first-episode psychosis: a two-year follow-up study. Actas Esp Psiquiatr 2002; 30:142–152.

22. Udina Abello C, Roca Bennasar M, Octavio Del Valle I. Long-term relapse prevention with risperidone in 215 schizophrenic patients. Acta Esp Psiquiatr 2001; 29:243–249.

23. Davidson M, Harvey PD, Vervarcke J, Gagiano CA, De Hooge JD, Bray G, Dose M, Barak Y, Haushofer M. A long-term, multicenter, open-label study of risperidone in elderly patients with psychosis. Int J Geriatr Psychiatry 2000; 15:506–514.

24. Malla AK, Norman RM, Kotteda V, Zirul S. Switching from therapy with typical antipsychotic agents to risperidone: long-term impact on patient outcome. Clin Ther 1999; 21:806–817.

25. Kane J, Gharabawi G, Bossie CA, Zhu Y, Lasser R. Effect of novel long-acting antipsychotic formulation in stable patients with schizoaffective disorder. Presented at the American College of Neuropsychopharmacology. San Juan, Puerto Rico, December 2002.

26. Kane JM, Eerdekens M, Lindenmayer J, Keith SJ, Lesem M, Karcher K. Long-acting injectable risperidone: efficacy and safety of the first long-acting atypical antipsychotic. Am J Psychiatry 2003; 160:1125–1132.

27. Tran PV, Dellva MA, Tollefson GD, Wently AW, Beasley CM. Oral olanzapine versus haloperidol in the maintenance treatment of schizophrenia and related psychosis. Brit J Psychiatry 1998; 172:499–505.

28. Glick ID, Berg PH. Time to study discontinuation, relapse, and compliance with atypical or conventional antipsychotics in schizophrenia and related disorders. Int Clin Psychopharmacol 2002; 17:65–68.

29. Noordsy DL, O'Keefe C, Mueser KT, Xie H. Six-month outcomes for patients who switched to olanzapine treatment. Psychiatr Serv 2001; 52:501–507.

30. Mullen J, Jibson MD, Sweitzer D. A comparison of the relative safety, efficacy, and tolerability of quetiapine and risperidone in outpatients with schizophrenia and other psychotic disorders: the quetiapine experience with safety and tolerability (QUEST) study. Clin Ther 2001; 23(11):1839–1854.

31. Tariot PN, Salzman C, Yeung PP, Pultz J, Rak IW. Long-term use of quetiapine in elderly patients with psychotic disorders. Clin Ther 2000; 22(9):1068–1084.

32. Lynch J, Morrison J, Graves N, Meddis D, Drummond MF, Hellewell JS. The health economic implications of treatment with quetiapine: an audit of long-term treatment for patients with chronic schizophrenia. Eur Psychiatry 2001; 16(5):307–312.

33. Margolese HC, Chouinard G, Beauclair L, Belanger MC. Therapeutic tolerance and rebound psychosis during quetiapine maintenance monotherapy in patients with schizophrenia and schizoaffective disorder. J Clin Psychopharmacol 2002; 22:347–352.

34. Hirsch SR, Kissling W, Bauml J, Power A, O'Connor R. A 28-week comparison of ziprasidone and haloperidol in outpatients with stable schizophrenia. J Clin Psychiatry 2002; 63(6):516–523.

35. Meltzer HY. Ziprasidone's long-term efficacy and tolerability in schizophrenia. Presented at the 42th Annual New Clinical Drug Evaluation Unit Meeting, Boca Raton, FL, June 2002.

36. Arato M, O'Connor R, Meltzer HY, Zeus Study Group. A 1-year, double-blind, placebo controlled trial of ziprasidone 40, 80, and 160 mg/day in chronic

schizophrenia: the Ziprasidone Extended Use in Schizophrenia (ZEUS) study. Int Clin Psychopharmacol 2002; 17:207–215.

37. Simpson O, Horne RL, Weiden P, Pigott T, Bari M, Romano SJ. Ziprasidone vs olanzapine in schizophrenia: a 6-month extension study. Eur Psychiatry 2002; 17(suppl 1):186–187.

38. Carson W, Pigott T, Saha A, Ali M, McQuade RD, Torbeyns AF, Stock E. Aripiprazole vs. placebo in the treatment of stable, chronic schizophrenia. Presented at the 42nd Annual New Clinical Drug Evaluation Unit Meeting, Boca Raton, FL, June, 2002.

39. Kujawa M, Saha A, Ingenito GG, Mirza A, Luo X, Archibald DG, Carson WH. Aripiprazole for long-term maintenance treatment of schizophrenia. Collegium Internationale Neuro-Psychopharmacologium (CINP) 2002, Montreal, Quebec, Canada.

40. Voruganti L, Cortese L, Owyeumi L, Kotteda V, Cernovsky Z, Zirul S, Awad A. Switching from conventional to novel antipsychotic drugs: results of a prospective naturalistic study. Schizophr Res 2002; 57:201.

41. Davis JM, Chen N, Glick ID. A meta-analysis of the efficacy of second-generation antipsychotics. Arch Gen Psychiatry 2003; 60:553–564.

42. Doering S, Muller E, Kopcke W, et al. Predictors of relapse and rehospitalization in schizophrenia and schizoaffective disorder. Schizophr Bull 1998; 24:87–98.

43. Haywood TW, Kravitz HM, Grossman LS, et al. Predicting the "revolving door" phenomenon among patients with schizophrenic, schizoaffective, and affective disorders. Am J Psychiatry 1995; 152:856–861.

44. Kent S, Yellowlees P. Psychiatric and social reasons for frequent hospitalization. Hosp Community Psychiatry 1994; 45:347–350.

45. Sullivan G, Wells KB, Morgenstern H, et al. Identifying modifiable risk factors for rehospitalization: a case-control study of seriously mentally ill persons in Mississippi. Am J Psychiatry 1995; 152:1749–1756.

46. Perkins DO. Adherence to antipsychotic medications. J Clin Psychiatry 1999; 60 supp 21:25–30.

47. Fleischhacker WW, Meise U, Gunther V, et al. Compliance with antipsychotic drug treatment: influence of side effects. Acta Psychiatr Scand 1994; 89(suppl 382):11–15.

48. Valenstein M, Copeland LA, Blow FC, McCarthy JF, Zeber JE, Gillon L, Bingham CR, Stavenger T. Pharmacy data identify poorly adherent patients with schizophrenia at increased risk for admission. Med Care 2002; 40:630–639.

49. Dolder CR, Lacro JP, Dunn LB, Jeste DV. Antipsychotic medication adherence: is there a difference between typical and atypical agents? Am J Psychiatry 2002; 159:103–108.

50. Gaebel W, Janner M, Frommann N, Pietzcker A, Kopcke W, Linden M, Muller P, Muller-Spahn F, Tegeler J. First vs multiple episode schizophrenia: two-year outcome of intermittent and maintenance medication strategies. Schizophr Res 2002; 53:145–159.

51. Satterlee W, Dellva MA, Beasley C, Tran P, Tollefson G. Effectiveness of olanzapine in long-term continuation treatment. Presented at the 36th Annual New Clinical Evaluation Unit Program, Boca Raton, FL, 1996.

52. Conley RR, Love RC, Kelly DL, Bartko JJ. Rehospitalization rates of patients recently discharged on a regimen of risperidone or clozapine. Am J Psychiatry 1999; 156:863–868.

53. Hogarty GE. Prevention of relapse in chronic schizophrenic patients. J Clin Psychiatry 1993; 54(suppl 3):18–23.

54. Rabinowitz J, Licthenberg P, Kaplan Z, Mark M, Nahon D, Davidson M. Rehospitalization rates of chronically ill schizophrenic patients discharged on a regimen of risperidone, olanzapine, or conventional antipsychotics. Am J Psychiatry 2001; 158:266–269.

55. Conley RR, Kelly DL, Love RC, McMahon RP. Rehospitalization risk with second-generation and depot antipsychotics. Ann Clin Psychiatry 2003; 15:23–31.

56. Remington G, Khramov I. Health care utilization in patients with schizophrenia maintained on atypical versus conventional antipsychotics. Prog Neuro-Psychopharmacol Biol Psychiatry 2001; 25:363–369.

57. Aronne LJ. Epidemiology, morbidity and treatment of overweight and obesity. J Clin Psychiatry 2001; 62(suppl 23):13–22.

58. Allison DB, Casey DE. Antipsychotic-induced weight gain: a review of the literature. J Clin Psychiatry 2001; 62(suppl 7):22–31.

59. Hummer M, Kemmler G, Kurz M, Kurzthaler I, Oberbauer HJ, Fleischhacker W. Weight gain induced by clozapine. Eur Neuropsychopharmacol 1995; 5: 437–440.

60. Henderson DC, Cagliero E, Gray C, Nasrallah RA, Hayden DL, Schoenfeld DA, Goff DC. Clozapine, diabetes mellitus, weight gain, and lipid abnormalities: a five-year naturalistic study. Am J Psychiatry 2000; 157:975–981.

61. Hong CJ, Lin CH, Yu YW, et al. Genetic variants of the serotonin system and weight change during clozapine treatment. Pharmacogenetics 2001; 11: 265–268.

62. Baymiller SP, Ball P, McMahon RP, Buchanan RW. Weight and blood pressure change during clozapine treatment. Clin Neuropharmacol 2002; 25:202–206.

63. Spivak B, Musin E, Mester R, Gonen N, Talmon Y, Guy N, Roitman S, Kupchik M, Kotler M, Weizman A. The effect of long-term antipsychotic treatment on the body weight of patients suffering from chronic schizophrenia: clozapine versus classical antipsychotic agents. Int Clin Psychopharmacol 1999; 14:229–232.

64. Nemeroff CB. Dosing the antipsychotic medication olanzapine. J Clin Psychiatry 1997; 58(suppl 10):45–49.

65. Kinon BJ, Basson BR, Gilmore JA, et al. Long-term olanzapine treatment: weight change and weight-related health factors in schizophrenia. J Clin Psychiatry 2001; 62:92–100.

66. Volavka J, Czobor P, Sheitman B, Lindenmayer JP, Citrome L, McEvoy JP, Cooper TB, Chakos M, Lieberman JA. Clozapine, olanzapine, risperidone, and haloperidol in the treatment of patients with chronic schizophrenia and schizoaffective disorder. Am J Psychiatry 2002; 159:255–262.

67. Brecher M, Rak IW, et al. The long-term effect of quetiapine (Seroquel) monotherapy on weight in patients with schizophrenia. Int J Psychiatry Clin Pract 2000; 4:287–292.

68. Jones AM, Rak IW, Raniwalla J, et al. Weight changes in patients treated with quetiapine. In: New Research Abstracts of the 153rd Annual Meeting of the American Psychiatric Association, Chicago, IL, May 18, 2000.

69. Fertig MK, Brooks VC, Shelton PS, English CW. Hyperglycemia associated with olanzapine. J Clin Psychiatry 1998; 59:687–689.

70. Ober SK, Hudak R, Rusterholtz A. Hyperglycemia and olanzapine. Am J Psychiatry 1999; 156:970.

71. Lindenmayer JP, Patel R. Olanzapine-induced ketoacidosis with diabetes mellitus. Am J Psychiatry 1999; 156:1471.

72. Rigalleau V, Gatta B, Bonnaud S, Masson M, Suourgeois ML, Vergnot V, et al. Diabetes as a result of atypical antipsychotic drugs: a report of three cases. Diabet Med 2000; 17:484–486.

73. Bettinger TL, Mendelson SC, Dorson PG, Crismon ML. Olanzapine-induced glucose dysregulation. Ann Pharmacother 2000; 34:865–867.

74. Melkerson KI, Hulting AL, Brismar KE. Elevated levels of insulin, leptin, and blood lipids in olanzapine-treated patients with schizophrenia or related psychoses. J Clin Psychiatry 2000; 31:742–749.

75. Biswas PN, Wilton LV, Pearce GL, Freemantle S, Shakir SAW. The pharmacovigilance of olanzapine: results of a post-marketing surveillance study on 8858 patients in England. J Psychopharmacol 2001; 15:265–271.

76. Koro CE, Fedder DO, Weiss SS, Magder LS, Kreyenbuhl J, Revicki DA, Buchanan RW. Assessment of independent effect of olanzapine and risperidone on risk of diabetes among patients with schizophrenia: population based nested case-control study. Brit Med J 2002; 325–331.

77. Koller E, et al. Clozapine-associated diabetes. Am J Med 2001; 111:716–723.

78. Koller E, Doraiswamy PM. Olanzapine-associated DM. Pharmacotherapy 2002; 22(7):841–852.

79. Ghaeli P, Dufresne RL. Serum triglyceride levels in patients treated with clozapine. Am J Health Syst Pharm 1996; 53:79–81.

80. Sheitman BB, Bird PM, Binz W, Akinli L, Sanchez C. Olanzapine-induced elevation of plasma triglyceride levels. Am J Psychiatry 1999; 156:1471–1472.

81. Osser DN, Najarian DM, Dufresne RL. Olanzapine increases weight and serum triglyceride levels. J Clin Psychiatry 1999; 60:767–770.

82. Meyer JM. Novel antipsychotics and severe hyperlipidemia. J Clin Psychopharmacol 2001; 21:369–374.

83. Koro CE, Fedder DO, Weiss S, Magder LS, I'talien GJ, Kreyenbuhl J, Revicki D, Buchanan RW. An assessment of independent effect of olanzapine and

risperidone exposure on the risk of the hyperlipidemia in schizophrenic patients. Arch Gen Psychiatry 2002; 59:1021–1026.

84. Meyer JM. A retrospective comparison of weight, lipid, and glucose changes between risperidone- and olanzapine-treated inpatients: metabolic outcomes after 1 year. J Clin Psychiatry 2002; 63(5):425–433.

85. Casey DE, Carson WH, Saha AR, Liebeskind A, Ali MW, Jody D, Ingenio GG. Psychopharmacology 2003; 166:391–399.

86. Yassa R, Lal S. Impaired sexual intercourse as a complication of tardive dyskinesia. Am J Psychiatry 142:1514–1515, 1985.

87. Meston CM, Gorzalka BB. Psychoactive drugs and human sexual behaviour: the role of serotonergic activity. J Psychoactive Drugs 1992; 24:1–40.

88. Pollack MH, Rosenbaum JF. Management of antidepressant-induced side effects: a practical guide for the clinician. J Clin Psychiatry 1987; 48:3–8.

89. Tamminga CA, Mack RJ. Granneman GR, et al. Sertindole in the treatment of psychosis in schizophrenia: efficacy and safety. Int Clin Psychopharmacol 1997; 12(suppl 1):S29–S35.

90. Pollack MH, Reiter S, Hammerness P. Genitourinary and sexual adverse effects of psychotropic medication. Int J Psychiatry Med 1992; 22; 305–327.

91. Halbreich U, Kinon BJ, Gilmore JA, Kahn LS. Elevated prolactin levels in patients with schizophrenia: mechanisms and related adverse effects. Psychoneuroendocrinology 2003; 28 (suppl 1):53–67.

92. Maguire GA. Prolactin elevation with antipsychotic medications: mechanisms of action and clinical consequences. J Clin Psychiatry 2002; 63(suppl 4):56–62.

93. Naidoo U, Goff DC, Klibanski A. Hyperprolactinemia and bone mineral density: the potential impact of antipsychotic agents. Psychoneuroendocrinology 2003; 28(suppl 2):97–108.

94. Turrone P, Kapur S, Seeman MV, Flint AJ. Elevation of prolactin levels by atypical antipsychotics. Am J Psychiatry 2002; 159:133–135.

95. Peacock L, Solgard T, Lublin H, Gerlach, J. Clozapine versus typical antipsychotics: effects and side effects. Neuropsychopharmacology 1994; 10: 223–354.

96. Aizenberg D, Modai I, Landa A, Gil-Ad I, Weizman A. Comparison of sexual dysfunction in male schizophrenic patients maintained on treatment with classical antipsychotics versus clozapine. J Clin Psychiatry 2001; 62:541–544.

97. Hummer M, Kemmler G, Kurz M, Kurzthaler I, Oberbauer H, Fleischhacker WW. Sexual disturbances during clozapine and haloperidol treatment for schizophrenia. Am J Psychiatry 1999; 156(4):631–633.

98. Mullen B, Brar JS, Vagnucci AH, Ganguli R. Frequency of sexual dysfunction in patients with schizophrenia on haloperidol, clozapine, or risperidone. Schizophrenia Res 2001; 48:155–158.

99. Compton MT, Miller AH. Priapism associated with conventional and atypical antipsychotic medications: a review. J Clin Psychiatry 2001; 62(5):362–366.

100. Kleinberg DL, Davis JM, de Coster R, Van Baelen B, Brecher M. Prolactin levels and adverse events in patients treated with risperidone. J Clin Psychopharmacol 1999; 19:57–61.

101. Conley RR, Mahmoud R. A randomized double-blind study of risperidone and olanzapine in the treatment of schizophrenia or schizoaffective disorder. Am J Psychiatry 2001; 158(5):765–774.

102. Bobes J, Garcia-Portilla MP, Rejas J, Hernandez G, Garcia-Garcia M, Rico-Villademoros F, Porras A. Frequency of sexual dysfunction and other reproductive side-effects in patients with schizophrenia treated with risperidone, olanzapine, quetiapine, or haloperidol: the results of the EIRE group. J Sex Marital Ther 2003; 29:125–147.

103. Shiwach RS, Carmody TJ. Prolactogenic effects of risperidone in male patients – a preliminary study. Acta Psychiatr Scand 1998; 98:81–83.

104. Mabini R, Wegowske G, Baker FM. Galactorrhea and gynecomastia in a hypothyroid male being treated with risperidone. Psychiatr Serv 2000; 51: 983–985.

105. Benazzi F. Gynecomastia with risperidone-fluoxetine combination. Pharmacopsychiatry 1999; 32:41.

106. Kaneda, Y. Risperidone-induced ejaculatory dysfunction: a case report. Eur Psychiatry, 16(2):134–135, 2001.

107. Raja M. Risperidone-induced absence of ejaculation. Int Clin Psychopharmacol 1999; 14(5):317–319.

108. Nicholson R, McCurley R. Risperidone-associated priapism. J Clin Psychopharmacol 1997; 7(2):133–134.

109. Emes CE, Millson RC. Risperidone-induced priapism. Can J Psychiatry 1994; 39(5):315–316.

110. Dickson RA, Dalby JT, Williams R, Edwards AL. Risperidone-induced prolactin elevations in premenopausal women with schizophrenia. Am J Psychiatry 1995; 152:1102–1103.

111. Kim Y-K, Kim L, Lee M-S. Risperidone and associated amenorrhea: a report of 5 cases. J Clin Psychiatry 60:315–317, 1999.

112. Tran PV, Hamilton SH, Kuntz AJ, Potvin JH, Anderson SW, Beasley C Jr, Tollefson GD. Double-blind comparison of olanzapine versus risperidone in the treatment of schizophrenia and other psychotic disorders. J Clin Psychopharmacol 1997; 17:407–418.

113. Crawford AMK, Beasley CM Jr., Tollefson GD. The acute and long-term effect of olanzapine compared with placebo and haloperidol on serum prolactin concentrations. Schizophr Res 1997; 26:41–54.

114. Markianos M, Hatzimanolis J, Lykouras L. Neuroendocrine responsiveness of the pituitary dopamine system in male schizophrenic patients during treatment with clozapine, olanzapine, risperidone, sulpiride, or haloperidol. Eur Arch Psychiatry Clin Neurosci 2001; 251:141–146.

115. Arvenitis L, Miller B, Study Group. Multiple fixed doses of Seroquel (quetiapine) in patients with acute exacerbation of schizophrenia: a comparison with haloperidol and placebo. Biol Psychiatry 1997; 42(4):233–246.

116. Small JG, Hirsch SR, Arvanitis LA, et al. Quetiapine in patients with schizophrenia: a high- and low-dose double-blind comparison with placebo. Arch Gen Psychiatry 1997; 54(6):549–557.

117. King DJ, Link CGG, Kowalcyk B. A comparison of bid and tid dose regimens of quetiapine (Seroquel) in the treatment of schizophrenia. Psychopharmacology 1998; 37:139–146.

118. Borison RL, Arvanitis LA, Miller BG. ICI 204,636, an atypical antipsychotic: efficacy and safety in a multicenter, placebo-controlled trial in patients with schizophrenia. J Clin Psychopharmacol 1996; 16(2):158–169.

119. Goldstein JM, Cantillon M. Low incidence of reproductive/hormonal side effects with Seroquel (quetiapine) is supported by its lack of elevation of plasma prolactin concentrations. Presented at the American College of Neuropsychopharmacology, Hawaii, December 7–12, 1997.

120. Pais VM, Ayvazian PJ. Priapism from quetiapine overdose: first report and proposal of mechanism. Urology 2001; 58(3):462.

121. Physician's Desk Reference. 56th edition. Montvale, NJ: Medical Economics Company, Inc, 2003.

122. Oenanthe J, Burgoyne K, Smith M, Gadasally R. Prolactin levels and new antipsychotics. Presented at the European College of Neuropsychopharmacology, Glasgow, Scotland 1998:PT 10064.

123. Reeves RR, Kimble R. Prolonged erections associated with ziprasidone treatment: a case report. J Clin Psychiatry 2003; 64:97–98.

124. Reeves RR, Mack JE. Priapism associated with two atypical antipsychotic agents. Pharmacotherapy 2002; 22:1070–1073.

125. Kane JM, Carson WH, Saha AR, McQuade RD, Ingenito GG, Zimbroff DL, Ali MW. Efficacy and safety of aripiprazole and haloperidol versus placebo in patients with schizophrenia and schizoaffective disorder. J Clin Psychiatry 2002; 63:763–771.

126. Llorca PM, Chereau I, Bayle FJ, Lancon C. Tardive dyskinesias and antipsychotics: a review. Eur Psychiatry 2002; 17:263–264.

127. Yovtcheva SP, Stanley-Tilt C, Moles JK. Reemergence of tardive dyskinesia after discontinuation of clozapine treatment. Schizophr Res 2000; 46:107–109.

128. Uzun O, Cansever A, Ozsahin A. A case of relapsed tardive dyskinesia due to clozapine dose reduction. Int Clin Psychopharmacol 2001; 16:369–371.

129. Caroff SN, Mann SC, Campbell EC, Sullivan KA. Movement disorders associated with atypical antipsychotic drugs. J Clin Psychiatry 2002; 63(suppl 4):12–19.

130. Beasley CM, Dellva MA, Tamura RN, Morgenstern H, Glazer WM, Ferguson K, Tollefson GD. Randomized double-blind comparison of the incidence of tardive dyskinesia in patients with schizophrenia during long-term treatment with olanzapine or haloperidol. Brit J Psychiatry 1999; 174:23–30.

131. Jeste DV, Lacro JP, Bailey A, Rockwell E, Harris MJ, Caliguiri MP. Lower incidence of tardive dyskinesia with risperidone compared with haloperidol in older patients. J Am Geriatr Soc 1999; 47:716–719.

132. Faber TS, Zehender M, Just H. Drug-induced torsades de pointes: incidence, management and prevention. Drug Saf 1994; 11:463–476.

133. Lazzara R. Antiarrhythmic drugs and torsades de pointes. Eur Heart J 1993; 14:88–93.

134. Reilly JG, Ayis SA, Ferrier IN, Jones SJ, Thomas SHL. QTc-interval abnormalities and psychotropic drug therapy in psychiatric patients. Lancet 2000; 355:1048–1052.

135. Food and Drug Administration Center for Drug Evaluation Research. Transcript of Psychopharmacological Drugs Advisory Committee July 19, 2000. Ziprasidone Briefing Document. Available at http://www.fda.gov/ohrms/dockets/ac/00/backgrd/3619b1a.pdf.

136. Ravin DS, Levenson JW. Fatal cardiac event following initiation of risperidone therapy. Ann Pharmacother 1997; 31:867–870.

137. Biswas AK, Zabrocki LA, Mayes KL, Morris-Kukoski CL. Cardiotoxicity associated with intentional ziprasidone and buproprion overdose. J Toxicol Clin Toxicol 2003; 41:101–104.

138. Dineen S, Withrow K, Voronovitch L, Munshi R, Nawbary MW, Lippmann S. QTc prolongation and high-dose olanzapine. Psychosomatics 2003; 44: 174–175.

139. Hustey FM. Acute quetiapine poisoning. J Emerg Med 1999; 17: 995–997.

140. Beelen AP, Yeo KT, Lewis LD. Asymptomatic QTc prolongation associated with quetiapine fumarate overdose in a patient being treated with risperidone. Hum Exp Toxicol 2001; 20:215–219.

141. Furst BA, Champion KM, Pierre JM, Wirshing DA, Wirshing WC. Possible association of QTc interval prolongation with coadministration of quetiapine and lovastatin. Biol Psychiatry 2002; 51:264–265.

142. Warner B, Hoffmann P. Investigation of the potential of clozapine to cause torsade de pointes. Adverse Drug React Toxicol Rev 2002; 21:189–203.

143. Miceli JJ, Smith M, Robarge L, Morse T, Laruent A. The effects of ketoconazole on ziprasidone pharmacokinetics – a placebo-controlled cross-over study in healthy volunteers. Brit J Clin Pharmacol 2000; 49(suppl 1): 71S–76S.

144. Oberg K, Bauman JL. QT prolongation and torsades de pointes due to erythromycin lactobionate. Pharmacotherapy 1995; 15:687–692.

145. Lai D, Brown G, MacDonald I. Clarithromycin-induced prolonged QT syndrome. Can J Hosp Pharm 1996; 49:33–35.

146. Kamochi H, Nii T, Eguchi K, Mori T, Yamamoto A, Shimoda K, Ibaraki K. Clarithromycin associated with torsades de pointes. Jpn Circ J 1999; 63: 421–422.

147. Thomas SHL. Drugs, QT abnormalities, and ventricular arrhythmias. Adverse Drug React Toxicol Rev 1994; 13:77–102.

148. Dekker JM, Feskens EJ, Schouten EG, Klootwijk P, Pool J, Kromhout D. QTc duration is associated with levels of insulin and glucose intolerance. The Zuphen Elderly Study. Diabetes 1996; 45:376–380.

149. Haverkamp W, Breithardt G, Camm AJ, Janse MJ, Rosen MR, Antzelevtich C, Escande D, Franz M, Malik M, Moss A, Shah R. The potential for QT prolongation and proarrhythmia by non-antiarrhythmic drugs: clinical and regulatory implications. Eur Heart J 2000; 21:1216–1231.

150. Welch R, Chue P. Antipsychotic agents and QT changes. J Psychiatry Neurosci 2000; 25(2):154–160.

151. Marfella R, Napo F, De Angelis L, Siniscalchi M, Rossi R, Giugliano D. The effect of acute hyperglycemia on QTc duration in healthy man. Diabetologia 2000; 43:571–575.

152. Peralta V, Cuesta MJ, Caro F, et al. Neuroleptic dose and schizophrenic symptoms. A survey a prescribing practices. Acta Psychiatr Scand 1994; 90(5):354–357.

153. Citrome L, Volavka J. Optimal dosing of atypical antipsychotics in adults: a review of the current evidence. Harv Rev Psychiatry 2002; 10:280–291.

154. Love RC. Novel versus conventional antipsychotic drugs. Pharmacotherapy 1996; 16:6–10.

155. Marder SR, Meibach RC. Risperidone in the treatment of schizophrenia. Am J Psychiatry 1994; 151:825–835.

156. Muller-Spahn F. Risperidone in the treatment of chronic schizophrenic patients: an international double-blind parallel-group study versus haloperidol. Clin Neuropharm 1992; 12(1):90.

157. Klieser E, Lehmann E, Kinzler E, et al. Randomized, double-blind controlled trial of risperidone versus clozapine in patients with chronic schizophrenia. J Clin Psychopharmacol 1995; 15(1):45–51.

158. Moller HJ, Bauml J, Ferrero F, et al. Risperidone in the treatment of schizophrenia: results of a study of patients from Germany, Austria and Switzerland. Eur Arch Psychiatry Clin Neurosci 1997; 246(6):291–296.

159. Ho BC, Miller D, Nopoulos P, Andreasen NC. A comparative effectiveness study of risperidone and olanzapine in the treatment of schizophrenia. J Clin Psychiatry 1999; 60:658–663.

160. Love RC, Conley RR, Kelly DL, Bartko JJ. A dose-outcome analysis of risperidone. J Clin Psychiatry 1999; 60:771–775.

161. Beasley CM Jr, Tollefson G, Tran P, Satterlee W, Sanger T, Hamilton S. Olanzapine versus placebo and haloperidol: acute phase results of the North American double-blind olanzapine trial. Neuropsychopharmacology 1996; 14:111–123.

162. Kinon BJ, Gilmore JA, Wang L. Exploration of a dose-response relationship in schizophrenia with the novel antipsychotic drug olanzapine. Presented at the 13th Annual US Psychiatric & Mental Health Congress, San Diego, November 2000.

163. Perry PJ, Lund BC, Sanger T, Beasley C. Olanzapine plasma concentrations and clinical response: acute phase results of the North American Olanzapine Trial. J Clin Psychopharmacol 2001; 212:14–20.

164. Kelly DL, Conley RR, Tamminga CA. Differential olanzapine plasma concentrations by sex in a fixed dose study. Schizophrenia Research 1999; 40(2):101–104.

165. Conley RR, Kelly DL, Richardson CM, Tamminga CA, Carpenter WT. The efficacy of high-dose olanzapine versus clozapine in treatment-resistant

schizophrenia: a double-blind crossover study. J Clin Psychopharmacol 2003; 23:668–671.

166. Kelly DL, Conley RR, Richardson CM, Tamminga CA. High-dose olanzapine vs. clozapine in treatment-resistant schizophrenia: adverse effects and laboratory results. Presented at the 42nd Annual New Clinical Drug Evaluation Unit Meeting, Boca Raton, FL, June 2002.

167. Perry PJ, Miller DD, Arndt SV, Cadoret RJ. Clozapine and norclozapine plasma concentrations and clinical response of treatment-refractory schizophrenic patients. Am J. Psychiatry 1991; 148:231–235.

168. Arvanitis LA, Miller BG. Multiple fixed doses of Seroquel™ (quetiapine) in patients with acute-exacerbation of schizophrenia: a comparison with haloperidol and placebo. Biol Psychiatry 1997; 42:233–246.

169. Small JG, Hirsch SR, Arvenitis LA, Miller BG, Link CG. Quetiapine in patients with schizophrenia: a high- and low-dose double-blind comparison with placebo. Arch Gen Psychiatry 1997; 54:549–557.

170. Emsley RA, Raniwalla J, Bailey PJ, Jones AM. A comparison of the effects of quetiapine (Seroquel™) and haloperidol in schizophrenic patients with a history of and a demonstrated, partial response to conventional antipsychotic treatment. PRIZE study group. Int Clin Psychopharmacol 2000; 15:121–131.

171. Keck P Jr, Buffenstein A, Ferguson J, Feighner J, Jaffe W, Harrigan EP, et al. Ziprasidone 40 and 120 mg/day in the acute exacerbation of schizophrenia and schizoaffective disorder: a 4-week placebo-controlled trial. Psychopharmacology 1998; 140:173–184.

172. Daniel DG, Zimbroff DL, Potkin SG, Reeves KR, Harrigan EP, Lakshminarayanan M. Ziprasidone 80 mg/day and 160 mg/day in the acute exacerbation of schizophrenia and schizoaffective disorder: a 6-week placebo-controlled trial. Neuropsychopharmacology 1999; 20:491–505.

173. Marder SR, Essock SM, Miller AL, Buchanan RW, Davis JM, Kane JM, Lieberman J, Schooler NR. The Mount Sinai conference on the pharmacotherapy of schizophrenia. Schizophr Bull 2002; 28:5–16.

174. Texas Medication Algorithm Progect (TMAP) for schizophrenia. http://www.mhmr.state.tx.us/centraloffice/medicaldirector/timascz1algo.pdf.

175. Weiden PJ, Olfson M. Cost of relapse in schizophrenia. Schizophr Bull 1995; 21(3):419–429.

9

Assessing the Effects of Atypical Antipsychotics on the CNS Utilizing Neuroimaging

Laura M. Rowland and Juan R. Bustillo

University of New Mexico,
Albuquerque, New Mexico, U.S.A.

I. INTRODUCTION

There is little question that brain structure and function are abnormally affected in schizophrenia independent of the effects of antipsychotic medications. Many studies using high resolution magnetic resonance imaging (MRI) have consistently found increased ventricular volume, and reduced cortical and subcortical volumes in various brain regions very early in the illness, before any exposure to antipsychotic drugs (1–3). Likewise, abnormal patterns of brain activation in unmedicated schizophrenia patients, carefully matched for task performance, have been reported with positron emission tomography (PET) and functional MRI techniques (4–6). Whether these activation abnormalities are traits of the illness or states related to clinical exacerbations of some components of the disorder is less clear. To characterize systematic brain changes directly linked to antipsychotic drugs, these trait and state illness-related effects must be considered. Antipsychotic medications, the mainstay of the modern treatment for schizophrenia, have been found to be reliably efficacious in improving psychotic symptoms. These agents also have the propensity to induce neuromotoric side effects, hence their original term neuroleptic ("to seize the neuron"). Not surprisingly, neurobiological correlates for both the beneficial and deleterious neuromotoric effects have been identified with neuroimaging techniques. With the introduction over the past decade of atypical antipsychotic agents, effective medications that are less likely to induce extrapyramidal side effects, a variety of studies have attempted to identify the structural and functional brain correlates of the antipsychotic and the extrapyramidal effects. In this chapter we present a selective review of the literature addressing these important issues. A general overview of findings from studies utilizing the following methodologies will be discussed: MRI, magnetic resonance spectroscopy (MRS), functional MRI (fMRI), magnetoencephalography (MEG), and PET (glucose metabolism, blood flow, and receptor ligand).

II. MRI VOLUME

Macrostructural brain changes have been documented in schizophrenia resulting from treatment with typical antipsychotic drugs. The best documented of these changes is enlargement of the caudate nucleus (7,8), which reverts with clozapine treatment (9,10). In addition, several studies have shown caudate volumes to decrease when patients with schizophrenia were treated with atypical agents (8,11). Interestingly, Tauscher et al. (12) showed caudate volumes to decline in first-episode patients treated with either atypicals or low dose typicals for 5 years; however, this reduction in caudate volumes was shown to correspond with normal aging effects.

Investigations of early schizophrenia with longitudinal MRI follow-up consistently document some reduction of brain volume early in the illness (13–17). The large majority of subjects in these studies were chronically treated with typical antipsychotics (with exception of the childhood-onset schizophrenia sample studied by Rappaport et al. (14), most of whom responded poorly to typical agents and were switched to clozapine). Nevertheless, medication status was not controlled and only Gur et al. (13) reported a relationship between length of antipsychotic exposure and reduction of frontal tissue. Another naturalistic longitudinal study compared computed tomography (CT) scans in antipsychotic-naïve subjects and after 5 years of treatment with typical medications. Cumulative dose of medication, but not illness-related factors, directly predicted the presence of frontal atrophy (18). Although these structural imaging studies cannot demonstrate specific changes in the neuronal component of brain tissue, their findings challenge a strict neurodevelopmental model of schizophrenia that assumes an early static lesion (19). The possibility that these early reductions in brain volumes in schizophrenia patients may be in part related to antipsychotic *class* cannot be excluded. For instance, Lieberman et al. (20) showed whole brain and cerebral gray matter volume to be significantly smaller in first-episode patients following 12 weeks of haloperidol treatment compared to first-episode patients following 12 weeks of olanzapine treatment. However, extensive human post-mortem and animal data have failed to document that antipsychotic medications (typical or atypical) cause neuronal death.

III. MAGNETIC RESONANCE SPECTROSCOPY

A. Proton (^{1}H) MRS Studies

Magnetic resonance spectroscopy (MRS), using the same basic hardware as MRI, can quantify concentrations of biochemical compounds in brain structures. Hence, MRS provides some of the advantages of both post-mortem tissue examination (i.e., location-specific chemical analysis) and in-vivo, noninvasive neuroimaging (i.e., safe, repeated assessments during the course of illness). There are two basic types of MRS acquisition techniques, single-voxel and chemical shift imaging or spectroscopic imaging (^{1}H-MRSI). ^{1}H-MRS allows the measurement of metabolites such as N-acetylaspartate (NAA), choline (Cho), creatine (Cre), glutamate (Glu), glutamine (Gln), and GABA, with the latter three comprising the component "Glx" at lower field strengths. NAA is among the most abundant amino acids in the brain – up to 0.1% wet weight of brain (21) – second only to glutamate. NAA is produced in the neuronal mitochondria, found almost exclusively in the neuron (lower concentrations are found in oligodendrocyte progenitor and immature oligodendrocyte cells), and more concentrated in gray than white matter (21). Once thought to be a relatively stable marker of neuronal density, NAA is now considered a marker of neuronal integrity and function, and predicts severity of illness in various neurodegenerative disorders (22–24). NAA as an index of neuronal integrity has underscored much of the ^{1}H-MRS research in schizophrenia. Much less is known about the significance of the ^{1}H-MRS assessed Cho and Cre. The Cho peak is comprised of glycerophosphocholine and phosphocholine, which are involved in lipid membrane turnover and elevated in active inflammatory processes, such as multiple sclerosis (25) and cerebral lupus erythematosus (26). Hence, increases in Cho with reductions in NAA are usually interpreted as evidence of an active process of neuronal death with glial reaction. The Cre peak is comprised of creatine and phosphocreatine, which are involved in energy metabolism; however, the clinical and physiological significance of changes in Cre is not fully understood. The

Glx peak is comprised of glutamate, glutamine, and GABA, which can be quantified separately at higher field strengths (27,28). Many researchers believe that glutamine reflects mostly glutamate concentrations that are involved in neurotransmission (29,30).

To date, over 50 ^{1}H-MRS studies of schizophrenia have been conducted, and only a few have considered the impact of antipsychotic medication on concentrations of NAA. The majority of such studies have primarily focused on frontal brain regions. Choe et al. (31) investigated frontal lobe spectra (8 cc voxel) in control subjects ($n = 20$) and in antipsychotic-free (at least 6 months) and naïve patients ($n = 34$) with schizophrenia both before and after 1 to 6 months of treatment with various typical and atypical antipsychotic medications. Results indicated frontal NAA/Cre to be decreased in patients compared to controls, with no apparent effect of antipsychotic treatment on frontal NAA/Cre; however, this analysis was not broken down by drug class.

Ende et al. (32) have shown decreased anterior cingulate NAA in patients ($n = 19$) compared to controls ($n = 16$), with greater reductions in those treated with typical ($n = 9$) compared to atypical ($n = 10$) medications with ^{1}H-MRSI. In a follow-up study, this group found anterior cingulate NAA to be greater in chronic patients treated with atypical antipsychotics ($n = 9$ clozapine, $n = 2$ risperidone) for at least 6 months compared to patients ($n = 10$) treated with typical antipsychotics (4). In addition, a significant correlation was revealed for length of time on atypical medication, higher NAA levels, and better performance on test of frontal lobe function, the Wisconsin Card Sorting Test (WCST).

We have also shown a differentiation in frontal lobe (12 cc voxel) NAA concentrations in patients treated with either the atypical, clozapine, or the typical, haloperidol (33). Here, it was shown that patients treated with haloperidol ($n = 18$) but not clozapine ($n = 17$) exhibited significantly less frontal NAA than controls ($n = 17$). Furthermore, frontal NAA was directly related to a measure of motor dexterity, a proxy for parkinsonian side effects but not related to any illness measures such as psychopathology or chronicity. This is consistent with an NAA reducing effect of haloperidol linked to neuromotoric disturbances. More recently, we studied 10 minimally treated (less than 3 weeks lifetime exposure) schizophrenia patients and 10 normal controls with single-voxel ^{1}H-MRS of the left frontal and occipital lobes (34). Patients then were treated in a randomized-controlled, double-blind design with either haloperidol or quetiapine, and ^{1}H-MRS was repeated within a year. There were no differences in frontal or occipital NAA between patients and controls at baseline. However, frontal NAA was reduced in all but one patient with schizophrenia within the first year of treatment. In addition, patients had a clear clinical response to treatment but changes in frontal NAA were not correlated with symptom improvement. We were not able, however, to determine if drug class had an effect on NAA because unblinded data are not currently available. The results of this preliminary study are in contrast to a study that reported higher NAA/Cre in the dorsolateral prefrontal cortex (DLPFC) in 23 schizophrenia patients treated with antipsychotic medication compared to when the subjects had been medication free for at least 2 weeks (35). Of these subjects, seven patients had their first scan off drugs while the other 16 were initially on medications (there is no report of the interval between scans or evidence of symptomatic changes with treatment). Bertolino et al. (35) suggested that antipsychotic medications tend to normalize DLPFC NAA/ Cre ratios. It is important to emphasize that Bertolino et al. (35) assessed small voxels that encompassed only the DLPFC using the technique of chemical shift imaging, and their findings suggest increases in NAA/Cre with antipsychotic treatment. Bustillo et al. (34) used a much larger (12.6 cc) single voxel region of interest. It is possible that the impact of antipsychotic medication differs regionally within the frontal lobe, with some areas having increases and others reductions in NAA.

One study sought to determine if the anterior cingulate Glx/Cr, measured with MRSI, changed when 11 patients taking typical drugs were switched to olanzapine and if such alterations relate to changes in symptoms (36). Results revealed a 12.5% increase in Glx/Cr when patients were switched to olanzapine, which was not statistically significant. However, when the group was broken down into six responders (negative symptom improvement) and five nonresponders (negative symptom worsening), responders had a mean increase of 45.8% in Glx/Cr versus a decrease of 20.8% for nonresponders. These results provide evidence that in a subgroup of patients with schizophrenia, atypical antipsychotics, in contrast to typical agents, may alter the glutamatergic system, which may play a role in improving negative symptoms.

Two studies investigated the possible effects of antipsychotic medication on the striatum. A single-voxel study of the left striatum (8 cc) found no differences in metabolite concentrations between patient ($n = 18$) and control ($n = 31$) groups, but did find reduced Cho in patients on atypical ($n = 7$) versus typical ($n = 6$) antipsychotics (37). Bustillo et al. (33) found lower NAA in the caudate nuclei in patients treated with haloperidol ($n = 18$), but not clozapine ($n = 17$), when compared to controls ($n = 17$). However, correction of the CSF fraction in the spectroscopic voxels (6 cc) resulted in similar caudate NAA concentrations among the three groups.

Although findings across studies are mixed, it appears that atypical antipsychotic drugs are more favorably associated with NAA and Glx concentrations or changes compared to typical antipsychotics. However, future investigations should focus on the effects of typical and atypical drug agents on ^{1}H metabolites in normal volunteers as well as carefully controlled studies of both chronic and drug-naïve persons with schizophrenia. In addition, studies conducted at higher field strengths could help elucidate whether antipsychotic class has effects on metabolites that are difficult to quantify at lower field strengths (e.g., glutamate, glutamine, GABA) in very specific brain regions of interest.

B. [31]Phosphorus (^{31}P) MRS Studies

^{31}P-MRS allows for the measurement of metabolites that are involved in tissue metabolism. Of main interest are phosphocreatine (PCr), inorganic orthophosphate (Pi), and adenosine triphosphate (ATP), which are involved in high-energy metabolism; and phosphomonoesters (PMEs), which are involved in phospholipid membrane synthesis, and phosphodiesters (PDEs), which are involved in phospholipid breakdown. Intracellular pH and magnesium (Mg^{++}) can also be indirectly determined.

One of the first studies to investigate the influence of antipsychotic medications on ^{31}P spectra was conducted by Volz et al. (38). This study compared ^{31}P frontal lobe spectra in patients with schizophrenia on antipsychotic medication (drug class not specified; $n = 50$) and off antipsychotic medication ($n = 10$), and normal volunteers ($n = 36$). Results revealed elevated PCr and PCr/ATP, which reportedly reflects decreased ATP consumption, in patients treated with antipsychotics but not in antipsychotic-free patients compared to controls.

In a series of follow-up studies, Riehemann et al. (39) sought to determine if frontal lobe intracellular pH varies with different antipsychotics. Intracellular pH can affect biochemical processes, such as cellular respiration. In the first study, patients taking the atypical, clozapine ($n = 14$), were shown to have lower pH values than schizophrenics taking haloperidol ($n = 29$) and no medication ($n = 14$), and normal controls ($n = 32$). The second study revealed no difference in frontal intracellular pH when eight patients were assessed off medication and then following treatment with the atypical, olanzapine. Consistently, the third study showed no difference in frontal intracellular pH when 13 patients were assessed off medication, then following a 2-week treatment with the typical, haloperidol, and then following a 2-week treatment with the atypical, olanzapine.

There have been no published ^{31}P-MRS studies investigating the effects of atypical antipsychotics on brain regions other than frontal. However, one study investigated the effects of the typical, haloperidol, on ^{31}P spectra of the temporal lobe (40). Sixteen first-episode, drug-naïve patients were scanned prior to and following a 12-week treatment with haloperidol. Thirteen normal controls were assessed twice with 12 weeks between scans. Elevated bilateral temporal lobe PDE, reflective of abnormal metabolism or structure of phospholipid membranes, was observed in patients prior to haloperidol treatment when compared to controls. However, this elevation was found to decrease in the left temporal lobe following treatment, and thus, did not differ from the control group.

The few studies that investigated the effects of antipsychotics on ^{31}P spectra have not produced consistent findings. It appears that antipsychotics influence ^{31}P spectra, but the specific metabolite(s) and drug class cannot be determined from these studies. Future studies are necessary.

IV. FUNCTIONAL MRI (fMRI)

fMRI is a technique that allows for the assessment of blood oxygen level-dependent contrast (BOLD), reflective of oxygen consumption and perfusion rates. fFMRI is an advantageous functional neuroimaging technique in that it is noninvasive, provides good spatial resolution, and temporal information superior to PET. Thus, fMRI is an ideal technique to utilize for assessing the effects of antipsychotic class on brain function underlying cognitive processing.

Several fMRI studies have utilized fingertapping tasks to investigate the differential effects of atypical and typical antipsychotics. One of the first fMRI schizophrenia studies to consider antipsychotic medication class was conducted by Braus et al. (41). In this study, patients with schizophrenia who were first-episode drug-naïve ($n = 14$), patients treated with various typicals ($n = 17$) and atypicals ($n = 13$), and normal controls ($n = 15$) were assessed with fMRI while performing a left-handed, fingertapping task (sequential finger opposition (SFO)). Results revealed that patients treated with typical antipsychotics had decreased overall BOLD response and decreased activation in sensorimotor cortices than normal controls, drug-naïve patients, and patients treated with atypicals. In addition, normal controls and drug-naïve patients had greater activation in the sensorimotor areas than the two treated groups.

Muller and Klein (42) investigated the effects of haloperidol and olanzapine on BOLD responses associated with fingertapping performance in six patients with schizophrenia and in three healthy controls. An additional patient was assessed on two separate occasions while being treated with olanzapine and then with haloperidol. Contralateral sensorimotor and basal ganglia, as well as ipsilateral cerebellar regions were activated with fingertapping in all groups. However, the ventral thalamus was activated only in the patients treated with olanzapine. In a similar fMRI study, Muller et al. (43) studied unmedicated patients ($n = 10$), patients treated with either olanzapine ($n = 10$) or haloperidol ($n = 10$), and normal controls ($n = 10$) while performing a fingertapping task. As with the preceding study, all groups showed activations in the contralateral sensorimotor and basal ganglia, and ipsilateral cerebellar regions. Unmedicated patients showed greater activation in the ipsilateral pallidum than controls and treated patients. However, the significant difference between the olanzapine- and haloperidol-treated groups was that the olanzapine-treated group had greater thalamic activation than the haloperidol-treated group.

In another fingertapping study, Stephan et al. (44) investigated six unmedicated patients with schizophrenia before and following a 3-week treatment with olanzapine. Results revealed increased activation associated with olanzapine treatment in vast brain regions with the greatest changes in the orbito–medial prefrontal cortex, thalamus, and cerebellum.

Other fMRI studies have investigated the differential effects of atypical and typical antipsychotics on higher cognitive processes. One study investigated 10 healthy controls and 20 chronic patients with schizophrenia treated with various typical medications and following 6 weeks of treatment with risperidone in half of the patients (45). Subjects with schizophrenia were assessed with fMRI while performing a verbal version of the N-back working memory task at baseline and following a 6-week time period while continuing treatment with typical medications or switching to risperidone. Healthy controls were assessed once. All subjects showed activation of frontal, motor, and parietal regions with performance on the working memory task. Interestingly, patients that were switched to risperidone showed increased activation in the right dorsolateral prefrontal cortex, supplementary motor association area, and posterior parietal cortex. However, it is important to note that there was no improvement in working memory performance in the patients switched to risperidone.

Ramsey et al. (46) utilized fMRI to study patients with schizophrenia that were medication-naïve ($n = 10$) or treated with either olanzapine ($n = 5$) or clozapine ($n = 5$), and normal controls ($n = 10$) while performing a logical reasoning task. Since patients with schizophrenia tend to perform poorer than normal controls on tasks that tap executive function, brain activity was corrected for performance on the task. Brain activity was not different between medicated patients and controls. However, brain activity, overall, was greater in unmedicated patients than medicated patients and normal controls. These findings are not consistent with the previous studies of schizophrenia that often showed hypofrontal activity associated with cognition tasks that did not correct for performance. However, these findings are consistent with studies that carefully controlled for performance.

V. MAGNETOENCEPHALOGRAPHY

MEG is a noninvasive neuroimaging technique that provides excellent temporal resolution of neuronal activity. MEG primarily measures the magnetic field that is generated by the intracellular current flowing in the pyramidal neurons that are parallel to the skull. MEG only measures the magnetic field that is tangential to the scalp (47,48). Therefore, it mainly measures activity from the sulci of the cortex. To record MEG, sensors are placed around the head. The magnetic field induces a current in the detection coils of the sensors, which are connected to a superconduction quantum interference device (SQUID) that measures the current and infers the magnetic field (47,48). The result is a signal that appears very similar to EEG. MEG is analyzed by applying dipole modeling techniques to localize the source and spatial extent of activity. Source localization is much easier and more accurate with MEG than EEG because MEG is not affected by the properties of the skull, scalp, and CSF. Also, MEG is measured in units that are independent of reference level and the spatial resolution is higher for MEG than EEG.

Few studies have investigated the effects of atypical antipsychotic agents on MEG. One study assessed five patients with schizophrenia with no treatment and following 8 weeks of aripiprazole and 10 normal controls with resting MEG (49). Results revealed patients to have increased spontaneous delta and theta activity during the washout period. In addition, patients also showed paraxosymal bitemporal slow waves, which were localized to the superior temporal plane in two patients with dipole modeling. Patients also showed decreased alpha activity when compared to controls. Interestingly, treatment with aripiprazole appeared to normalize the delta and theta, but not the alpha activity.

Another study sought to determine if spontaneous MEG activity differed between patients treated for at least 4 weeks with haloperidol or clozapine, and normal controls (50). Three frequency bands, delta/theta (2–6 Hz), alpha (7.5–12 Hz), and beta (12.5–30 Hz) were examined during the resting state. Results revealed an increase in left-hemisphere beta activity in the patients treated with clozapine. In addition, source localization revealed concentrations in the temporoparietal region in clozapine-treated patients, in contrast to localization of sources in the central region in patients treated with haloperidol and normal controls. There were no other differences noted between the clozapine- and haloperidol-treated groups. However, there was a significant difference between patients overall and normal controls in dipole localization of delta/theta activity. Delta/theta activity was predominantly localized to the temporoparietal region in patients and in the central region for normal controls.

Rosburg et al. (51) sought to determine if there were differences in N100 habituation between male patients with schizophrenia and normal controls. N100 is an auditory event-related potential (ERP) or evoked potential (EP), and is a particular waveform component that is commonly studied with auditory processing. N100 habituation was investigated over three blocks of 90 trials of auditory tones. Habituation is reflected in a decrease in mean global field power (MGFP) and an increase in latency. Results revealed patients to have a greater decrease in N100 MGFP only in the right hemisphere from block 1 to 2. However, this finding was explained as a medication effect related to clozapine. Overall, patients did not show impairments in N100 habituation.

MEG is a noninvasive technique that shows great promise in that it allows great temporal assessment of neuronal activity. However, the investigation of atypical antipsychotic activity through the utility of MEG has been minimal and to this point not very enlightening. As more technological advances are made in this field, MEG hopefully will prove useful in elucidating atypical antipsychotic effects on neuronal activity.

VI. POSITRON EMISSION TOMOGRAPHY

A. Receptor Studies

The dopaminergic (DA) neurotransmitter system, with focus on the D_2 receptor, has been studied intensely with respect to antipsychotic drug action. Numerous PET studies have provided consistent evidence that both typical and atypical antipsychotic drugs block D_2 receptors but vary according to the degree and time-course (for review see refs. 52–54). The earliest PET studies showed high striatal D_2 receptor occupancy with a variety of typical antipsychotic agents (55). Proceeding studies have consistently replicated this finding. These studies reinforced the idea that clinical efficacy coincided with D_2 blockade in a linear fashion, whereby an average of 60–80% of D_2 blockade was necessary for clinical efficacy. However, proceeding studies proved the relationship between receptor occupancy and clinical response to be much more complex.

Clozapine was the first atypical antipsychotic agent to be assessed with PET D_2 receptor occupancy studies. These initial studies showed clozapine to have a low D_2 receptor occupancy compared to traditional antipsychotics. Farde et al. (56) attempted to elucidate the atypical mechanism by which clozapine acts by investigating D_1, D_2, and 5-HT$_2$ receptor occupancy with PET [^{11}C]SCH 23390, [^{11}C]raclopride, and [^{11}C]NMSP, respectively. Patients with schizophrenia treated with clozapine were assessed, and the regions of interest for D_1 and D_2 receptor occupancy were putamen and cerebellum, and for $5\text{-}HT_2$ were frontal cortex and the cerebellum. For the putamen, D_2 receptor occupancy was a mean of 47%, and a mean of 44% for D_1 receptor occupancy. For the frontal cortex, $5\text{-}HT_2$ receptor occupancy was a mean of 89%. Thus, this initial study revealed that clozapine is unique compared to traditional antipsychotics in that it has low D_2, high D_1, and high $5\text{-}HT_2$ receptor occupancies. In addition, other studies confirmed the low striatal D_2 blockade with clozapine (57,58).

To investigate if clozapine preferentially blocks D_2 receptors in extra-striatal (thalamus, frontal, temporal) as opposed to striatal regions, Talvik et al. (58) used [11C]raclopride to assess striatal D_2 occupancy and [11C]FLB 457 for extra-striatal D_2 occupancy. Subjects were three patients treated with haloperidol for 5–7 weeks and four patients treated with clozapine for 1–5 years. PET scans were performed on the same day. Consistent with previous studies, haloperidol-treated patients had greater striatal D_2 occupancy (78–85%) than clozapine-treated patients (32–63%). For extra-striatal regions, D_2 occupancy was higher for the haloperidol- than clozapine-treated patients, but had similar occupancy levels compared to the striatum for both groups. These findings suggest that clozapine does not have a regional specificity for D_2 blockade.

More recent evidence points to the idea that atypicals may occupy D_2 receptors at levels comparable to that of typical antipsychotics, but that they dissociate from the D_2 receptor more rapidly (59). For instance, it has been shown that clozapine and quetiapine occupy approximately 65–75% of D_2 receptors about 2 hours following oral dose, but dramatically drop off within a 24-hour period (for review, see ref. 53).

The newer atypical antipsychotic aripiprazole also has been studied in 15 normal, healthy males (60). Aripiprazole has been shown to have a high affinity for D_2 and D_3 receptors, lower affinity for D_4 receptors, and insignificant affinity for D_1 receptors. In addition, aripiprazole has a high affinity for presynaptic DA autoreceptor, and also acts as a DA agonist at the D_2 receptor and autoreceptor. In this study, D_2 receptor occupancy was measured with PET [11C]raclopride in the striatum and cerebellum at baseline and following 14 days of 30 mg, 10 mg, 2 mg, 1 mg, or 0.5 mg aripiprazole administration. Results revealed a linear relationship between striatal D_2 receptor occupancy and aripiprazole dose with a range of about 40% for the 0.5 mg dose to 95% for the 30 mg dose. Aripiprazole appears to be unique because even with D_2 occupancy values of greater than 90% no EPS were observed. This is attributable to its D_2 partial agonist properties.

Another study investigated the atypical antipsychotic, sertindole. D_2 receptor occupancy of the striatum, thalamus, temporal cortex, and frontal cortex was studied in four stabilized patients with schizophrenia (61). Two

PET radioligands, [^{11}C]raclopride for striatal D_2 quantification and [^{11}C] FLB 457 for extra-striatal D_2 quantification, were utilized. Four patients with schizophrenia were treated with sertindole (titrated to 20 mg per day) for 7–9 weeks following a 1-week placebo if previously treated with antipsychotic medication. A 2-week placebo washout phase followed sertindole treatment. PET scans were acquired following the treatment and washout phases. Results revealed D_2 striatal occupancy with sertindole to be moderate (52–68%), and extra-striatal region occupancy was similar. Patients had no marked EPS or changes in psychopathology during the treatment phase. These results suggest that sertindole, like clozapine, has low D_2 receptor occupancy properties while being effective with low EPS.

PET receptor studies of antipsychotic action have been very informative at revealing the differential effects of typical and atypical agents. Typical agents, such as haloperidol, prove to have great striatal D_2 affinity, which corresponds with EPS in a linear fashion. In contrast, atypical agents have been shown to have less striatal D_2 affinity. To further investigate atypical antipsychotic action, recent studies have elucidated the time-course of D_2 occupancy in typical and atypical agents. Results suggest that atypical agents moderately occupy D_2 receptors directly following dosage administration, but dramatically drop off with time. This quick striatal D_2 dissociation characterizes the unique properties of atypical antipsychotic action. The question as to whether a high or moderate striatal D_2 occupancy is necessary for antipsychotic action, albeit brief as with the case of atypical agents, remains to be determined.

B. Glucose Metabolism and Blood Flow Studies

There have been numerous studies investigating the effects of typical antipsychotic medications on brain glucose metabolism and regional cerebral blood flow (rCBF) assessed with positron emission tomography (PET)-[^{18}F]fluorodeoxyglucose (FDG) and -[^{15}O]H$_2$O, respectively. The most consistent finding among these studies is increased metabolism or blood flow in the basal ganglia. Many studies also showed decreased metabolism or blood flow in frontal regions with typical antipsychotics. For example, a within-subject PET study found lower frontal glucose metabolism during haloperidol treatment compared to a drug-free state in schizophrenia patients who did not relapse (62), and another reported that this hypofrontal effect occurs after a single dose of haloperidol (63).

There have been few studies that have examined the effects of atypical antipsychotic medications on either brain blood flow or glucose metabolism. One study sought to compare the effects of risperidone and haloperidol on PET-rCBF in patients with schizophrenia (64). Patients were first scanned in a drug-free state (17 antipsychotic-naive, 15 antipsychotic-free for 3 weeks) and then following a 3-week treatment phase with either risperidone or haloperidol. Subjects were scanned during a resting state. Haloperidol had a greater decrease on blood flow in the frontal lobe and a greater increase in the left putamen and posterior cingulate than risperidone. In addition, risperidone decreased cerebellar blood flow more than haloperidol.

One of the first studies to compare the effects of atypical and typical antipsychotic medications on glucose metabolism with PET-FDG was conducted by Buchsbaum et al. (65). Patients with schizophrenia were assessed in a drug-free state of at least 2 weeks and following 4–6 weeks treatment with clozapine ($n = 7$) or the typical agent, thiothixene ($n = 5$). Subjects performed a visual Continuous Performance Task (CPT) during FDG uptake. Results revealed basal ganglia glucose metabolism to increase with clozapine and, in contrast, to decrease with thiothixene. Another study by the same research group found corroborating results (66). Patients with schizophrenia ($n = 18$) participated in a double-blind (placebo or clozapine) within-subject study and were scanned during each condition. FDG uptake was obtained while subjects performed a visual CPT. Results revealed increased glucose metabolism in the striatum (greater on the right side), and decreased metabolism in frontal regions (more on the left side) and the anterior nucleus of the thalamus associated with clozapine. Past research showed patients with schizophrenia to have lower metabolism in the basal ganglia compared to healthy subjects and to lack greater right than left basal ganglia metabolism. Thus, the authors concluded that clozapine appeared to normalized metabolism in the basal ganglia.

Cohen et al. (67) sought to determine the effects of clozapine compared to the typical, fluphenazine, in patients with schizophrenia. With two studies, four groups of male subjects were assessed with PET-FDG while performing an auditory discrimination task: 1) healthy controls, 2) unmedicated patients, 3) patients treated with clozapine, and 4) patients treated with fluphenazine. Results showed normal controls and unmedicated patients to have greater overall cortical metabolism when compared to patients treated with either medication. Also, lower superior frontal metabolism and greater limbic metabolism was seen with both medications compared to normal controls and unmedicated patients. Furthermore, when the clozapine-treated group was compared to the fluphenazine-treated group, greater basal ganglia metabolism was seen with fluphenazine, and lower inferior frontal metabolism was seen with clozapine. The studies that compared typical versus atypical medications revealed minor differential effects on glucose metabolism and blood flow. Both classes of medications tended to decrease frontal and increase basal ganglia metabolism and blood flow, with the typicals producing a greater effect. These results may reflect differences in side effect and therapeutic profiles between typical and atypical antipsychotics.

VII. CONCLUSION

The marked increase in usage of atypical antipsychotic medications to treat schizophrenia has sparked a variety of studies in an attempt to identify the structural and functional brain action that accompanies atypical antipsychotic efficacy and side effects. Findings from studies employing neuroimaging techniques such as MRI, MRS, fMRI, and PET, have revealed differences in actions of atypicals and typical antipsychotics on brain structure, blood flow, metabolism, and receptor occupancy. MEG studies are very few and no consistent differential drug effects have been found. With respect to volumetric MRI studies, atypical agents, in contrast to typicals, do not appear to be associated with an increase in caudate volume. The most notable finding from ^{1}H-MRS studies is that a higher level of NAA, a marker of neuronal integrity, is associated with atypical antipsychotics when compared to typical antipsychotic usage. At this time, ^{31}P-MRS studies have not provided consistent differences across antipsychotic class. The few fMRI studies that have explored atypical antipsychotic action have mainly focused on BOLD response underlying motor function. These studies have been consistent in revealing increased BOLD response in thalamic regions associated with atypical antipsychotic treatment as compared to an unmedicated state or typical antipsychotic treatment. In addition, with fMRI studies of cognition, increased BOLD response in frontal and parietal cortices has also been noted with atypical antipsychotic treatment. Probably, the most informative studies that have led to the understanding of antipsychotic drug action have been PET D_2 receptor studies. Numerous studies have provided corroborating evidence that typical agents have great striatal D_2 affinity, with clinical efficacy levels at 60–80%. In contrast, atypical agents may have less striatal D_2 affinity or more correctly, may have moderate D_2 occupancy directly following dosage administration, but this dramatically drops off with time. This striatal D_2 quick dissociation seems to characterize the unique properties of atypical antipsychotic action. Lastly, PET-FDG and PET-rCBF studies of antipsychotic class drug action have revealed only minor differential effects on glucose metabolism and blood flow. It appears that both classes of drugs decrease frontal and increase basal ganglia metabolism and blood flow but that typical antipsychotics do so to a greater extent.

REFERENCES

1. Gur RE, Turetsky BI, Cowell PE, Finkelman C, Maany V, Grossman RI, Arnold SE, Bilker WB, Gur RC. Temporolimbic volume reductions in schizophrenia. Arch Gen Psychiatry 2000; 57:769–775.
2. Gur RE, Cowell PE, Latshaw A, Turetsky BI, Grossman RI, Arnold SE, Bilker WB, Gur RC. Reduced dorsal and orbital prefrontal gray matter volumes in schizophrenia. Arch Gen Psychiatry 2000; 57:761–768.
3. Cahn W, Pol HE, Bongers M, Schnack HG, Mandl RC, Van Haren NE, Durston S, Koning H, Van der Linden JA, Kahn RS. Brain morphology in antipsychotic-naïve schizophrenia: a study of multiple brain structures. Brit J Psychiatry 2002; 43(suppl 1):s66–s72.
4. Braus DF, Ende G, Weber-Fahr W, Demirakca T, Tost H, Henn FA. Functioning and neuronal viability of the anterior cingulate neurons following antipsychotic treatment: MR-spectroscopic imaging in chronic schizophrenia. Eur Neuropsychopharmacol 2002; 12:145–152.
5. Barch DM, Carter CS, Braver TS, Sabb FW, MacDonald A 3rd, Noll DC, Cohen JD. Selective deficits in prefrontal cortex function in medication-naïve patients with schizophrenia. Arch Gen Psychiatry 2001; 58:280–288.
6. Holcomb HH, Lahti AC, Medoff DR, Weiler M, Dannals RF, Tamminga CA. Brain activation patterns in schizophrenic and comparison volunteers during a matched-performance auditory recognition task. Am J Psychiatry 2000; 157:1634–1645.
7. Chakos M, Lieberman J, Bilder R, Borenstein M, Lerner G, Bogerts B, Houwei W, Kinon B, Ashtari M. Increase in caudate nuclei volumes of first-episode schizophrenic patients taking antipsychotic drugs. Am J Psychiatry 1994; 151:1430–1436.
8. Corson PW, Nopoulos P, Miller DD, Arndt S, Andreasen NC. Change in basal ganglia volume over 2 years in patients with schizophrenia: typical versus atypical neuroleptics. Am J Psychiatry 1999; 156:1200–1204.
9. Chakos M, Lieberman J, Alvir J, Bilder R, Ashtari M. Caudate nuclei volumes in schizophrenic patients treated with typical antipsychotics or clozapine. Lancet 1995; 345:456–457.
10. Keshavan MS, Bagwell WW, Haas GL, Sweeney JA, Schooler NR, Pettegrew JW. Changes in caudate volume with neuroleptic treatment [letter]. Lancet 1994; 344:1434.
11. Scheepers FE, Gispen de Wied CC, Hulshoff Pol HE, Kahn RS. Effect of clozapine on caudate nucleus volume in relation to symptoms of schizophrenia. Am J Psychiatry 2001; 158:644–646.
12. Tauscher-Wisniewski S, Tauscher J, Logan J, Christensen BK, Mikulis DJ, Zipursky RB. Caudate volume changes in first episode psychosis parallel the effects of normal aging: a 5-year follow-up study. Schizophr Res 2002; 58:185–188.
13. Gur RE, Cowell P, Turetsky BI, Gallagher F, Cannon T, Bilker W, Gur RC. A follow-up magnetic resonance imaging study of schizophrenia. Arch Gen Psychiatry 1998; 55:145–152.

14. Rappaport JL, Giedd J, Kumra S, Jacobsen L, Smith A, Lee P, Nelson J, Hamburger S. Childhood-onset schizophrenia. Progressive ventricular change during adolescence. Arch Gen Psychiatry 1997; 54:897–903.

15. DeLisi LE, Sakuma M, Tew W, Kushner M, Hoff AL, Grimson R. Schizophrenia as a chronic brain process: a study of progressive brain structural change subsequent to the onset of schizophrenia. Psychiatry Res Neuroimaging 1997; 74:129–140.

16. Lieberman J, Chakos M, Wu H, Alvir J, Hoffman E, Robinson D, Bilder R. Longitudinal study of brain morphology in first episode schizophrenia. Biol Psychiatry 2001; 49:487–499.

17. Mathalon DH, Sullivan EV, Lim KO, Pfefferbaum A. Progressive brain volume changes and the clinical course of schizophrenia in men: a longitudinal magnetic resonance imaging study. Arch Gen Psychiatry 2001; 58:148–157.

18. Madsen AL, Keiding N, Karle A, Esbjerg S, Hemmingsen R. Neuroleptics in progressive structural brain abnormalities in psychiatric illness. Lancet 1998; 352:784–785.

19. Woods BT. Is schizophrenia a progressive neurodevelopmental disorder? Towards a unitary pathogenetic mechanism. Am J Psychiatry 1998; 155:1661–1670.

20. Lieberman J, Charles HC, Sharma T, Zipursky R, Kahn R, Gur R, Tohen M, Green AI, McEvoy J, Perkins D, Hamer RM, Nemeroff C, Rothschild A, Kuldau J, Strakowski S, Tollefson GD. Antipsychotic treatment effects on progression of brain pathomorphology in first episode schizophrenia. Schizophr Res 2003; 60(1):293.

21. Tsai G, Coyle JT. N-acetylaspartate in neuropsychiatric disorders. Prog Neurobiol 1995; 46:531–540.

22. Brooks WM, Wesley MH, Kodituwakku P, et al. ^{1}H-MRS differentiates white matter hyperintensities in subcortical arteriosclerotic encephalopathy from those in normal elderly. Stroke 1997; 28:1940–1943.

23. Brooks WM, Jung RE, Ford CC, et al. Relationship between neurometabolite derangement and neurocognitive dysfunction in systemic lupus erythematosus. J Rheumatol 1999; 26:81–85.

24. Friedman SD, Brooks WM, Jung R, et al. Proton MR spectroscopic findings correspond to diffuse neuropsychological function in traumatic brain injury. Am J Neuroradiol 1998; 19:1879–1885.

25. Simone IL, Tortorella C, Federico F. The contribution of (1) H-resonance spectroscopy in defining the pathophysiology of multiple sclerosis. Ital J Neurol Sci 1999; 20(5s):241–245.

26. Friedman SD, Stidley CA, Brooks WM, et al. Brain injury and neurometabolic abnormalities in systemic lupus erythematosus. Radiology 1998; 209:79–84.

27. Gruetter R, Weisdorf SA, Rajanayagan V, Terpstra M, Merkle H, Truwit CL, Garwood M, Nyberg SL, Ugurbil K. Resolution improvements in in vivo 1H NMR spectra with increased magnetic field strength. J Magn Reson 1998; 135:260–264.

28. Petroff OA, Mattson RH, Rothman DL. Proton MRS: GABA and glutamate. Adv Neurol 2000; 83:261–271.
29. Magistretti PJ, Pellerin L. Cellular mechanisms of brain energy metabolism and their relevance to functional brain imaging. Phil Trans R Soc Lond 1999; 354:1155–1163.
30. Rothman DL, Sibson NR, Hyder F, Shen J, Behar KL, Shulman RG. In vivo nuclear magnetic resonance spectroscopy studies of the relationship between the glutamate-glutamine neurotransmitter cycle and functional neuroenergetics. Phil Trans R Soc Lond B Biol Sci 1999; 354:1165–1177.
31. Choe BY, Suh TS, Shinn KS, et al. Observation of metabolic changes in chronic schizophrenia after neuroleptic treatment by in vivo hydrogen magnetic resonance spectroscopy. Invest Radiol 1996; 6:345–352.
32. Ende G, Braus DF, Walter S, Weber-Fahr W, Soher B, Maudsley AA, Henn FA. Effects of age, medication, and illness duration on the N-acetylaspartate signal of the anterior cingulate region in schizophrenia. Schizophr Res 2000; 41:389–395.
33. Bustillo JR, Lauriello J, Rowland LM, Jung RE, Petropoulos H, Hart B, Blanchard J, Keith SJ, Brooks WM. Effects of chronic haloperidol and clozapine treatments on frontal and caudate neurochemistry in schizophrenia. Psychiatry Res 2001; 107:135–149.
34. Bustillo JR, Lauriello J, Rowland LM, Thomson LM, Petropoulos H, Hammond R, Hart B, Brooks WM. Longitudinal follow-up of neurochemical changes during the first year of antipsychotic treatment in schizophrenia patients with minimal previous medication exposure. Schizophr Res 2002; 58:313–321.
35. Bertolino A, Callicott JH, Mattay VS, Weidenhammer KM, Rakow R, Egan MF, Weinberger DR. The effect of treatment with antipsychotic drugs on brain N-acetylaspartate measures in patients with schizophrenia. Biol Psychiatry 2001; 49:39–46.
36. Goff DC, Hennen J, Lyoo IK, Tsai G, Wald LL, Evins AE, Yurgelun-Todd DA, Renshaw PF. Modulation of brain and serum glutamatergic concentrations following a switch from conventional neuroleptics to olanzapine. Biol Psychiatry 2002; 51:493–497.
37. Heimberg C, Komoroski RA, Lawson WB, Cardwell D, Karson CN. Regional proton magnetic resonance spectroscopy in schizophrenia and exploration of drug effect. Psychiatry Res 1998; 83:105–115.
38. Volz H-P, Rzanny R, Robger G, Hubner G, Kreitschmann-Andermahr I, Kaiser WA, Sauer H. Decreased energy demanding processes in the frontal lobes of schizophrenics due to neuroleptics? A 31P-magneto-resonance spectroscopy study. Psychiatry Res 1997; 76:123–129.
39. Riehemann S, Hubner G, Smesny S, Volz H-P, Sauer H. Do neuroleptics alter the cerebral intracellular pH value in schizophrenics?: a ^{31}P-MRS study on three different patient groups. Psychiatry Res 2002; 114:113–177.
40. Fukuzako H, Fukuzako T, Kodama S, Hashiguchi T, Takigawa M, Fujimoto T. Haloperidol improves phospholipid abnormalities in temporal lobes of schizophrenic patients. Neuropsychopharmacology 1999; 21:542–549.

41. Braus DF, Ende G, Weber-Fahr W, Sartorius A, Krier A, Hubrich-Ungureanu P, Ruf M, Stuck S, Henn FA. Antipsychotic drug effects on motor activation measured by functional magnetic resonance imaging in schizophrenic patients. Schizophr Res 1999; 39:19–29.
42. Muller JL, Klein HE. Neuroleptic therapy influences basal ganglia activation: a functional magnetic resonance imaging study comparing controls to haloperidol- and olanzapine-treated inpatients. Psychiatry Clin Neurosci 2000; 54:653–658.
43. Muller JL, Roder C, Gerhardt S, Klein HE. Subcortical overactivation in untreated schizophrenic patients: a functional magnetic resonance image finger-tapping study. Psychiatry Clin Neurosci 2002; 56:77–84.
44. Stephan KE, Magnotta VA, White T, Arndt S, Flaum M, O'Leary DS, Andreasen NC. Effects of olanzapine on cerebellar functional connectivity in schizophrenia measured by fMRI during a simple motor task. Psychol Med 2001; 31:1065–1078.
45. Honey GD, Bullmore ET, Soni W, Varatheesan M, Williams SCR, Sharma T. Differences in frontal cortical activation by working memory task after substitution of risperidone for typical antipsychotic drugs in patients with schizophrenia. Proc Natl Acad Sci USA 1999; 96:13432–13437.
46. Ramsey NF, Koning HA, Welles P, Cahn W, van der Linden JA, Kahn RS. Excessive recruitment of neural systems subserving logical reasoning in schizophrenia. Brain 2002; 125:1793–1807.
47. Hamalainen M, Hari R, Llmoniemi RJ, Knuutil J, Lounasmaa OV. Magnetoencephalography: theory, instrumentation, and applications to non-invasive studies of the working human brain. Rev Modern Physics 1993; 65(2):413–498.
48. Lewine JD, Orrison WW. Magnetoencephalography and magnetic source imaging. In: Orrison WW Jr, Lewine JD, Sanders JA, Hartshorne MF, Orrison WW, eds. Functional Brain Imaging. St. Louis: Mosby-Year Book, 1995:369–417.
49. Canive JM, Lewine JD, Edgar JC, Davis JT, Miller GA, Torres F, Tsuag VB. Spontaneous brain magnetic activity in schizophrenia patients treated with aripiprazole. Psychopharmacol Bull 1998; 34:101–105.
50. Sperling W, Vieth J, Martus M, Demling J, Barocka A. Spontaneous slow and fast MEG activity in male schizophrenics treated with clozapine. Psychopharmacology 1999; 142:375–382.
51. Rosburg T, Kreitschmann-Andermahr I, Nowak H, Sauer H. Habituation of the auditory evoked field component N100m in male patients with schizophrenia. J Psychiatr Res 2000; 34:245–254.
52. Pilowsky LS. Probing targets for antipsychotic drug action with PET and SPECT receptor imaging. Nucl Med Commun 2001; 22:829–833.
53. Seeman P. Atypical antipsychotics: mechanism of action. Can J Psychiatry 2002; 47:27–38.
54. Talbot PS, Laruelle M. The role of in vivo molecular imaging with PET and SPECT in the elucidation of psychiatric drug action and new drug development. Eur Neuropsychopharmacol 2002; 12:503–511.

55. Farde L, Weisel F-A, Nordstrom A-L, Sedvall G. D1 and D2 dopamine receptor occupancy during treatment with conventional and atypical neuroleptics. Psychopharmacology 1989; 99:28–31.

56. Farde L, Nordstrom A-L, Nyberg S, Halldin C, Sedvall G. D1-, D2-, and 5-HT2-receptor occupancy in clozapine-treated patients. J Clin Psychiatry 1994; 55:67–69.

57. Nordstrom A-L, Farde L, Nyberg S, Karlsson P, Halldin C, Sedvall G. D1, D2, and 5-HT2receptor occupancy in relation to clozapine serum concentration: a PET study of schizophrenic patients. Am J Psychiatry 1995; 152: 1444–1449.

58. Talvik M, Nordstrom A-L, Nyberg S, Olsson H, Halldin C, Farde L. No support for regional selectivity in clozapine-treated patients: a PET study with [^{11}C]raclopride and [^{11}C]FLB 457. Am J Psychiatry 2001; 158:926–930.

59. Kapur S, Seeman P. Does fast dissociation from the dopamine D2 receptor explain the action of atypical antipsychotics?: a new hypothesis. Am J Psychiatry 2001; 158:360–369.

60. Yokoi F, Grunder G, Bizierre K, Stephane M, Dogan AS, Dannals RF, Ravert H, Suri A, Bramer S, Wong DF. Dopamine D2 and D3 receptor occupancy in normal humans treated with antipsychotic drug aripiprazole (OPC 14597): a study using positron emission tomography and [^{11}C]raclopride. Neuropsychopharmacology 2002; 27:248–259.

61. Nyberg S, Olsson H, Nilsson U, Maehlum E, Halldin C, Farde L. Low striatal and extra-striatal D2 receptor occupancy during treatment with the atypical antipsychotic sertindole. Psychopharmacology 2002; 162:37–41.

62. Holcomb HH, Cascella NG, Thaker GK, Medoff DR, Dannals RF, Tamminga CA. Functional sites of neuroleptic drug action in the human brain: PET/FDG studies with and without haloperidol. Am J Psychiatry 1996; 153:41–49.

63. Lahti AC, Holcomb HH, Weiler M, Parwani A, Machaelidis T, Medoff DR, Tamminga CA. Changes in rCBF after acute challenge with haloperidol and olanzapine in patients with schizophrenia. Schizophr Res 1999; 36:224.

64. Miller DD, Andreasen NC, O'Leary DS, Watkins GL, Ponto LL, Hichwa RD. Comparison of the effects of risperidone and haloperidol on regional cerebral blood flow in schizophrenia. Biol Psychiatry 2001; 49:704–715.

65. Buchsbaum MS, Potkin SG, Marshall JF, Lottenberg S, Teng C, Heh CW, Tafalla R, Reynolds C, Abel L, Plon L, Bunney WE Jr. Effects of clozapine and thiothixene on glucose metabolic rate in schizophrenia. Neuropsychopharmacology 1992; 6:155–163.

66. Potkin SG, Buchsbaum MS, Jin Y, Tang C, Telford J, Friedman G, Lottenberg S, Najafi A, Gulasekaram B, Costa J, Richmond GH, Bunney WE Jr. Clozapine effects on glucose metabolic rate in striatum and frontal cortex. J Clin Psychiatry 1994; 55:63–66.

67. Cohen RM, Nordahl TE, Semple WE, Andreason P, Litman RE, Pickar D. The brain metabolic patterns of clozapine- and fluphenazine-treated patients with schizophrenia during a continuous performance task. Arch Gen Psychiatry 1997; 54:481–486.

10

Evolving Use of Atypical Antipsychotic Medications in Childhood Psychiatric Conditions

Donna L. Londino, Lisa Wiggins, Jennifer Dallas, Edna Stirewalt, and Peter F. Buckley

*Medical College of Georgia,
Augusta, Georgia, U.S.A.*

I. OVERVIEW

A. Introduction

The past 5 years have witnessed a dramatic shift in the pharmacotherapy of adult schizophrenia. Following on the therapeutic success of clozapine in patients with treatment-refractory schizophrenia, there are now several agents available in the United States as first-line choices in the treatment of schizophrenia (Table 1). The evidence for superior efficacy of these agents over typical antipsychotics is substantial and continues to accrue (1). The evidence for a more favorable adverse-effect profile, especially with respect to extrapyramidal side effects (EPS) and tardive dyskinesia (TD), is compelling. Collectively, these data have supported a shift in clinical practice wherein most clinicians in the United States are prescribing atypical antipsychotics as the first-choice agents for new-onset schizophrenia as a maintenance therapy. The preferential role for typical antipsychotics remains in the management of acute agitation in

Table 1 Atypical Antipsychotic Medications Approved for Use in the
United States

Generic name[a]	Trade name	Year of FDA[b] approval	Indication for use beyond psychosis[c]
Clozapine	Clozaril	1990	None
Risperidone	Risperdal	1993	None
Olanzapine	Zyprexa	1996	Acute mania
Quetiapine	Seroquel	1997	None
Ziprasidone	Geodon	2001	None
Aripiprazole	Abilify	2002	None

[a]Clozapine but not any other atypical antipsychotic is also available in several generic forms.
[b]Food and Drug Administration.
[c]None of these agents has a recognized and approved indication in the childhood/adolescent population.

psychosis – by the use of acute intramuscular preparations – and in the management of patients who are persistently noncompliant with medication – by the use of long-acting (depot) injections. The coming on-line of both short-acting and depot forms of atypical antipsychotic medication is likely to further diminish the role of typical antipsychotics in clinical practice (2–4). The pace of this shift in treatment patterns and the ultimate equipoise between atypical and typical antipsychotic medications remains to be determined (5,6).

The practice pattern for adult schizophrenia is of importance to the consideration of the use of atypical antipsychotics in childhood schizophrenia and other conditions. This is particularly so because the evidence base for efficacy and tolerability of these agents overwhelmingly is derived from studies in adult populations. A recent review by Roberts et al. noted that "only one-third of drugs used to treat children have been studied adequately in the population in which they are being used and have appropriate use information on the product label. For the other two-thirds of drugs, information regarding safety and efficacy for pediatric patients is insufficient or absent" (7). The FDA has echoed similar sentiments and has attempted since the late 1970s to increase research by manufacturers on the safety and efficacy of their drugs in children. Recent legislation to give the FDA authority to require testing in children appears promising and research in this area has grown; however, at present, much of clinical practice is still guided by what is learnt from studies in adults more so than studies in children.

It is also important to note that the current use of atypical antipsychotics is more extensive in adult affective and nonpsychotic conditions than the prescription of these drugs for the treatment of schizophrenia (8). This practice is in part driven by the inadequate efficacy of primary treatments for these conditions, as well as accumulating evidence that atypical antipsychotics have potential thymoleptic, antiaggressive, and anxiolytic properties beyond the treatment of psychosis. In an attempt to evaluate clinician choice of atypicals, Buckley and colleagues administered a 12-item questionnaire to 284 general and specialist psychiatrists from Iowa and Ohio (9). The majority of respondents (86%) favored the use of atypical antipsychotics as first-line treatments for schizophrenia. They also, however, indicated their use of atypicals in dementia (80%), personality disorders (69%), developmental delay/mental retardation (65%), and autism (40%).

Similarly, these drugs are increasingly being prescribed for childhood conditions beyond psychosis. Examples include bipolar illness, psychotic depression, anxiety disorders, autism and other developmental disorders, Tourette's syndrome, disruptive behavior disorders, and childhood anorexia nervosa. Emerging evidence thus suggests that atypical antipsychotic medications offer important therapeutic advantages beyond their initial regulatory approval in several conditions and patient populations. Available information on the efficacy and tolerability of atypical antipsychotics in these conditions is reviewed in this chapter.

Toren and colleagues published a thorough review of the use of atypical neuroleptics in child and adolescent psychiatry in 1998 (10). At the time of that review, there were only five blind placebo-controlled clinical trials, 24 open-label trials, and 33 case series which encompassed research on the use of clozapine, risperidone, olanzapine, and several selective dopamine receptor blockers (i.e., sulpiride, tiapride, remoxipride) not currently approved for clinical use. A subsequent review by Malone et al. in 1999 and Findling et al. in 2000 again found most of the currently available data based on case reports and case series with a limited number of controlled prospective studies (11,12).

Given this context, the purpose of the present chapter is to provide an account of the evolving use of atypical antipsychotics in childhood conditions. As mentioned previously, the literature is in most circumstances sparse and there is a marked lack of randomized, controlled clinical trials of antipsychotics (both typicals and atypicals) in this population. Thus, this review was based upon a Medline search to retrieve current reports on atypical antipsychotics in childhood and adolescent disorders, a selective evaluation of recent information from pertinent major (child and adolescent) psychiatric meetings, as well as a review of the most current state of knowledge about the treatment of child and adolescent disorders derived from practice parameters that have been established by the American Academy of Child and Adolescent Psychiatry.

B. Basic Concepts

1. Pharmacokinetics in Children and Adolescents

Special precautions should be taken when administering medications to children and adolescents. This subset of patients responds differently than adults to psychotropic medications, secondary to differences in both pharmacokinetics and pharmacodynamics. Pharmacokinetics describes how the body handles a drug and is divided into drug absorption, distribution, metabolism, and excretion. Pharmacodynamics describes the effect that a drug has on the body and includes considerations of the receptor activities of medications.

Developmental issues are relevant to an understanding of both of these factors. Changes during development in drug absorption, distribution, metabolism, and excretion may affect the delivery of a drug to the target tissue. In addition, maturation of brain regions and neurotransmitter systems during development may alter the effect that a medication has at different ages. Early childhood is a time of tremendous change for the human brain. Visual processing, motor skills, and language are acquired during this sensitive period (13). Cortical synaptic density is substantially modified by pruning until the age of 10. Despite knowledge of the same, controlled studies of child and adolescent pharmacokinetics are limited. Grothe and colleagues found the pharmacokinetics of olanzapine in children and adolescents to be similar to the pharmacokinetics in adults (14). McConville et al. likewise noted similarities between the pharmacokinetics of quetiapine in adolescents and adults (15). Limited data are available about the effect of differing psychodynamics in children and its influence on drug response and safety.

The impact that absorption differences between adults and children have on the pharmacokinetics in the pediatric population is unclear. Stomach contents tend to be less acidic in younger populations, leading to a slower absorption of acidic drugs such as antidepressants and psychosti-mulants more than antipsychotics (16). Taylor proposed that children have fewer and less diverse intestinal microflora, and that this observation may explain why phenothiazines (absorbed or metabolized in the intestinal wall) have to be given at larger dosages to achieve a therapeutic effect (17). The absorption of oral doses of the atypical antipsychotic agents is often erratic, but peak serum concentrations typically occur 2 to 4 hours following a dose (18). Clinical observation has suggested that absorption of certain psychotropic medications may be even more rapid in children than in adults, contributing to greater fluctuations in blood levels and possible cardiac toxicity, oftentimes a function of peak plasma concentration.

Jatlow has done extensive work looking at the differences in drug distribution between adults, children, and adolescents (19). He has noted that infants, children, and adolescents are not a homogeneous group in terms of drug distribution patterns. These differences can be especially significant in adolescents going through puberty. Fat stores and the relative proportion of total body water to extra-cellular water change with development and affect the distribution of medications. Because of their high degree of lipophilicity, antipsychotic medications tend to accumulate in tissues. Overall, children have a proportion of body fat less than that in adults. The volume of distribution is therefore considered to be smaller, suggesting a larger plasma concentration of a lipophilic drug in a child as compared to an adult given the same weight-adjusted dose.

In general, children tend to break down and eliminate most drugs more rapidly and efficiently than adults and elderly persons. Metabolic pathways for many drugs function at a low level during the perinatal period, mature by about 6 months of age, peak between the ages of 1 and 5 years, and decline gradually to adult values by 15 years of age. Additionally, the liver is proportionally larger in children than in adults. The relatively higher dosage requirement of a majority of psychotropic drugs in children is most commonly explained by this disproportionate liver size and increased hepatic metabolism. The consideration of a larger liver size and increased hepatic metabolic rate suggest that higher ratios of milligram of drug to kilograms of body weight should be used to achieve comparable steady-state plasma levels as seen in adults. Similarly, the half-life of a medication may be shorter in a child, suggesting the use of divided doses for more consistent coverage of symptoms throughout the day.

The kidney is the most important organ for drug excretion. Renal functioning, even in infants, in contrast to hepatic function, approximates that of adults. In the 1987 study published by Jatlow, developmental changes in renal functions were not found to contribute substantially to age-related differences in psychotropic drug excretion, with the exception of lithium, whose clearance may be increased in children secondary to an increased GFR (19).

The use of antipsychotics in children and adolescents should be undertaken not only with consideration of the pharmacokinetic differences between children and adults, but also with consideration of differences in pharmacodynamics. Verghese and colleagues demonstrated that children actually require smaller weight-adjusted doses of antipsychotic medications than do adults in order to achieve the same therapeutic effect (20). Children have a greater density of dopamine D_1 and D_2 receptors than do adults, suggesting a greater sensitivity to the beneficial and adverse-effects of antipsychotic medications. To date there have been no studies of dopamine receptor occupancy using positron emission tomography to specifically determine the impact that this has on the response to antipsychotics in this age group. Smaller doses are recommended for the initial treatment, particularly if the child is very young. This conservative approach may offer beneficial effects on targeted symptoms with decreased risk of dystonias and EPS. In conclusion, when compared to adults, children require an increased milligram-to-kilogram dose to achieve the same plasma concentration but clinically require a lower milligram-to-kilogram dose to achieve the same therapeutic effect and to avoid unwanted side effects.

II. ANTIPSYCHOTIC USE IN CHILDHOOD AND ADOLESCENT DISORDERS

A. Childhood/Adolescent-Onset Schizophrenia (CAS)

It is often underappreciated that one-fourth of patients with schizophrenia develop their illness before age 15. Moreover, as research on early intervention intensifies, there is a growing awareness that more subtle manifestations of psychosis, including cognitive and social impairments are often observed early in childhood (21,22). In general, the symptomatic expression of schizophrenia in children/adolescents is comparable to the presentation in adults. However, childhood/adolescent-onset is, by definition, a more severe form of schizophrenia. Several recent follow-up studies are consistent with this observation (23,24).

In view of the poor course of childhood schizophrenia and the paucity of studies in this population, it is not surprising that the known efficacy of typical antipsychotics in this group is limited. There are several older studies of treatment of childhood/adolescent schizophrenia. Most are case series and/or open-labeled clinical trials of relatively short duration (25–29). Pool and colleagues compared loxapine with haloperidol in 75 adolescents and found comparable efficacy (which for both active drugs was superior to placebo), but adverse-effect profiles were problematic (27). The mean dose of loxapine (87 mg) was somewhat high for the patient population, especially in consideration of recent speculations that low dose loxapine may confer a "quasi-atypical" advantage. In a single arm, placebo-controlled trial of haloperidol in 16 children (ages between 5 and 12), haloperidol was effective but with substantial EPS (29). A similar high level of intolerance to EPS was demonstrated in another comparative trial of thioridazine and thiothixene in adolescents with schizophrenia (28). Although less is known about the incidence of TD in CAS, there is no reason to believe that the rate is any lower than that observed in adult schizophrenia (estimated at 5% per year for the first 5 years of treatment), inferring an increased risk for treatment of children or adolescents secondary to the projected long course of medication exposure.

There is emerging information on the efficacy and tolerability of atypical antipsychotic medications in CAS (10,25,26). To date, more information is available regarding clozapine; in part because of the more severe illness in CAS, and also as a consequence of the longer period of clinical experience with clozapine over other atypicals in clinical practice. The prototype atypical agent, clozapine (Clozaril) was introduced in 1990. It was the first agent to display both serotonin and dopamine antagonism. Clozapine is associated with little to no incidence of extrapyramidal reactions or increased prolactin concentrations. It is more effective against the negative symptoms compared to the conventional antipsychotics, making it very beneficial for patients who are refractory to conventional antipsychotics. Early case reports and small open-labeled trials confirmed that clozapine was an effective treatment option for patients with CAS who had failed prior antipsychotic treatments (26,30–32). The best information on clozapine (mean dose 176 mg/day) versus haloperidol (mean dose 16 mg/day) came from the childhood schizophrenia division of the National Institute of Mental Health (26). This was a 6-week treatment study in 21 severely ill adolescents with neuroleptic-resistant schizophrenia (mean age 14.0 years). The response rate to clozapine was superior to haloperidol for both positive and negative symptoms. The difference was assessed as clinically and statistically significant. Additionally, 62% of clozapine-treated patients were rated as very much improved on the Clinical Global Impression Scale. Clozapine treatment, however, was complicated by higher rates of adverse-effects in this population than typically observed in adult studies. One-third of the patients treated with clozapine had to have the medication discontinued. Sedation was common and reported in 90% of patients. Two of 10 patients developed a seizure during clozapine therapy. Five of the 10 subjects developed significant neutropenia and 2% developed agranulocytosis. This was disconcerting given the current rate of agranulocytosis in adults (0.38%) and the occurrence of a higher rate in CAS during a brief clinical trial. Since older age is also a known risk factor for clozapine-induced agranulocytosis, it may well be that the incidence of this adverse-effect is higher at both extremes of age. Of note, as well, are rare reports of stuttering induced by higher doses (300 mg/day or more) of clozapine in adults (33). It remains to be seen whether this side effect will be observed in children and adolescents. Despite the significant improvement in symptoms observed with clozapine treatment in CAS, the adverse-effect profile, particularly its association with rare, but occasionally fatal, agranulocytosis in up to 1% of treated patients, has limited its usefulness.

With the approval of risperidone by the Food and Drug Administration (FDA) in 1993, the first safer alternative to clozapine became available. Most of the information on risperidone therapy in CAS is derived from small case series (10,34–38). Grcevich et al. published a retrospective chart review of 16 youths treated with risperidone (39). Armenteros et al. published a prospective open pilot study of risperidone in 10 adolescents with schizophrenia (40). When taken in entirety, the available data suggest that risperidone is effective for both positive and negative symptoms of CAS. Additionally, recent work by McGorry and colleagues demonstrated a benefit for low-dose risperidone in the prodrome of schizophrenia in a cohort of study participants, a portion of which had CAS (41). The most common side effects seen early in the course of treatment include sedation and weight gain. Although EPS can occur in teen-agers with schizophrenia who are prescribed risperidone, the reported rates are smaller than those seen previously with high-potency neuroleptics. It appears as if a gradual dose-titration strategy might minimize the risk of EPS (39). In general, doses of 1–2 mg are appropriate for patients with CAS, depending on age. Higher dosages of risperidone above 5–6 mg begin to approximate haloperidol in mechanism of action and potential for EPS. Children are particularly sensitive to the EPS and hyperprolactinemia effects of risperidone necessitating close monitoring of these symptoms and efforts by the clinician to keep treatment at the lowest effective dose.

Olanzapine was approved by the FDA in September 1996. The drug has a high affinity for $5\text{-}HT_2$ receptors and a moderate affinity for D_2 receptors. It was initially tested as a possible treatment alternative to clozapine in adolescents with neuroleptic-resistant schizophrenia. Like clozapine, it also has affinity for muscarinic receptors contributing to similar problematic side effects of sedation and weight gain. In a 1998 pilot study, Kumra and colleagues examined the efficacy of olanzapine in 23 children with schizophrenia who had not previously responded to neuroleptic treatment (42). After 8 weeks of treatment, children receiving olanzapine showed improvements on the BPRS (Brief Psychiatric Rating Scale), the SANS (Scale for the Assessment for Negative Symptoms), and the PANSS (Positive and Negative Symptom Scale). In this trial, olanzapine did not appear to be as effective as clozapine in reducing psychotic symptomatology; however, an earlier study by Mandoki (1997) suggested that both drugs had equal efficacy in neuroleptic-resistant schizophrenia (43). Current work by Schulz et al. also suggests that olanzapine is safe and effective for adolescents with psychotic disorders (44). A recent pharmacovigilance study of olanzapine therapy in CAS demonstrated that the adverse-effect profile was overall similar to adult schizophrenia but that some effects were more common in children; notably weight gain, sedation, and dystonia. Cardiac arrhythmias were significantly less common in children than in adults (45).

Quetiapine was FDA approved for the treatment of schizophrenia in September 1997. Quetiapine is a potent $5-HT_2$ antagonist with weaker D_2 activity but also binds to several other receptors such as the alpha-1 adrenergic receptors. Its side effects include low blood pressure at high doses. Unlike clozapine, it is not linked to agranulocytosis, and unlike typical antipsychotics, it is not linked to EPS. McConville and colleagues have examined the use of quetiapine in CAS (46,15). They studied the efficacy and tolerability of quetiapine in 10 adolescents with chronic psychosis, seven who had schizoaffective disorder and three who had a diagnosis of bipolar disorder. Quetiapine was well tolerated, including dose titration to up to above 750 mg in several patients. In this 3-week study, patients showed a reduction in psychotic symptoms and demonstrated global improvement in functioning. The authors reported that the pharmacokinetic profile in adolescents was similar to that of adults. Overall, treatment was well tolerated, and no patients developed EPS. Two case reports suggest that youths who do not respond to another atypical agent may respond to quetiapine offering an additional pharmacological option for treatment-resistant patients poorly responsive to risperidone or olanzapine (47,48). Initial concerns over the development of cataracts in animal models have not conclusively been confirmed in humans. Further research will be needed to determine the exact role of quetiapine in the first-line management of CAS.

In February 2001, ziprasidone was approved by the FDA. Unlike earlier agents, it was studied in pediatric patients prior to its release; however, published data of extensive clinical trials examining the safety and efficacy of ziprasidone in CAS are limited (49). Concerns that children may be more susceptible to the effects of ziprasidone on cardiac function, most notably the prolongation of the QTc interval and subsequent potential for arrhythmias or sudden cardiac death, are understandable and may preclude the use of this drug in this population. One retrospective analysis, although limited due to small sample size, indicated that ziprasidone was well tolerated in children (50). Only one child in this analysis showed any QTc interval increase. The FDA has recently mandated new label warnings to indicate that ziprasidone is not to be used in patients with a history of cardiac arrhythmia due to the risk of QTc prolongation. As with olanzapine, quetiapine, and risperidone, a baseline ECG should be obtained in all patients, but most notably pediatric patients, especially those with cardiac complications at birth, family history of arrhythmias, or with known mitral valve prolapse, prior to the use of ziprasidone. Monitoring is recommended throughout the course of treatment.

The newest atypical antipsychotic to receive an FDA indication for use in adult schizophrenia is aripiprazole, approved on November 15 2002. It is so new that clinical experience with it, particularly in children, remains very limited. Aripiprazole is chemically different from other atypical antipsychotic agents and subsequently is believed to have unique pharmacological actions different from other atypicals, suggesting that it may be considered as a "next-generation" atypical antipsychotic (51,52). It is the first dopamine partial-agonist approved in the United States for clinical use in adult patients with schizophrenia, although other dopamine partial-agonists (e.g., bromocriptine) have been used to treat Parkinson's disease for many years. Partial agonism refers to the ability of a drug to block a receptor if it is overstimulated or in competition with a natural agonist, but also to stimulate a receptor when the natural agonist is unavailable. Aripiprizole acts as a weak stimulator at dopamine D_2 receptors, with the potential for exerting either antagonistic (inhibitory) or agonistic (stimulating) effects, depending on the sensitivity of the receptors and availability of dopamine, its natural agonist in the brain (53). Aripiprazole has similar actions at serotonin $5-HT_{1A}$ receptors. It is a $5-HT_{2A}$ antagonist. In short, aripiprazole may act to modulate or stabilize dopamine–serotonin systems in the brain (52).

Aripiprazole is effective in reducing both the positive and negative symptoms of schizophrenia, and is well tolerated by most patients (54–56). Promising results from recent clinical trials of aripiprazole in adult patients with bipolar disorder also suggest that this drug may be useful for other indications as well and will be discussed at length later (57). Kane and colleagues demonstrated the benefit of both 15 mg/day and 30 mg/day doses of aripiprazole over placebo in a published placebo-controlled 4-week trial of aripiprazole and haloperidol in 414 patients with schizoaffective disorder or schizophrenia. Superior efficacy was noted for aripiprazole over haloperidol on PANSS scores and significantly greater improvement than placebo in overall functioning was reported on the Clinical Global Impression Scale (CGI) (55). The improvements were comparable to the haloperidol-treated subjects. Additionally, the rate of discontinuation from the study due to adverse-effects was comparable between the two groups. Only the haloperidol-treated group had significantly greater extrapyramidal side effects than placebo, as like other atypical antipsychotics, aripiprazole has a low risk of producing EPS.

Aripiprazole has minimal antagonism at histaminergic and muscarinic receptors. Subsequently, unlike other atypical antipsychotics, particularly risperidone, olanzapine, and clozapine, patients treated with aripiprazole gain little if any weight. The drug seems to cause no changes in the plasma glucose levels that might suggest a risk for diabetes and the drug does not appear to have the propensity to increase prolactin levels that is problematic with the other atypical antipsychotic medications. Initial studies have even suggested that aripiprazole may decrease prolactin levels to a normal range (52,55). There have been no reports of cardiac abnormalities associated with its use. Although it is early to determine the incidence rates of these increasingly concerning side effects potentially associated with the other agents, aripiprazole may offer comparable benefits in the treatment of CAS without increased risk of side effects, particularly problematic in this patient population.

Much like the literature on the use of atypicals in adult schizophrenia, there is a paucity of information on the comparative efficacy of these drugs in CAS. Grcevich and colleagues have addressed the issue of comparative tolerability in a retrospective analysis of patients receiving risperidone, olanzapine, or quetiapine (58). Seventy-five patients received risperidone (mean maximum daily dose 13.3 mg/day), and 25 patients were treated with quetiapine (mean maximum daily dose 210.3 mg/day). Results found that after 3 months of treatment, patients gained 8.6 lb with risperidone, 7.2 lb with quetiapine, and 14.1 lb with olanzapine. Weight gain was noted as the most common side effect. In a similar trial conducted by Ratzoni and colleagues, olanzapine, risperidone, and haloperidol were compared in adolescent inpatients (59). Subjects treated with atypicals exhibited higher weight gain, an average of 7.2 lb for olanzapine and 3.9 lb with risperidone, as compared to haloperidol, which produced an average weight gain of 1.1 lb.

B. Bipolar Disorder

The principal categories of psychotic illness that affect children are schizophrenia and bipolar disorder, both chronic and disabling disorders. Typically, the illness emerges in mid to late adolescence or early adulthood. Bipolar I disorder is estimated to affect 0.6% of adolescents. Once thought to be rare in childhood, this disorder is now diagnosed even in the prepubertal age group. Traditionally, lithium, sodium valproate, carbamazepine, and adjunctive treatment with benzodiazapines have been used to treat bipolar I disorders in both adults and the pediatric population (60); however, as in the adult population, there has been substantial recent use of antipsychotic medications in children and adolescents with bipolar illness as well.

In treating bipolar illness, pharmacological intervention is twofold. Initial pharmacotherapy is instituted to target manic or mixed symptoms, and continued treatment is aimed at maintenance and the prevention of relapse. The new antipsychotics, particularly olanzapine, risperidone, and quetiapine, are particularly effective in treating agitated mania and disrupted sleep that may impair function and/or mandate inpatient stabilization. The highly sedative properties offer an acute benefit in restoring disrupted sleep. Likewise, the psychotic symptoms seen in mania may need to be targeted independent of the mood symptoms and would suggest the use of an antipsychotic for optimal benefit. Clearly, the newer atypical antipsychotics offer an improved side effect profile as compared to the older neuroleptics.

Information on the use of atypical antipsychotics for the treatment of adolescent bipolar disorder is beginning to emerge but is predominantly limited to open studies and case reports. In one early case report (1994), Fuchs noted benefit in a young adolescent bipolar patient treated with clozapine (61). More recently, Masi et al. (2002) noted that clozapine improved manic symptoms in pediatric patients, including those who had failed to respond to other treatments (62).

Frazier and colleagues published a retrospective chart review of 28 outpatient children and adolescents ages 4–17 with bipolar disorder (25 mixed and three hypomanic) treated adjunctively with risperidone (mean dose 1.7 ± 1.3 mg) for 6 months. Significant improvement in mania and aggression was seen in 82% of patients. Eight percent of the study cohort also showed improvement in ADHD symptoms (63). An open trial by Schreier likewise demonstrated therapeutic response to low-dose risperidone as adjunctive treatment for affective symptoms (predominantly suggestive of bipolar disorder), aggression, and violent behavior (64).

Recent interest in the thymoleptic properties of olanzapine has contributed to the frequent clinical use of this atypical antipsychotic in bipolar disorder, specifically psychotic mania, and the recent FDA approval for treatment of acute mania in adults. Interest in the use of olanzapine as long-term maintenance therapy in bipolar disorders continues to grow. Preliminary data by Tohen and colleagues demonstrated benefit of olanzapine over depakote in a 47-week, randomized, double-blind study (65). After 3 weeks, olanzapine showed a significantly greater improvement in the Young Mania Rating Scale (47%) as compared to depakote (34%). Both medications were effective over the course of the entire 47-week study.

There are two case series and one open trial of olanzapine as either primary or adjunctive treatment for children and adolescents with bipolar disorder. In an open study, Frazier and colleagues treated 23 children ages 5–14 years diagnosed with bipolar disorder with olanzapine 2.5–20 mg/day for 8 weeks (66). Response was based on a 30% or greater improvement on the Young Mania Rating Scale. A 61% response rate was noted in this sample. Weight gain was the predominant side effect with a mean increase in weight of 5 kg. Chang and Ketter demonstrated "marked improvement" on

CGI scores from the use of olanzapine as an adjunct to the current treatment regimen for three youths diagnosed with bipolar disorder (67). Similar findings were reported by Soutullo and colleagues in the treatment of a small cohort of youths presenting with acute mania (68). Because of olanzapine's broad affinity for both dopaminergic and serotonergic receptors, these results are not that surprising and may be related to the beneficial therapeutic outcome.

In the first double-blind, randomized, placebo-controlled study of adolescents with mania published by DelBello and colleagues, the benefit of quetiapine as adjunctive treatment for adolescent mania was noted (69). Thirty hospitalized adolescents with mania or mixed bipolar I disorder were treated with divalproex, either alone or in conjunction with quetiapine for 6 weeks. All patients were treated with divalproex at an initial dose of 20 mg/kg, thereafter adjusted to maintain a serum level between 80 and 130 md/dl. All patients were randomly administered either quetiapine at an initial dose of 25 mg bid, thereafter titrated to a maximum of 150 mg tid, or placebo. Patients in both the divalproex and divalproex plus quetiapine groups showed significant reduction from baseline to endpoint Young Mania Rating Scale (YMRS) scores. The improvement was significantly greater in the combination treatment group ($p = 0.03$) who were also significantly more likely to be reported as responders than those patients treated with divalproex only (87% and 53%, respectively). Weight gain was no greater with combination treatment than with divalproex sodium. Sedation was more problematic in the group treated with both divalproex and quetiapine.

Neither ziprasidone nor aripiprazole are approved by the FDA for the treatment of acute mania or bipolar disorder. Published studies that are randomized and placebo-controlled are limited in adults and almost nonexistent in the child and adolescent literature. A randomized, double-blind, placebo-controlled multicenter trial by Keck and colleagues (2003) demonstrated the efficacy and safety of ziprasidone in adult bipolar patients presenting with a manic or mixed manic episode (70). Ziprasidone (80 to 160 mg/day) was significantly more effective than placebo in the acute treatment of mania in hospitalized patients. It demonstrated a favourable tolerability profile with a low incidence of EPS and weight gain, and no clinically relevant changes in ECG parameters, vital signs, or laboratory values. Similarly, preliminary findings in a multicenter, double-blind, randomized, placebo-controlled trial of 262 adult patients presenting with acute manic or mixed manic states noted significant improvement in symptoms over placebo after only 4 days of treatment with aripiprazole (57). Targeted symptoms included irritability, euphoria, disturbed thinking, and disruptive-aggressive behavior.

These findings have prompted adult and child psychiatrists alike to prescribe both ziprasidone and aripipazole for adults with bipolar disorder and for early-onset bipolar disorder in children and adolescents, particularly those individuals who have not demonstrated efficacy from the mood stabilizers, or the more well-studied atypical antipsychotics (olanzapine, quetiapine, risperidone). There is an obvious need for more research in this area. It is still unclear whether the newer agents will be beneficial in maintenance therapy, but they do show promise in the acute stabilization of behavior in children and adolescents with mood lability, and certainly would be considered appropriate adjunctive therapy to the mood stabilizers in the treatment of psychotic mania. Adverse side effects must be monitored and discontinuation of the medicine considered if the apparent risks outweigh the noted clinical benefit. Although at present practice guidelines confirm the preferential role of lithium and anticonvulsant medications as the treatment of first choice for bipolar illness, these recommendations may change as more formal research is conducted in this area.

C. Psychotic Depression

Psychosis can complicate depression in both adults and adolescents. Gellar and colleagues demonstrated the benefit of conventional neuroleptics in combination with antidepressants in a small study of adolescents with psychotic depression (71). There are, however, no data on the use of atypical antipsychotics in childhood depression, and of some concern are published accounts of depression seen adversely in patients treated with atypical antipsychotics for bipolar illness. In a study by Mandoki (72), four of six patients with bipolar disorder developed dysphoric mood within 3 months of starting risperidone treatment. Two of them met the criteria for major depression and required the addition of an antidepressant. This finding was somewhat surprising given the antidepressant benefit of risperidone seen in some adults, most likely due to the 5-HT_2 antagonistic effect of the medication. Frazier and colleagues similarly noted that one patient discontinued treatment secondary to emerging depressive symptoms during an open-label trial examining the benefit of olanzapine in the treatment of bipolar-disorder in juveniles (73). These findings, albeit in the adolescent bipolar population, should not be ignored when considering the treatment of a primary depressive disorder with psychosis. Antipsychotics are often indicated for the treatment of psychotic depression, especially if command hallucinations are instructing the patient to engage in self harm or violence toward others, or severe paranoia is contributing to similar risks and distress. The newer atypical antipsychotics have consistently been proven to have a less adverse side effect profile and thus would be indicated in children and adolescents. Further research is needed in this area with particular attention to the possibility of worsening dysphoria with prolonged treatment.

D. Anxiety Disorders

Anxiety disorders comprise one of the most prevalent categories of psychopathology in the pediatric population. Treatment most often includes an integration of several interventions and these nonpharmacological interventions contribute to an overall more favorable outcome with a decreased occurrence of relapse, particularly after medication discontinuation. Pharmacological interventions, however, can offer an important adjunct to behavioral and other treatment modalities, particularly at the onset of illness and before behavioral techniques are learned.

In the 1997 Practice Parameters for anxiety disorders, "neuroleptics were not recommended in the absence of comorbid disorders," such as Tourette's disorder or psychosis (74). The lack of a recommendation for the use of neuroleptics without a comorbid disorder was due to a real concern about impaired cognitive functioning, tardive dyskinesia, and reports of "neuroleptic separation anxiety syndrome" described in children who developed school phobia in response to haloperidol or pimozide treatment for Tourette's disorder. Stein et al. suggested that risperidone might augment the benefit of serotonin reuptake inhibitors in obsessive-compulsive and related disorders (75); however, it is interesting to note that similar reports were published describing the emergence of separation anxiety in two adolescent boys and one prepubertal boy who were adjunctively treated with low-dose risperidone for obsessive-compulsive disorder (OCD), ADHD, and increasing behavioral disruption. Of note, two of the three patients in these reports were subsequently treated with olanzapine without a recurrence of anxiety.

At the present time, it is unclear what role the atypical antipsychotics will play in the management of pediatric anxiety disorders. Owing to the more tolerable side effect profile, clinicians may consider these drugs for treatment of severe obsessive-compulsive disorder, either monotherapy or as adjunct to other agents. The atypical antipsychotics may be preferable for use in severe anxiety as compared to the potentially habit forming benzodiazapines in this young population. Psychotic symptoms associated with post-traumatic stress would be a reasonable indication for antipsychotic use, but clearly more research is needed in this area.

E. Autism and Developmental Disorders

Autism and the pervasive developmental disorders (PDD) are defined by
the American Academy of Child and Adolescent Psychiatry as "neuropsychiatric disorders characterized by patterns of delay and deviance in
the development of social, communicative, and cognitive skills" (76). The
characteristic symptoms of autism and other pervasive developmental
disorders include abnormalities in social relatedness, communication, and
repetitive behavior. These conditions have their onset in the first years of life
and disrupt many areas of functioning. With the exception of Asperger's
disorder, autistic disorders are generally associated with mental retardation.
The expression of the disorders is diverse and may present a significant
challenge for the clinician.

The most effective treatment of autism and developmental disorders is
a multidisciplinary approach, which encompasses educational needs, social
relatedness with family and peers, communicative skills, and adaptive
functioning. Pharmacotherapy has been historically used to target
symptoms of aggression, irritability, stereotypic behavior, hyperactivity,
self-abusive behavior, and self-stimulatory behavior. The medications are
not specific to autism and have not traditionally been used to treat core
aspects of the disorder. Clinical trials have examined almost all classes of
medications targeting these problematic symptoms as they further impair
the individual's ability to benefit from educational and psychosocial
interventions. Antipsychotics, selective serotonin reuptake inhibitors,
tricyclic antidepressants, lithium, mood stabilizers, and anxiolytics have
been used in these patients with varying degrees of success.

Only recently have controlled studies begun to examine the benefit of
the new atypical antipsychotics on the disruptive symptoms associated with
autistic and developmental disorders. Early studies primarily examined the
benefit of haloperidol and have repeatedly demonstrated the efficacy in this
population. Anderson and colleagues noted that educational learning was
not impaired, but was facilitated (77). Concern has continued to exist,
however, over the long-term use of haloperidol (especially in children)
secondary to the concern of dyskinesia, including tardive dyskinesia. The
development of the newer atypical antipsychotics, which have consistently
demonstrated a lower risk of extrapyramidal symptoms, steered clinical
intervention towards these agents as first-line treatment to target disruptive
behavioral symptoms, and subsequently underscored the need for controlled
studies to formally evaluate the efficacy and safety profile of these agents in
this subpopulation. Research endeavors ensued rather quickly. Considering
the limited research on the use of atypical antipsychotics in other childhood
disorders, more double-blind, placebo-controlled studies are available

demonstrating the efficacy of these agents in the treatment of autistic and developmental disorders.

The most extensive research on the use of atypical antipsychotics in autism and other developmental disorders has focused on risperidone and olanzapine. Masi and colleagues conducted an open-label trial of risperidone in a small cohort of young children (3.6 to 6.6 years) with an optimal dose of 0.5 mg/day (78). Modest improvement was noted; at least 25% improvement on the Children's Psychiatric Rating Scale (CPRS) was seen in the majority of patients. Improvement was noted on the Childhood Autism Rating Scale (CARS) with greater than 25% improvement seen in symptoms of hyperactivity, fidgetiness, rhythmic motions, mood lability, and angry affect. Functional impairment, as determined on the Children's Global Assessment Scale (C-GAS), improved more than 25%. Two participants did not complete the study because of side effects even though risperidone was overall well tolerated at this low dose. Only three subjects had a weight gain of over 10%. Zuddis and colleagues published a semi-naturalistic prospective study investigating the safety and efficacy of the long-term use of risperidone in children and adolescents and to additionally ascertain the effects of drug withdrawal (79). Subjects with autism or pervasive developmental disorders not otherwise specified (PDD-NOS) were treated with risperidone for 6 months after which parents were given the option of continuing for an additional 6 months. Risperidone was reported to significantly ameliorate behavioral symptoms of PDD in 10 out of 11 subjects. There were mild improvements noted in the core symptoms of autism, but these effects were of slower onset and reported later in treatment. Weight gain was common, although the rate of increase lessened over a period of time. After drug withdrawal, considerable weight loss was observed in the patient who had previously shown the most significant increase. After 6 months of therapy, two patients developed facial dystonia (this disappeared after reducing the dose of risperidone in one case and discontinuing the medication in the other). Amenorrhea was also observed, but no changes in liver function, blood tests, or EEG were reported.

McDougle, Arnold, Posey, Nicolson, Rubin, and others have contributed greatly to our current understanding of atypical antipsychotic use in the treatment of autism and other developmental disorders (80–87). Posey and colleagues published a report on the use of risperidone in the treatment of two younger children with autistic disorder, a 29-month-old boy and a 23-month-old boy (85). In both cases, risperidone significantly reduced aggression and improved social relatedness. One patient's treatment was complicated by persistent tachycardia and QTc prolongation that was dose related. McDougle et al. conducted an initial prospective open-label study examining risperidone treatment in children and adolescents with pervasive developmental disorders followed by an 8-week double-blind, placebo-controlled study of risperidone in autistic disorders (not including Asperger's disorder). The study examined the benefit in a relatively young cohort (Tanner stage I and II). The mean dose was 2.1 mg/day (0.75 mg–3.5 mg/day) doses twice a day. The most significant response was seen in the improvement of irritability as determined by a greater than 25% improvement on the Aberrant Behavior Checklist. No benefit was noted on inappropriate speech patterns. Benefit was noted at 2 to 4 weeks of treatment and also included improvements in reducing stereotypic behavior. Improvement on social relatedness was inconclusive and limited instruments were implemented to evaluate this symptom, however, anecdotal reports suggested improvement in this behavioral realm. Extrapyramidal symptoms (as evaluated by the Simpson Angus EPS score) were mild and were predominantly seen early in treatment. Side effects included increased appetite, weight gain, decreased energy, and sedation (80).

Because of its later introduction into the field, most current studies on olanzapine are open label. Potenza and colleagues conducted an open-label pilot study examining the efficacy and tolerability of olanzapine in the treatment of children, adolescents, and adults with pervasive developmental disorders (88). Eight patients were treated with olanzapine (mean dose 7.8 mg/day ± 4.7 mg/day) for 12 weeks. Seven of the eight patients completed the study. Six were noted to be "much improved" or "very much improved" on the global improvement item of the Clinical Global Impression Scale. Significant improvements were noted in symptoms of hyperactivity, aggression, anger, self-injurious behavior as well as the overall symptoms of autism, including social relatedness, affectual reactions, sensory responses, and language usage. The drug was well tolerated with the most significant side effect being increased appetite and weight gain (mean increase of 8.3 kg). Malone and colleagues likewise noted improvements in autistic children treated with olanzapine (89). In an open-label pilot study comparing olanzapine and haloperidol, 12 children (mean age 7.8 ± 2.1 years) were randomized to 6 weeks of open treatment with olanzapine (mean final dose 7.9 ± 2.5 mg/day) or haloperidol (mean final dose 1.4 ± 0.7 mg/day). Both groups had symptom reduction. Five of six children in the olanzapine group and three of six children in the haloperidol group were observed to be positive responders based on changes in CGI scores and improvements on the Children's Psychiatric Rating Scale (CPRS) Autism Factor. Side effects seen with olanzapine included drowsiness and weight gain. Kemner and colleagues demonstrated similar results with significant improvements noted on irritability, hyperactivity, and excessive speech as evaluated by the Abberant Behavior Checklist (90,91).

It is beyond the scope of this chapter to mention all of the current studies, although an attempt has been made to give the reader an appreciation of the active research in this area. It is without doubt that the new atypical antipsychotics appear to be effective and well tolerated in children and adolescents with autistic and developmental disorders. Double-blind, placebo-controlled studies confirm the benefit of risperidone. Open-label trials likewise suggest the benefit of olanzapine, and are likely to be confirmed by double-blind studies. Limited research is available on quetiapine, ziprasidone, and aripiprazole. The use of these agents will need more investigation. Weight gain appears to be most problematic and should be monitored. Recommendations for early dietary education and a clear discussion of this side effect with the parents and family as well as the patient have demonstrated benefit in keeping weight gain to a minimum. More studies are certainly indicated and hold future promise in not only treating the behavioral symptoms of autism which interfere with functioning, but also in addressing more core symptoms of the disorder itself.

F. Tourette's Disorder

Tourette's disorder, as well as simple motor or vocal tics, have traditionally been treated with good success using the older neuroleptics, particularly haloperidol and pimozide. These agents have increasingly fallen out of favor because of the risk of short- and long-term side effects, including EPS and tardive dyskinesia. In addition, there were reports of cognitive blunting (potentially disabling to a child's school performance) and emergence of school phobia during treatment which concerned child practitioners and educators (92). Clinicians subsequently turned to alternative agents such as clonidine and guanfacine (alpha-2 agonists) to treat tic disorders, including Tourette's. With the development of the newer atypical antipsychotics, with reported less risk of extrapyramidal side effects, there has recently been renewed interest in the use of antipsychotics to treat tics.

Review of the literature, including open and controlled studies of the new atypical antipsychotics, has demonstrated predominantly moderate improvement in Tourette's disorder. In a study by Scahill and colleagues (2000), the newer antipsychotic agents failed to show benefits comparable to haloperidol-treated patients who had a 66% improvement as compared to placebo (93). Sallee and colleagues performed a pilot study of ziprasidone in adolescent patients with Tourette's disorder. Patients treated with ziprasidone had a 35% improvement rate when compared to placebo (94). In a later double-blind study by Bruggeman and colleagues (2001), risperidone was shown to have a 44% improvement rate measured by change in baseline as compared to placebo in 17 pediatric patients (95). Scahill and colleagues did not demonstrate any benefit of clozapine use on the symptoms of Tourette's disorder, and the response to olanzapine was reported to be modest to moderate, but somewhat less effective than risperidone or ziprasidone (93). Results of a double-blind study conducted by Gaffney noted a 21% improvement in the Yale Global Tic Severity Scale in children aged 7–17 treated with risperidone as compared to a 26% improvement from baseline in children prescribed the alpha-2 agonist clonidine. The observed benefit for both cohorts was comparable; however, the reduced risk of EPS of the atypical antipsychotic compared to the problematic side effects of sedation seen with the use of clonidine made the use of risperidone more desirable (96).

Sedation can also be a problematic side effect associated with the use of the new atypical antipsychotics. In the study published by Scahill and colleagues (93), a clear interpretation of the benefit of risperidone, ziprasidone, and olanzapine on tic symptoms in the pediatric population was confounded by a low sample size and the inclusion of adult patients. Sedation was a common side effect seen with all three medications. Olanzapine use, in particular, was also associated with problematic weight gain. Of good report, no EKG abnormalities were noted in an open study of 28 children treated with ziprasidone (94). Studies on efficacy and safety of aripiprazole in this population of patients are not available.

Thus, evidence exists for the use of atypical antipsychotics in Tourette's syndrome. In general, these drugs are better tolerated than typical antipsychotics in pediatric populations who are particularly prone to the secondary negative symptoms and EPS induced by typical agents. It is unlikely that atypicals of lower D_2 blockade (e.g., clozapine, quetiapine, $\pm$ olanzapine) will be beneficial, but certainly risperidone, and potentially ziprasidone and/or olanzapine hold promise. The generally good response of tic symptoms to low doses of antipsychotics will be helpful in keeping the total daily dosage to a minimum, thus further decreasing the risk of extrapyramidal symptoms, and perhaps in keeping weight gain to a minimum.

G. Disruptive Behavior Disorders

The disruptive behavior disorders of childhood and adolescence include conduct disorder and oppositional defiant disorder. FDA approval for treatment of behavioral symptoms currently exists for only two antipsychotic medications, chlorpromazine and thioridazine; and this approval from the 1980s is based on limited study trials with poor use of statistical comparison and controlled study groups. Moreover, thioridazine has now been "black boxed" by the FDA secondary to concerns regarding cardiac complications from QTc prolongation. Therefore, the likelihood of currently using these drugs in this patient group is markedly diminished.

Much of the research on typical antipsychotics in disruptive behavior disorders has centered on haloperidol, which is not FDA approved for this indication. Studies have demonstrated the efficacy of haloperidol in decreasing destructive and aggressive behavior, oppositionality, and hostility, as well as improving scores on children's psychiatric rating scales and CGI severity (97). More recent studies have examined the role of atypical antipsychotics in this patient group. Findling and colleagues conducted a double-blind study comparing the response to risperidone versus placebo in 20 children, 5 to 15 years old, diagnosed with conduct disorder and demonstrated improvement in measures of aggression and delinquent behavior (98). In another larger study, Aman and colleagues presented findings from a U.S. multisite study of risperidone examining the benefit in 118 children with conduct problems and borderline intellectual functioning (99). Sixty percent of the children had oppositional defiant disorder, 40% had conduct disorder, and 60% had comorbid attention-deficit/hyperactivity disorder. Improvements were seen on subscales of anxious, hyperactive, self-injurious, isolative, and stereotypic behavior, as well as on subscales of prosocial behavior such as adaptive skills. The most common side effects seen with the use of risperidone were sedation, gastrointestinal distress, weight gain, hyperprolactinemia, rhinitis, and headaches. Turgay and colleagues replicated this study with similar findings (101).

Holford and colleagues have presented findings from an extension study of the treatment of conduct disorder in 34 children, ages 5–14 years, with comorbid borderline intellectual functioning (101). Subjects were treated for approximately 1 year with doses of risperidone ranging from 0.02 to 0.06 mg/kg/d (mean dose 1.48 mg). Clinical benefit was noted throughout the study. Prolactin levels were elevated after 3 months of treatment, but declined thereafter. No controlled studies are yet available for the other antipsychotics in this subpopulation. Since other medications are available for symptomatic treatment of disruptive behavioral disorders (lithium, anticonvulsants, and psychostimulants), the question remains as to whether the antipsychotics are the best class of medication for this purpose and whether antipsychotics should be prescribed prior to other agents. Few comparison studies are available to determine efficacy between antipsychotics with other pharmacological options.

H. Anorexia Nervosa

In the 1960s, Dally and Sargant performed the earliest work on the use of antipsychotics in anorexia nervosa, using chlorpromazine as high as

1600 mg/day, often in combination with insulin (102,103). Short-term monitoring revealed faster weight gain and subsequent decreased hospital stays, but side effects, including seizures (five of 30 patients) substantially complicated treatment (102). Moreover, with longer follow-up, there was no significant improvement in weight gain in patients receiving antipsychotic medication and, interestingly, there was even observation of the emergence of purging behavior in those patients treated with the neuroleptic (103). Vandereycken and Pierloot conducted a double-blind, placebo-controlled, cross-over design study of pimozide in 17 hospitalized patients and a similar study design using sulpiride (104). There was a trend towards increased weight gain in the patients receiving pimozide; however, overall treatment outcomes were unclear.

There is now considerable interest in the use of atypical antipsychotics as an adjunct in the treatment of anorexia nervosa. Case reports by Hansen and by La Via et al. describe the efficacy of olanzapine for weight gain and also on psychological improvement in patients with severe anorexia nervosa (105,106). These preclinical findings may have important implications in this challenging disorder. The first and most essential step in treatment is to focus on weight restoration, and paradoxically, as a beneficial exploitation of their side effect profile, the atypical antipsychotics can offer adjunctive benefit in this area. Additionally and consistent with the potential of the broader therapeutic profile of atypical antipsychotics (7), these agents may decrease relapse rates by treating comorbid mood disorders and by offering benefit on target personality traits seen in anorexia patients (e.g., rigidity and obsessionality). They may offer long-term benefits in restoring distorted cognitions which may approach delusional magnitude in many patients. Such claims are at present speculative, but are worthy of rigorous scientific investigation.

I. Other Disorders

1. Stuttering

Numerous arrays of medications have been used, with limited success, to manage stuttering. Haloperidol and risperidone are the only two medications that have shown efficacy in double-blind studies with this population (107). Lavid and colleagues have examined the efficacy of olanzapine in the management of stuttering in three cases, a 10-year-old boy, a 16-year-old adolescent male with developmental stuttering, and a 9-year-old boy with medication-induced stuttering (107). All three patients in this study demonstrated improvement in symptoms. These studies, albeit very limited, suggest that antipsychotics may be an appropriate pharmacological option in the management of this impairing disorder.

III. CURRENT ISSUES IN PEDIATRIC USE OF ATYPICALS

It is clear that our field is only just learning the extent and pattern of side effects with atypical antipsychotic medications. Most pronounced among these are weight gain (108), metabolic disturbances such as diabetes mellitus (109), hyperprolactinemia (110), and cardiac conduction abnormalities (111). The side effects of typical antipsychotics are well known and have appropriately curtailed the use of these agents in childhood conditions. However, the use of atypicals has expanded and at a pace that outstrips our knowledge base empirically with respect to side effects. All of the side effects of these agents (weight gain, metabolic dysfunction, hyperprolactinemia, cardiac conduction disturbances) are a real concern for the younger population. This is particularly so because of the potential of developmental/growth interactions and because of the likelihood that patients will require lengthy (lifelong) exposure to these drugs. The long-term impact is unknown and understudied.

For example, is the effect of weight gain with atypicals more pronounced in younger patients? We examined this issue in a study of weight gain and atypicals in a state hospital population. In this study, a strong inverse relationship between age and weight gain was observed, which suggests that the younger patients may be particularly susceptible to weight gain when treated with atypicals (112). If this is so, then what are the implications of this? Will children have greater difficulties losing weight over time? Will they stop their medications over time? Will they stop their medications due to this effect? Will they be further stigmatized at school because of their obesity? Are they more likely to develop diabetes mellitus? And what will be the long-term consequences of antipsychotic-induced obesity and metabolic disturbances for this patient population? The answers to these questions are unknown at this stage.

There is increasing concern about the consequences of hyperprolactinemia in children and adolescents. Breast enlargement and galactorrhea are particularly distressing in this patient population. There is evidence that sustained elevation of prolactin is accompanied by dysregulation of other hormones (in particular low estrogen and low testosterone) as well as preliminary evidence that antipsychotic-induced hyperprolactinemia may be associated with reduction in bone density (113,114). Finally, there is concern regarding cardiac conduction abnormalities that may be associated with antipsychotic therapy (115). Thioridazine has recently received a "black box" label warning from the FDA because of sudden deaths and prolonged QTc interval on electrocardiogram (EKG). There is EKG evidence that several other antipsychotics cause small rises in QTc prolongation, the most notable agent in this being ziprasidone (111,115). While these effects may still be of doubtful clinical significance in the adult population, they should be borne in mind when considering the use of atypical antipsychotic medications in this patient population.

Secondary to these multiple concerns, the physician should be aware of the possible side effects and their particular impact on the still incomplete physical, hormonal, and developmental growth of the child and adolescent. The clinical practice of "start low, go slow" is of particular benefit in this population. Early onset of side effects has been linked to medication noncompliance, as has poor understanding of the expected benefit and possible side effects associated with a recommended medication. The clinician should always obtain a comprehensive history to include past history of seizures, head trauma, and cardiac or endocrine problems (often best elicited with questions about fatigue, temperature intolerance, or weight concerns). The perinatal history (apnea, apgar scores, days in hospital), as well as good family history, including significant medical problems in the family will give the clinician a good understanding of potential vulnerabilities to side effects prior to the recommendation of a particular agent. Prior to the implementation of not only antipsychotic medications, but ideally with other medications as well, a complete physical including blood pressure, pulse, assessment of current body weight and habitus, and laboratory tests including a complete blood count (CBC), comprehensive metabolic profile, including liver function tests, and cholesterol/triglyceride levels in already obese patients will provide a baseline for comparison after the medication is begun. The parent and the child or adolescent should clearly be educated on the possible side effects, whether the effect is likely to be transient or more persistent, and ways to minimize the side effect (for example, dosing at night to prevent daytime sedation, and dietary recommendations to lessen weight gain). The child or adolescent should be monitored throughout the course of treatment with documentation of weight changes (growth curves can be beneficial), appropriate laboratory tests, and inquiry about side effects in a way that is understood by the patient ("have you had leakage from your breasts?"). Continually weighing the benefits versus the risks of treatment and discussing this with the parent and child will increase compliance and decrease the risks associated with antipsychotic use.

IV. SUMMARY

This chapter has provided some evidence for a role of atypical antipsychotics in several childhood conditions beyond schizophrenia. However, it must be borne in mind that pharmacotherapy of childhood conditions is complex and is an extremely underdeveloped area of psychiatric research. Consequently, there are ample (opportunistic) circumstances where new medications may be used on a trial-and-error basis or as an adjunct to other medications. Zito and colleagues have drawn attention to these practices and they have highlighted a disproportionate growth in the use of psychotropic drugs in children (116). Federal attention has subsequently focused on appropriate labeling with warnings surrounding the possible long-term risk of antipsychotics, not only to include tardive dyskinesia, but endocrine changes, including diabetes, as well. The FDA is close to receiving federal authority to mandate research studies in children and adolescents which will assist in providing controlled studies of efficacy and tolerability in this population. President Bush acknowledged the overwhelming need for further work in this area as well with his 2001 "New Freedom Initiative." A report from that commission in October 2002 (117) noted that:

> Research is our best hope for the future. Scientists have made breakthrough discoveries on how the brain works and this has resulted in new medications that help the brain work better at regulating emotions and thought. These medicines, when combined with cognitive behavioral therapies and community-based services, family education, wrap-around services, and respite care give children and adolescents with mental illnesses the chance to recover from illnesses and enjoy a full and normal childhood. We must continue to invest in the support of research on early-onset mental illnesses. This includes research on the psychopharmacology for children and adolescents with mental illnesses.

Subsequent designations in the FY 2004 budget have been made to further research in mental illness, including child and adolescent, and to assist with mental health service programs.

It is clear that there is substantial use of atypical antipsychotic medications in conditions beyond psychosis, both for adult and childhood psychiatric conditions. It remains to be determined whether such use in the pediatric population is excessive or whether the trend reflects better detection and management of psychiatric morbidity in children/adolescents. This is clearly an important distinction, although discerning the differences will be difficult because it is juxtaposed with the evolution of clinical practice of child and adolescent psychiatry. While there is (variable) evidence of efficacy to support this trend, the evidence-base is thin and needs to be augmented with well-controlled clinical trials for the main conditions under review. Judicious use of atypicals, with an even more conservative approach to polypharmacy than in adult populations, is warranted because of the potential long-term consequences of side effects of these agents.

The interaction with developmental processes and the unique drug pharmacokinetics of childhood are also an important consideration. Nevertheless, these issues must be held in balance with the potential of atypical antipsychotic medications to improve behavioral control and functioning among intractable childhood conditions.

REFERENCES

1. World Psychiatric Association. The usefulness and use of second-generation antipsychotic medications. Curr Opin Psychiatry 2002; 15(suppl):51–551.
2. Kane JM, Eardekens M, Keith SJ, Lesem M, Karcher K, Lindenmayer JP. Efficacy and safety of a novel long-acting risperidone microspheres formulation. Schizophr Res 2002; 53:174.
3. Lesem MD, Zajecka JM, Swift RH, Reeves KR, Harrigan EP. Intramuscular ziprasidone, 2 mg versus 10 mg, in the short-term management of agitated psychotic patients. J Clin Psychiatry 2001; 62:12–18.
4. Wright P, Birkett M, David S, et al. Double-blind, placebo-controlled comparison of intramuscular olanzapine and intramuscular haloperidol in the treatment of acute agitation in schizophrenia. Am J Psychiatry 2001; 158: 1149–1151.
5. Davis JM. Meta-analysis of atypical antipsychotics. Presentation at the Winter Workshop on Schizophrenia Research, Davos, Switzerland, 2002.
6. Geddes J, Freemantale N, Harrison P, et al. Atypical antipsychotic in the treatment of schizophrenia: systematic overview and regression analysis. Brit Med J 2001; 321:1371–1376.
7. Roberts R, Rodriquez W, Murphy D, Crescenzi T. Pediatric drug labelling: improving the safety and efficacy of pediatric therapies. JAMA 2003; 290: 905–911.
8. Buckley, PF. Broad therapeutic uses of atypical medications. Biol Psychiatry 2001; 50:912–924.
9. Buckley PF, Miller DD, Singer B, Donnenwirth K. The evolving clinical profile of atypical antipsychotic medications. Can J Psychiatry 2001; 46:285.
10. Toren P, Laor N, Weizman R. Use of atypical neuroleptics in child and adolescent psychiatry. J Clin Psychiatry 1998; 58:644–656.
11. Malone RP, Sheikh R, Zito JM. Novel antipsychotic medications in the treatment of children and adolescents. Psychiatr Serv 1999; 50(2):171–174.
12. Findling RL, McNamara NK, Gracious BL. Paediatric uses of atypical antipsychotics. Expert Opin Pharmacother 2000; 1(5):935–945.
13. Harris JW. Developmental Neuropsychiatry. Vol 1. New York: Oxford University Press, 1995.
14. Grothe DR, Calis KA, et al. Olanzapine pharmacokinetics in pediatric and adolescent inpatients with childhood-onset schizophrenia. J Clin Psychopharmacol 2000; 20:220–225.

15. McConville B, Arvanitis L, et al. Pharmacokinetics, tolerability and clinical effectiveness of quetiapine fumarate in adolescents with selected psychotic disorders. J Clin Psychiatry 2000; 61:252–260.
16. Janicak PG, Davis JM, Preskorn SH, et al. Pharmacokinetics. In: Janicak PG, Davis JM, Preskorn SH, et al., eds. Principles and Practice of Psychopharmacotherapy. Baltimore: Williams & Wilkins, 1993:59–79.
17. Taylor E. Physical treatments. In: Child and Adolescent Psychiatry. Cambridge: Blackwell Scientific, 1994:880–899.
18. Olin BR. Drug Facts and Comparisons. St. Louis: Facts and Comparisons, Inc., 2001:933–950.
19. Jatlow PI. Psychotropic drug disposition during development. In: Popper C, ed. Psychiatric Pharmacosciences of Children and Adolescents. Washington, DC: American Psychiatric Publishing, 1987:29–44.
20. Verghese C, Kessel JB, Simpson GM: Pharmacokinetics of neuroleptics. Psychopharmacol Bull 1991; 27(4):551–563.
21. Hollis C. Child and adolescent (juvenile onset) schizophrenia: a case control study of premorbid development impairments. Brit J Psychiatry 1995; 166: 489–495.
22. Lieberman JA, Perkins D, Belgar A, Chakos M, Jarskog F, Boteva K, Gilmore J. The early stages of schizophrenia: speculations on pathogenesis, pathophysiology, and therapeutic approaches. Biol Psychiatry 2001; 50: 884–897.
23. Asarnow JR, Tompson MC, Goldstein MJ. Childhood onset schizophrenia: a follow-up study. Schizophr Bull 1994; 20:599–617.
24. Eggers C, Bunk D. The long-term course of childhood-onset schizophrenia: a 42-year follow up study. Schizophr Bull 1997; 23:105–117.
25. Franqu S, Kumra S. Treatment of childhood-onset schizophrenia. In: Buckley PF, Waddington JL, eds. Schizophrenia and Mood Disorders: The New Drug Therapies in Clinical Practice. Oxford,England: Arnold, 2000.
26. Kumra S, Frazier JA, Jacobsen LK, et al. Childhood onset schizophrenia: a double-blind clozapine-haloperidol comparison. Arch Gen Psychiatry 1996; 53: 1090–1097.
27. Pool D, Bloom W, Mielke DH, et al. A controlled evaluation of loxitane in seventy-five adolescent schizophrenia patients. Curr Ther Res Exp 1976; 19: 99–104.
28. Realmuto GM, Erikson WD, Yellin AM, et al. Clinical comparison of thiothixene and thioridazine in schizophrenia adolescents. Am J Psychiatry 1984; 141:440–442.
29. Spencer EK, Kafantaris V, Padron-Gayol MV, et al. Haloperidol in schizophrenia children: early findings from a study in progress. Psychopharmacol Bull 1992; 28:183–186.
30. Mozes T, Toren P, Chernauzan N. Case study: clozapine treatment in very early onset schizophrenia. J Am Acad Child Adolesc Psychiatry 1994; 33:65–70.
31. Remschmidt H, Schultz E, Martin M. An open trial of clozapine in thirty-six adolescents with schizophrenia. J Child Adolesc Psychiatry 1994; 4:31–41.

32. Turetz M, Mozes T, Toren P, et al. An open trial of clozapine in neuroleptic-resistant childhood-onset schizophrenia. Brit J Psychiatry 1997; 170:507–510.
33. Duggal HS, Jagadheean K, Nizamie SH. Clozapine-induced stuttering and seizures. Am J Psychiatry 2002; 159(2):315.
34. Sourander A. Risperidone for treatment of childhood schizophrenia. Am J Psychiatry 1997; 154(10):1476.
35. Simeon JG, Carrey NJ, Wiggins DM, et al. Risperidone effects in treatment-resistant adolescents: preliminary case reports. J Child Adolesc Psychopharmacol 1995; 5:69–79.
36. Lykes WC, Cueva JE. Risperidone in children with schizophrenia. J Am Acad Child Adolesc Psychiatry 1996; 35(4):405–406.
37. Sternlicht HC, Wells SR. Risperidone in childhood schizophrenia. J Am Acad Child Adolesc Psychiatry 1995; 34(5):540.
38. Quintanna H, Keshavan M. Case study: risperidone in children and adolescents with schizophrenia. J Am Acad Child Adolesc Psychiatry 1995; 34(10): 1292–1296.
39. Greevich SJ, Findling RL, Rowane WA, et al. Risperidone in the treatment of children and adolescents with schizophrenia: a retrospective study. J Child Adolesc Psychopharmacol 1996; 6(4):251–257.
40. Armenteros JL, Whitaker AH, Welikson M, et al. Risperidone in adolescents with schizophrenia: an open pilot study. J Am Acad Child Adolesc Psychiatry 1997; 36(5):694–700.
41. McGorry P, et al. Risperidone for prodrome of schizophrenia. Arch Gen Psychiatry 2002.
42. Kumra S, Jacobsen LK, Lanane M, et al. Childhood-onset schizophrenia: an open-label study of olanzapine in adolescents. J Am Acad Adolesc Psychiatry 1998; 37:377–385.
43. Mandoki M. Olanzapine in the treatment of early onset schizophrenia in children and adolescents. Biol Psychiatry Abstracts 1997; 41:22S.
44. Schulz SC, Findling RL, Branicky LA, et al. Olanzapine in adolescents with a psychotic disorder. Schizophr Res 1999; 36(1–3):297.
45. Wood SC, McGlashan TH. Adverse effects of olanzapine in adolescents and adults. Schizophr Res 2002; 53:170.
46. McConville B. Seroquel does not elevate prolactin levels in adolescents with selected psychotic disorders. Schizophr Res 2000; 41:206.
47. Szigethy E, Brent S, Findling RL. Quetiapine for refractory schizophrenia. J Am Acad Child Adolesc Psychiatry 1998; 37(11):1127–1128.
48. Healy E, Subotsky F, Pipe R. Quetiapine in adolescent psychosis. J Am Adolesc Psychiatry 1999; 38(11):1329.
49. Buck ML. Using the aypical antipsychotic agents in children and adolescents. pediatric pharmacotherapy: A Monthly Newsletter for Health Care Professionals from the Children's Medical Center at the University of Virginia, 2001; 7(8).
50. Patel NC, Sierk P, Dorson PG, Crismon ML. Experience with ziprasidone. J Am Acad Child Adolesc Psychiatry 2002; 41(5):495.
51. Papolos J, Papolos DF. The Bipolar Child Newsletter 2003; 13.

52. Buckley PF. Drugs of Today 2003; 39(2):145–151.
53. Burris KD, Molski TF, et al. Aripiprazole, a novel antipsychotic is a high-affinity partial agonist at human dopamine D2 receptors. J Pharmacol Exp Ther 2002; 302–389.
54. Goodnick PJ, Jerry JM. Aripiprazole: profile on efficacy and safety. Expert Opin Pharmacother 2002; 12:1773–1781.
55. Kane JM, Carson WH, Saha AR, et al. Efficacy and safety of aripiprazole and haloperidol versus placebo in patients with schizophrenia and schizoaffective disorder. J Clin Psychiatry 2002; 63:763–771.
56. Carson WH, Stock E, Saha AR, et al. Metaanalysis of the safety and tolerability of aripiprazole. Schizophr Res 2002; 53:186–187.
57. Keck P, Carson WH, Saha RA, et al. A placebo controlled trial of aripiprazole for the treatment of acute mania. Presentation at the Annual Meeting of the American Psychiatric Association, Philadelphia, May 2002.
58. Grcevich S, Melamed L, Richards R. Comparative side effects of atypical antipsychotics in children and adolescents. Poster presented at the International Congress on Schizophrenia Research. Whistler, British Columbia, April 2001.
59. Ratzoni G, Gothelf D, Brand-Gothelf A, Reidman J, Kikinzon L, Gal G, Phillip M, Apter A, Wietmen R. Weight gain associated with olanzapine and risperidone in adolescent patients: a comparative prospective study. J Am Acad Child Adolesc Psychiatry 2002; 41(3):337–343.
60. American Academy of Child and Adolescent Psychiatry. AACAP official action: practice parameters for the assessment and treatment of children and adolescents with bipolar disorder. J Am Acad Child Adolesc Psychiatry 1997; 36:138–157.
61. Fuchs DC. Clozapine treatment of bipolar disorder in a young adolescent. J Am Acad Child Adolesc Psychiatry 1994; 33:1299–1302.
62. Masi G, Mucci M, Millepiedi S. Clozapine in adolescent patients with acute mania. J Child Adolesc Psychopharmacol 2002; 1(2):93–99.
63. Frazier JA, Meyer MC, Biederman J, et al. Risperidone treatment for juvenile Bipolar disorder: a retrospective chart review. J Am Acad Child Adolesc Psychiatry 1999; 38:960–965.
64. Schreier HA. Risperidone for young children with mood disorders and aggressive behavior. J Child Adolesc Psychopharmacol 1998; 8:49–59.
65. Tohen M, Baker RW, Altshuler L, et al. Olanzapine versus divalproex sodium for bipolar mania: a 47-week study. Indianopolis, Indiana: Lilly Research Laboratories, Eli Lilly and Company.
66. Frazier JA, Biederman J, Jacobs TG, et al. Olanzapine in the treatment of bipolar disorder in juveniles. New Clin Eval Unit 2000, Program Abstracts: Washington DC: New Clinical Drug Evaluation Unit.
67. Chang KD, Ketter TA. Mood stabilizer augmentation with olanzapine in acutely manic children. J Child Adolesc Psychopharmacol 2000; 10:45–49.
68. Soutullo CA, Sorter MT, Foster KD, et al. Olanzapine in the treatment of adolescent acute mania: a report of seven cases. J Affect Dis 1999; 53: 279–283.

69. DelBello MP, Schwiers ML, Rosenberg HL, Strakowski SM. A double-blind, randomised, placebo-controlled study of quetiapine as adjunctive treatment for adolescent mania. J Am Acad Child Adolesc Psychiatry 2002; 41(10): 1216–1223.

70. Keck PE, Versiani M, Potkin S, West SA, et al. Ziprasidone in the treatment of acute bipolar mania: a three-week, placebo-controlled, double-blind, randomized trial. Am J Psychiatry 2003; 160:741–748.

71. Gellar B, Cooper TB, Farooki ZQ, et al. Dose and plasma levels of nortriptyline and chlorpromazine in delusionally depressed adolescents and of nortriptyline in nondelusionally depressed adolescents. Am J Psychiatry 1985; 142:336–338.

72. Mandoki MW. Risperidone treatment of children and adolescents: increased risk of extrapyramidal side effects? J Clin Adolesc Psychopharmacol 1995; 5: 49–67.

73. Frazier JA, Biederman J, Jacobs TG, et al. Olanzapine in the treatment of bipolar-disorder in juveniles. Schizophr Res 2000; 41(1 S1):194.

74. American Academy of Child and Adolescent Psychiatry. AACAP official action: practice Parameters for the assessment and treatment of children and adolescents with anxiety disorders. J Am Acad Child Adolesc Psychiatry 1997; 36:69–84.

75. Stein et al.

76. American Academy of Child and Adolescent Psychiatry. AACAP official action: practice Parameters for the assessment and treatment of children and adolescents with autistic disorder. J Am Acad Child Adolesc Psychiatry 1997; 36.

77. Anderson LT, Campbell M, Grega DM, et al. The effects of haloperidol on discrimination learning and behavioral symptoms in autistic children. Am J Psychiatry 1984; 141(10):1195–1202.

78. Masi G, Cosenza A, Mucci M, Brovedani P. Open trial of risperidone in 24 young children with pervasive developmental disorders. J Am Acad Child Adolesc Psychiatry 2001; 40(10):1206–1214.

79. Zuddis A, Di Martino A, Muglia P, et al. Long-term risperidone for pervasive developmental disorder: efficacy, tolerability, and discontinuation. J Child Adolesc Psychopharmacol 2000; 10(2):79–90.

80. McDougle CJ, Homes JP, Bronson MR, et al. Risperidone treatment of children and adolescents with pervasive developmental disorders: a prospective open-label study. J Am Acad Child Adolesc Psychiatry 1997; 36:685–693.

81. McDougle CJ, Holmes JP, Carlson DC, et al. A double-blind, placebo-controlled study of risperidone in adults with autistic disorder and other pervasive developmental disorders. Arch Gen Psychiatry 1998; 55:633–641.

82. McDougle CJ, Scahill L, McCracken JT, et al. Research units on pediatric psychopharmacology (RUPP) autism network. Background and rationale for an initial controlled study of risperidone. Child Adolesc Psychiatr Clin North Am 2000; 9(1):201–224.

83. Arnold LE, Aman MG, Marin A, et al. Assessment in multi-site randomized clinical trials of patients with autistic disorder. The autism RUPP network. Research units of pediatric psychopharmacology. J Autism Devel Disorders 2000; 30(2):99–111.

84. Posey DJ, McDougle CJ. The pharmacotherapy of target symptoms associated with autistic disorder and other pervasive developmental disorders. Harvard Rev Psychiatry 2000; 8(2):45–63.

85. Posey DJ, Walsh KH, Wilson GA, McDougle CJ. Risperidone in the treatment of two very young children with autism. J Child Adolesc Psychopharmacol 1999; 9:273–276.

86. Nicolson R, Awad G, Sloman L. An open trial of risperidone in young autistic children. J Am Acad Child Adolesc Psychiatry 1998; 37(4): 372–376.

87. Rubin M. Use of atypical antipsychotics in children with mental retardation, autism, and other develomental disabilities. Psychiatric Annals 1997; 27: 219–221.

88. Potenza MN, Holmes JP, Kanes SJ, McDougle CJ. Olanzapine treatment of children, adolescents, and adults with pervasive developmental disorders: a open-label pilot study. J Clin Psychopharmacol 1999; 19:37–44.

89. Malone RP, Cater J, Sheikah RM, et al. Olanzapine versus haloperidol in children with autistic disorder: an open pilot study. J Am Acad Child Adolesc Psychiatry 2001; 40:887–894.

90. Kemner C, van Engeland H, Tuynman-Que H. An open-label study of olanzapine in children with Pervasive Developmental Disorder. Eur Neuropsychopharmacol 1999; 9(suppl 5):S287–S288.

91. Kemner C, van Engeland H, Tuynman-Qua H. An open-label study of olanzapine in children with PDD. Schizophr Res 2000; 41(1 S1): 194.

92. Shapiro E, Shapiro AK, Fulop G, et al. Controlled study of haloperidol, pimozide, and PLA for the treatment of Gilles de la Tourette's syndrome. Arch Gen Psychiatry 1989; 46:722–730.

93. Scahill L, Chappell PB, King RA, et al. Pharmacologic treatment of tic disorders. Child Adolesc Clin North America 2000; 9:99–117.

94. Sallee FR, Kurlan R, Goetz CG, et al. Ziprasidone treatment of children and adolescents with Tourette's syndrome: a pilot study. J Am Acad Child Adolesc Psychiatry 2000; 39:292–299.

95. Bruggeman R, ver der Linden C, Buitelaar JK, et al. Risperidone versus pimozide in Tourette's disorder: a comparative double-blind parallel-group study. J Clin Psychiatry 2001; 50:912–924.

96. Gaffney GR. Risperidone versus clonidine in the treatment of children and adolescents with Tourette's syndrome. J Am Acad Child Adolesc Psychiatry 2002; 41(3):330–336.

97. Campbell M, Small AM, Green WH, et al. Behavioral efficacy of haloperidol and lithium carbonate: a comparison of hospitalized aggressive children with conduct disorder. Arch Gen Psychiatry 1984; 41:650–656.

98. Findling RL, McNamar NK, Branicky LA, et al. A double-blind pilot study of risperidone in the treatment of conduct disorder. J Am Acad Child Adolesc Psychiatry 2000; 39:509–516.

99. Aman MG, Findling RL, Derican A, et al. Safety and efficacy of risperidone in children with significant conduct problems and borderline IQ or mental retardation. 22nd Collegium Internationale Neuro-Psychopharmacologicum Congress, Brussels, July 2000.

100. Turgay A, Snyder R, Fishman S, et al, and the Conduct Research Group (Simeon J, Mahoney W, Yogel W, et al). Risperidone versus placebo for conduct and other disruptive behavior disorders in children with subaverage IQ. Poster presented at the Annual Meeting of the Canadian Psychiatric Association, Victoria, British Columbia, Canada, Oct 2000.

101. Holford LE, Peter E, Van der Walt A. Risperidone for behavior disorders in children with mental retardation. Poster presented at the Annual Meeting of the American Academy of Child and Adolescent Psychiatry, New York, Oct 24–29, 2000.

102. Dally P, Sargant W. A new treatment of anorexia nervosa. Brit Med J 1960; 1:1770–1773.

103. Dally P, Sargant W. Treatment and outcome of anorexia nervosa. Brit Med J 1966; 2:793–795.

104. Vandereycken W, Pierloot R. Pimozide combined with behavior therapy in the short-term treatment of anorexia nervosa. Acta Psychiatr Scand 1982; 66: 445–450.

105. Hanson L. Olanzapine in the treatment of anorexia nervosa. Brit J Psychiatry 1999; 175:592.

106. La Via MC, Gray N, Kaye WH. Case reports of Olanzapine treatment of anorexia nervosa. Intl J Eating Dis 2000; 27:363–366.

107. Lavid N, Franklin DL, Maquire GA. Management of child and adolescent stuttering with olanzapine: three case reports. Ann Clin Psychiatry 1999; 11(4):233–236.

108. Allison DB, Mentore JL, Heo M, et al. Antipsychotic induced weight gain: a comprehensive research synthesis. Am J Psychiatry 1999; 156:1686–1696.

109. Henderson DG, Calliero E, Gray C, et al. Clozapine, diabetes mellitus, weight gain, and lipid abnormalities. Am J Psychiatry 2000; 157:975–981.

110. Kinon B, Gilmore JA, Liu H. Potential clinical consequences of hyperprolactinemia on reproductive hormones and menstrual function in premenopausal female patients with schizophrenia. Schizophr Res 2002; 53:168.

111. Glassman AH, Bigger JT Jr. Antipsychotic drugs: prolonged QTC interval, torsade de pointes, and sudden death. Am J Psychiatry 2001; 158:1774–1782.

112. Singer B, Buckley PF, Freidman L, et al. Weight gain, diabetes mellitus, and the pharmacotherapy of schizophrenia. Schizophr Res 2001; 49:276.

113. Kaye WH, Ebert MH, Raleigh L, et al. Abnormalities in CNS monoamine metabolism in anorexia nervosa. Arch Gen Psychiatry 1984; 41:350–355.

114. Meaney AM, et al. Elevated prolactin levels and the effects with atypical antipsychotics. Presentation at the Winter Workshop on Schizophrenia Research. Davos, Switzerland, Feb 2002.
115. Reilly JG, Ayis S, Ferrier IN, et al. QTC interval abnormalities and psychotropic drug therapy in psychiatric patients. Lancet 2000; 355: 1048–1052.
116. Zito JM, Safer D, dosReis S, et al. Trends in the prescribing of psychotropic medications to preschoolers. JAMA 2000; 283:1025.
117. Gruttadaro DE. Child and teen mental illnesses and the national health crisis. www.nami.org.

11

Use of Atypical Antipsychotic Drugs for the Treatment of Affective Disorders

Martha Sajatovic and Melvin Shelton

*Case Western Reserve University School of Medicine,
Cleveland, Ohio, U.S.A.*

I. INTRODUCTION

There is a substantial body of literature on the use of antipsychotic medications in the management of mood disorders. Most of the older literature addresses use of the conventional antipsychotic or typical compounds (1). Controlled studies have shown that typical antipsychotics are superior to placebo in the treatment of acute mania, and that typical antipsychotics may have a relatively rapid onset of action (2,3). However, while use of these older drugs was widespread in the past, particularly in situations where acute psychotic mania was the focus of treatment, typical antipsychotic treatment was also frequently associated with a number of problematic adverse effects. Adverse effects associated with typical antipsychotic drugs include neurological adverse effects such as acute dystonias, drug-induced parkinsonism, akathisia and tardive dyskinesia as well as non-neurological adverse effects such as sedation, othostatic hypotension, anticholinergic symptoms, and endocrine abnormalities (4). It has been suggested that individuals in treatment for mood disorders may be particularly vulnerable to medication associated dyskinesias (5). Moreover, it has been reported that the older, neuroleptic compounds may exacerbate post-manic major depressive episodes, and induce rapid cycling in some patients with bipolar illness (6). For the most part, the utilization of older antipsychotic medications in the treatment of mood disorders has been limited by the common occurrence of adverse effects, and concerns about negative effects on mood illness outcome.

In contrast, the second generation or atypical antipsychotics have shown promise in the management of mood disorders (7–10). The atypical antipsychotics have a low incidence of extrapyramidal side effects, improved tardive dyskinesia profiles, and have a broad range of therapeutic efficacy (11). It has been reported that more than 70% of prescriptions for atypical antipsychotic medications are being used for conditions other than schizophrenia, such as bipolar disorder and geriatric agitation (12,13). Additionally, there is emerging evidence that atypical antipsychotic medications may have favorable effects on mood illness outcome. This is particularly true for bipolar disorder, where atypical compounds have substantially changed the recommended treatment guidelines for bipolar illness (7). The atypical antipsychotic medications olanzapine, risperidone and quetiapine have been demonstrated to be superior to placebo in the treatment of acute bipolar mania (14,15,38,87) and currently have FDA indications for the treatment of acute mania (4). There is growing evidence that other atypical antipsychotic medications also have a beneficial role in the management of bipolar illness (9,17).

In addition to improvement in acute symptomatology, use of atypical antipsychotics may offer individuals with bipolar illness improved quality of life and improved clinical outcomes. For example, one recent study of individuals with bipolar disorder treated in a community psychiatry system, found that there was a significant reduction in rates of emergency room visits with atypical agents compared to conventional neuroleptics (8). Miller et al. (18) found that hospitalized individuals with acute mania who were treated with atypical antipsychotics had significantly greater clinical improvement and fewer adverse effects than a comparison group of patients treated with typical antipsychotics.

The specific mechanisms as to how atypical antipsychotic drugs may enhance mood disorder outcomes remain unclear. It has been speculated that since the atypical agents seem to rely much less exclusively on dopaminergic blockade for their therapeutic action they may avoid the mechanism of neuroleptic-induced dysphoria that appears to contribute to depressive syndrome in some individuals (19). Also, it has been reported that atypical antipsychotic medications bind to a number of 5-HT (serotonergic) receptors in common with some of the antidepressant compounds (20,21). For example, Roth et al. (22) have noted that clozapine has high affinity for the 5-HT_{2A}, 5-HT_{2C}, 5-HT_{6}, and 5-HT_{7} sites, while other investigators (21,23) found that 5-HT_{7}, 5-HT_{2A}, and 5-HT_{2C} receptors had high affinity for tricyclic antidepressant compounds. However, receptor profiles among the atypicals differ, and it is probable that the atypicals' mechanisms of action on mood states may differ as well.

Until the introduction of the atypical antipsychotic compounds, the utilization of typical antipsychotics in unipolar depression was primarily confined to psychotic depression. However, this situation is changing with reports on the use of atypical antipsychotic medications as beneficial agents in the treatment of major depression with or without psychotic features (10). It has been suggested that the atypical antipsychotics in general may possess mild to moderate adjunctive antidepressant properties (24), and the majority of the current reports on use of atypical antipsychotics in non-psychotic depression involve atypicals as add-on therapy to antidepressant medications. It is speculated that the $5\text{-HT}_{2A/2C}$ antagonist properties of the atypical antipsychotics may provide additional efficacy when combined with the Selective Serotonin Reuptake Inhibitor (SSRI) antidepressants by contributing to improved affective and anxiety symptoms and minimization of side effects such as sexual dysfunction and sleep disturbance (10). Some atypicals appear to inhibit reuptake of norepinephrin as well (25) although it is not clear how this might interact with effects of antidepressant drugs.

II. SPECIFIC ATYPICAL ANTIPSYCHOTIC MEDICATIONS IN THE MANAGEMENT OF MOOD DISORDERS

A. Clozapine

Clozapine has maintained its place as a unique agent for the management of treatment-refractory schizophrenia and is used for severe bipolar illness in clinical settings. A number of investigators have noted that clozapine appears to have beneficial effects on primary mood disorders with and without psychosis (26,27,29). At this time, there are no blinded, placebo-controlled studies utilizing clozapine in affective disorders, and it is likely given clozapine's adverse effect profile, that it will remain reserved for individuals who are refractory to standard treatments.

1. Bipolar Disorder

A number of open trials suggest that clozapine is useful in treatment of refractory bipolar illness (17,28–30). Suppes et al. (28) reported on a randomized 1-year trial, which included individuals with refractory bipolar disorder. Clozapine therapy was compared to treatment as usual, and was superior in symptom control and in reducing hospitalizations during the

1-year treatment period. Although interpretation of the Suppes et al. (28) study is complicated by use of concomitant mood stabilizing medication, it is notable that polypharmacy in the clozapine-treated group decreased substantially during the study period compared to the treatment as usual group.

Barbini et al. (30) completed a randomized 3-week trial of clozapine vs. chlorpromazine among 30 individuals hospitalized for mania. Although clozapine-treated subjects had a more rapid response compared to individuals treated with chlorpromazine, by the end of the study there were no significant differences between treatment groups. It is possible that low dosing of clozapine (mean 166 mg/day) may have contributed to the negative findings in this trial.

A more recent trial by Green et al. (17) assessed effects of clozapine monotherapy in 22 individuals with treatment-resistant mania. During this 12-week trial, 77% of subjects had a 20% or greater improvement on the Young Mania Rating Scale (YMRS), Clinical Global Impression (CGI), and Brief Psychiatric Rating Scale (BPRS), while 46% had at least 50% improvement on all three scales.

Overall, clozapine appears to be effective in treatment-resistant bipolar illness, both in acute (particularly antimanic) and long-term (mood stabilizing/prophylaxis) phases. Clozapine may be utilized as a monotherapeutic agent in bipolar disorder, however optimal dosing of clozapine in bipolar illness has not been clearly determined. Frye et al. (26) noted that average daily dose of clozapine in mood disorder studies was 315 mg/day and suggested that this may be lower than average dosing in schizophrenia treatment for a variety of reasons, including differing therapeutic needs in mood disorder, lower dosing requirements due to concomitant mood stabilizing medication, or changes in U.S. practice patterns. Target clozapine serum levels have not been identified in the treatment of bipolar disorder (26).

2. Unipolar Disorder

Use of clozapine in major depression has not been well studied, with only limited case reports/case series available. Banov et al. (31) cited a 46% response rate in the treatment of 13 individuals with unipolar depression. Ranjan and Meltzer (32) reported on a case series of individuals with refractory major depression who were maintained on clozapine for 4–6 years. In this report there was good response to both mood and psychotic symptoms with improvements in tardive dyskinesia and tardive dystonia.

An extremely understudied area concerns issues of atypical antipsychotic/antidepressant concomitant therapy. Polypharmacy is common in clinical practice, and the effects of combined therapy on atypical antipsychotic medication levels and antidepressants may be significant. For example, Spina et al. (33) has reported that clozapine coadministration with either paroxetine or sertraline is well tolerated, but there may be differences in clozapine metabolism in relation to antidepressant compounds. Metabolism of clozapine does not appear to be affected by sertraline treatment, while paroxetine, a potent inhibitor of CYP2D6 appears to inhibit the metabolism of clozapine. This suggests a need for careful clinical observation and monitoring of plasma clozapine levels whenever paroxetine is coadministered with clozapine.

B. Risperidone

There are a number of reports and studies which involve the use of risperidone and affective disorders. Most of these reports focus on bipolar illness, and are open-label trials or retrospective reviews, however, there are numerous double-blind trials as well. Keck et al. (34) examined clinical predictors of acute risperidone response among individuals with schizophrenia, schizoaffective disorder, and bipolar disorder. Good response to risperidone appeared to be more likely in individuals who were younger, had a diagnosis of bipolar disorder or schizoaffective disorder, of depressed type and were less likely to have a diagnosis of schizophrenia (34).

1. Bipolar Disorder

There have been a number of double-blind trials conducted with risperidone in bipolar illness (35–39). Hirschfeld et al. (38) recently reported on a 3-week, randomized, double-blind, placebo-controlled study of risperidone monotherapy in acute mania. In this report, 262 patients were randomized, 134 to risperidone and 128 to placebo. Risperidone was administered orally, once daily, in a flexible range of 1–6 mg/day; lorazepam was allowed during washout and the first 10 days of treatment. The primary measure of efficacy was change in baseline to endpoint in mean Young Mania Rating Scale (YMRS) total score. All patients at study entry had a baseline YMRS score of 20 or greater. The trial was completed by 56% of the risperidone group and 42% of the placebo group. Mean dose of risperidone was 4.1 mg/day. Significantly greater improvements in YMRS total scores were seen in the risperidone group than in the placebo group at day 3 and at each subsequent time point ($p < 0.001$). A treatment response (defined as 50% or greater reduction in YMRS score) at endpoint was achieved by 43% of risperidone-treated patients, and 24% of placebo-treated patients ($p < 0.01$). Additionally, antimanic effect of risperidone was independent of the presence or absence of psychotic features. Gopal et al. (39) reported on a double-blind, randomized, placebo-controlled, 3-week trial of risperidone therapy conducted at eight clinical sites in India. In this study, 291 hospitalized patients with bipolar I disorder experiencing a manic or mixed episode were randomized to receive risperidone ($n = 146$) or placebo ($n = 145$). All patients had a YMRS of 20 or greater at study entry; however, it is notable that participants in this study had YMRS baseline scores that were substantially higher (mean for all patients 37.2 ± 7.9, 37.4 ± 7.9 for placebo, 36.9 ± 8.0 for resperidone) compared to baseline YMRS scores seen in many U.S. trials. The primary outcome variable tested was the presence or absence of sustained remission, defined as maintenance of YMRS score of 8 or less for the duration of the trial. Sustained remission was achieved by 41.7% of the risperidone patients and 12.5% of the placebo patients. Acutely manic patients treated with risperidone as monotherapy had odds approximately 5 times higher of achieving remission compared to manic patients receiving placebo. Unadjusted and adjusted analysis confirmed that treatment with risperidone was associated with statistically greater odds and relative risk of achieving remission compared with placebo. Segel et al. (35) compared the efficacy and tolerability of risperidone monotherapy to lithium and haloperidol for the treatment of acute mania in a 4-week double-blind, randomized, controlled study involving 54 subjects. Primary outcome measure was the Mania Rating Scale (MRS). Subjects received either risperidone 6 mg/day, haloperidol 10 mg/day, or lithium 800–1200 mg/day (serum levels 0.6–1.2 mmol/L). Results of the study showed improvement in all groups ($p < 0.001$) with no significant differences between treatment groups. Secondary measures of tolerability also showed no differences between treatment groups.

Sachs et al. (36) compared add-on risperidone therapy to mood stabilizer in a 3-week, randomized, double-blind, placebo-controlled trial. Subjects were 158 individuals hospitalized with acute manic or mixed bipolar illness. A haloperidol treatment arm was used as an internal reference. Primary outcome measure was change from baseline in YMRS score, while secondary measures were change in BPRS, CGI, and Hamilton Depression Scale (HAM-D). Extrapyramidal Symptoms Rating Scale (ESRS) scores were also evaluated as well as a series of basic safety parameters. Results of the study showed a significant change in symptoms from baseline with risperidone compared to placebo. In the intent to treat (ITT) population, change in YMRS score with risperidone was -14.3 vs. -8.2 with placebo ($p = 0.009$). Mean dose of risperidone at study end was 3.83 mg/day. Mean dose of haloperidol was 6.23 mg/day. The overall incidence of adverse events was similar in the risperidone-treated group compared to the placebo-treated group, and lower than the haloperidol-treated group.

Yatham (37) compared risperidone add-on therapy to placebo in a randomized, double-blind, 3-week study involving 154 subjects with mania or mixed mania. All subjects received a mood stabilizer, either lithium, valproate, or carbamazepine. Mean modal dose of risperidone was 3.68 mg/day. Outcome measures were the YMRS, BPRS, and CGI. Results were not significantly different between risperidone vs. placebo ($p = 0.098$) on YMRS change. However, change from baseline was significantly greater for risperidone compared to placebo on BPRS ($p = 0.006$) and on CGI ($p = 0.022$). Risperidone was efficacious in subjects with and without psychotic features.

There are numerous open-label trials (40–44) that primarily involve treatment of bipolar illness not responsive to mood stabilizer monotherapy. In these trials risperidone was effective to moderately effective and generally well tolerated. Adverse effects of risperidone included sedation, dizziness, extrapyramidal symptoms, and weight gain. Vieta et al. (45) conducted a large, long-term, open-label study with 541 patients with bipolar disorder or schizoaffective disorder. Individuals had a diagnosis of acute mania, hypomania, or mixed symptoms and were treated with a mood stabilizer plus risperidone for 6 months. By end of study, 111 subjects withdrew for a variety of reasons including lost to follow-up (4%), adverse events (3%), hospitalization (3%), lack of response (3%), non-adherence with treatment (1%), and patient choice (1%). Mean dose of risperidone was 3.9 mg/day. After 6 months there were significant improvements on rating scales including the YMRS, HAM-D, CGI, Positive and Negative Symptom Scale for Schizophrenia (PANSS), and the Udvalg for Kliniske Undersogelser (UKU) subscale for neurological side effects ($p < 0.001$).

There are few reported studies on use of risperidone in either bipolar depression or in rapid cycling illness. Shelton et al. (46) completed a double-blind trial comparing risperidone, paroxetine, and risperidone/paroxetine combination in 25 subjects with bipolar depression. At the end of the 12-week study there were no significant differences between the treatment groups. Vieta et al. (47) reported that 8/10 patients with refractory rapid cycling illness had significant improvement on YMRS and HAM-D scores with risperidone therapy 2–6 mg/day.

There are a number of case reports and case series, which cite apparent precipitation or exacerbation of manic symptoms associated with risperidone therapy (48–50). It has been suggested that in these reports of apparent mania precipitation, several factors may have contributed to or caused mood exacerbation including: discontinuation of mood stabilizers, natural fluctuation in cyclical course, high dosing of risperidone, and risperidone monotherapy (51). In some case reports mania resolved with risperidone continued at a lower dose or with addition of a mood stabilizer

(48,52). It must be noted that apparent mania precipitation has been reported with nearly all of the atypical antipsychotic medications, including risperidone, olanzapine, sertindole, quetiapine, and amisulpride (52–56).

2. Unipolar Disorder

There are a limited number of reports of use of risperidone for major depressive disorder. Jacobsen (57) described four patients with major depression treated with risperidone 1.0–6.0 mg/day. All patients had reductions in CGI scores and all were treated for greater than 12 weeks. Two of four individuals were treated with concomitant antidepressant medications, and one individual received concomitant thyroid hormone. Keck et al. (34) reported on three cases of patients with major depression with psychotic features who received risperidone, all in conjunction with antidepressants. All three were noted to have "moderate to marked" improvement based upon interview with the primary treating psychiatrist and review of hospital records. Hirose and Ashby (58) recently reported that the combination of risperidone and fluvoxamine from the beginning of antidepressant therapy enhanced the therapeutic response in depression. Finally, investigators have reported that risperidone may be a treatment option in non-psychotic major depression refractory to antidepressants alone. Ostroff and Nelson (59) reported on eight patients who had clinical improvement when risperidone therapy was added to SSRI treatment, and Stoll and Haura (60) recently cited that the addition of risperdone to tranylcypromine led to improvement in depressive symptoms.

C. Olanzapine

The largest body of data on use of atypical antipsychotic medication in the treatment of mood disorders is with the agent olanzapine. The available evidence suggests that use of olanzapine monotherapy is efficacious in the treatment of bipolar mania, and that olanzapine therapy in combination with SSRIs or other mood stabilizers may constitute a powerful new weapon in the armamentarium of treatments for bipolar disorder.

1. Bipolar Disorder

There are a number of published uncontrolled studies of olanzapine in the treatment of bipolar disorder (24,61–69). In a study of 150 olanzapine-treated patients, Zarate et al. (61) found moderate to marked improvement in CGI-I score in 83% of bipolar patients ($n = 47$), 74% of schizoaffective bipolar subtype patients ($n = 23$), 47% of depressed schizoaffective patients ($n = 17$), and 76% of schizophrenic patients ($n = 29$). McElroy et al. (62)

administered olanzapine as add-on therapy to 14 consecutive bipolar patients already on standard mood stabilizers, reporting much or very much improvement in 8/14 (57%). Guille et al. (63) also examined patients treated with add-on olanzapine ($n = 20$), and also with risperidone ($n = 25$), and clozapine ($n = 5$). All three agents showed significant improvement in CGI-I scores; there was no significant difference in the improvements shown by the three experimental groups.

The efficacy of olanzapine in the treatment of patients with acute manic and mixed state episodes has been addressed in two core multisite, parallel-group, randomized, placebo-controlled, double-blind studies of similar design. The first of these (14) was a 3-week evaluation of 139 patients assigned to olanzapine ($n = 70$) or to placebo ($n = 69$). All patients scored at least 20 on the YMRS at study entry. Olanzapine dosing began at 10 mg the first day, and could be raised as high as 20 mg daily, depending on clinical response. The primary efficacy measure was change from baseline on the YMRS. Response was defined as a decrease of 50% or more in the YMRS total score. Results indicated that roughly twice as many patients from the olanzapine cohort (43/70, 61.4%) as controls (24/69, 34.8%) completed the blinded phase of the study. In the primary efficacy analysis, the mean total YMRS Score was 5.3 points lower than that of the placebo group ($CI = 0.95$, -10.31 to -0.93). Olanzapine-treated patients displayed greater mean improvement (-10.26) on the YMRS total score than controls (-4.88; $F = 5.64$ (df = 1,108), $p < 0.02$). Compared to placebo, olanzapine showed as much efficacy in non-psychotic patients as in psychotics patients ($F = 0.02$ (df = 1,106), $p = 0.88$). Compared with 24.2% in controls, 48.6% of olanzapine-treated patients showed at least a 50% improvement in total YMRS score ($p < 0.004$). Last Observation Carried Forward (LOCF) analyses indicated that 80.9% of the improvement shown by the olanzapine cohort was achieved within the first week of treatment. There was no intergroup difference in the incidence of EPS. The responder analysis showed a significantly higher response rate ($p = 0.004$) in the olanzapine group (34/70, 48.6%) than in the placebo group (16/69, 23.2%). Of the 139 patients entering the original study, 114 continued in 49-week open-label extension (70), where median length of treatment was 6.6 months. It was found that 88.3% of patients experienced a remission of manic symptoms; 25.5% relapsed. Significant improvement over baseline was seen in depressive symptoms as well ($p = 0.001$), and 41% of the cohort was maintained on olanzapine monotherapy.

The second of the two core studies (15) was of identical design, save that the duration was 4 weeks, and the starting dose of olanzapine was 15 mg daily instead of 10 mg daily. In this study 115 manic or mixed state patients were randomized to olanzapine ($n = 55$) or placebo ($n = 60$).

At 4 weeks, LOCF analysis showed significantly greater improvement for the olanzapine group over placebo on Total YMRS score (olanzapine -14.78, placebo -8.13, $p = 0.001$). As in the previous study, change was detectable at week 1 and continued for the duration of the study. The responder analysis showed that subjects in the olanzapine group meeting response criteria had increased to 64.8% which was significantly greater than that of the placebo group ($p = 0.023$).

In the third controlled study of olanzapine in the treatment of acute mania, Berk and colleagues (71) randomly assigned 30 adult patients meeting DSM-IV criteria for mania to receive lithium carbonate (400 mg bid.; $n = 15$) or olanzapine (10 mg q day; $n = 15$) in a 4-week, double-blind parallel-group study. The primary outcome measures were scores on the MS, BPRS, CGI, and the Global Assessment of Functioning (GAF). Both groups showed highly significant ($p < 0.0002$) and roughly equal improvement from BPRS baseline score (53.3) to score at end of study (30.15). The olanzapine group showed significantly more improvement (2.29) than the lithium group (2.83, $p < 0.025$). The authors concluded that lithium and olanzapine are equally efficacious in the treatment of mania, however noted that the study was weakened by small sample sizes and the absence of a placebo control group.

Two 3-week, head-to-head comparisons of olanzapine and valproate have been completed (72,73). In the first study, the trial duration was 21 days; 120 bipolar inpatients were enrolled. Valproate was loaded at 20 mg/kg/day to a maximum of 20 mg/kg + 1000 mg, and olanzapine started at 10 mg q day with a maximum of 20 mg daily. On the primary outcome measure, the Mania Rating Scale (MRS), olanzapine-treated and valproate-treated patients were not significantly different. Drop-out rates due to adverse events were equivalent. Weight gain, slurred speech, and somnolence were significantly more frequent in the olanzapine cohort. In the second study, 251 bipolar I inpatients were started on olanzapine at 15 mg q day, while valproate was started at 750 mg daily. An additional open-label extension phase was completed after the 3-week acute phase of the study. On the primary outcome measure (the YMRS total score), the olanzapine cohort ($n = 125$) showed significantly greater improvement (13.4 points) than the valproate cohort ($n = 123$, 10.4 points, $p = 0.05$). The study concluded that the agents were both effective, but that the olanzapine cohort was more likely to achieve remission. At the conclusion of the 47-week extension phase, the median time to manic relapse was 270 days in the olanzapine cohort, and 74 days in the valproate cohort, but the difference did not achieve statistical significance ($p = 0.392$). In short, the two studies produced similar findings: both agents were effective and well tolerated.

Tohen et al. (74) recently reported on a randomized double-blind, 12-month comparison of olanzapine and lithium in the prevention of relapse into a manic, mixed, or depressed bipolar episode. In this study 543 patients with bipolar mania received open-label combination therapy of olanzapine and lithium for 6–12 weeks. Of these, 431 patients met symptomatic remission criteria (YMRS total score of 12 or less and Hamilton Depression Scale (HAM-D 21) score of 8 or less) and were randomized to monotherapy with either olanzapine ($n = 217$) or lithium ($n = 214$) for 52 weeks of double-blind treatment. Olanzapine was dosed in a range of 5–20 mg/day while lithium was dosed in a range of 300–1800 mg/day, serum level 0.6–1.2 mEq/L. Significantly more olanzapine-treated patients completed the 52-week trial (46.5%) compared to patients on lithium (32.7%, $p < 0.004$). Olanzapine-treated patients had a statistically significantly lower incidence of relapse into a manic episode compared to lithium-treated patients (14.3% vs. 28.0% respectively, $p < 0.001$), while both groups had similar incidences of relapse into a depressive episode (16.1% vs. 15.4% respectively). Rates of drug discontinuation were similar between treatment groups. Weight gain across open-label and double-blind phases was significantly greater in the olanzapine group compared to the lithium group (1.79 kg vs. −1.38 kg, respectively, $p < 0.001$).

A similarly designed study (75) compared olanzapine to placebo in a randomized, double-blind 12-month trial evaluating time to relapse in bipolar disorder. There were 731 patients entered into this study which began with 6–12 weeks of open-label olanzapine therapy until remission criteria were met (YMRS of 12 or less and HAM-D 21 of 8 or less). There were 370 patients who completed the open label phase, followed by a 52-week, double-blind phase of randomization to either olanzapine monotherapy or placebo (361 patients entering, 295 discontinued, Sixty-six patients completed the entire double-blind phase. Mean daily dose of olanzapine during the open-label phase was 11.8 mg/day, and mean daily dose of olanzapine during the double-blind phase was 12.5 mg/day. Time to relapse to a mood episode (defined as need for hospitalization and/or YMRS score of 15 or greater and/or HAM-D 21 score of 15 or greater) was significantly prolonged by olanzapine-treatment ($p < 0.001$). Relapse to a mood episode occurred in 46.7% of olanzapine-treated patients compared to 80.1% of patients who received placebo ($p < 0.001$). Common (>5%) and significant adverse events occurring in the olanzapine group compared to placebo were weight gain, fatigue, and akathisia.

An intramuscular (IM) formulation of olanzapine is currently under study for possible FDA approval. Meehan and colleagues (76) recently published a double-blind, randomized comparison of IM olanzapine, lorazepam, and placebo in acutely agitated manic patients. In this study

201 such patients were randomly assigned to receive one to three injections of olanzapine (10 mg for each of the first two injections, 5 mg for the third), lorazepam (2 mg for each of the first two injections, 1 mg for the third), or placebo (placebo for the first two injections, olanzapine 10 mg for the third) within a 24-hour period. Assessments of the severity of agitation were made using the PANSS Excited Component Subscale (PANSS-EC), the Agitated Behavior Scale (ABS), and the Agitation-Calmness Evaluation Scale (ACES). Measurements were taken at baseline, q 30 minutes for the first 2 hours, and at 24 hours after the injection. The olanzapine cohort achieved separation from the placebo and lorazepam cohorts by 30 minutes after the first injection ($p = 0.004$). At 2 hours after the first injection, the olanzapine cohort showed greater improvement, as measured by all three instruments. Fifty-three percent of lorazepam-treated patients received 2 or 3 injections; only 26% of the olanzapine-treated patients required more than one.

Recently, olanzapine co-therapy with lithium and valproate has also been examined for efficacy in prevention of recurrence of bipolar depression (77). The study examined 99 patients randomized to olanzapine plus lithium or valproate in a 6-week stabilization phase. Responders in remission were re-randomized to 18 months of continued mood stabilizer therapy plus olanzapine ($n = 51$) or placebo ($n = 48$). The primary response variable was time to recurrence. Significantly more patients in the co-treatment group than in the monotherapy group completed the study (31.4% vs. 10.4%, $p = 0.014$). Patients in the olanzapine co-therapy group were significantly improved over the monotherapy group in time to recurrence of mania following symptomatic remission of mania ($p = 0.005$; estimated 25th percentile = 362 vs. 63 days, respectively). There was a similar trend that did not reach statistical significance in time to recurrence of depression after symptomatic remission of depression and mania ($p = 0.071$; estimated 25th percentile = 155 vs. 27 days, respectively). Time to recurrence into either pole, depression or mania, after remission of depression and mania was similarly longer for the co-treatment group than the placebo group ($p = 0.023$; estimated 25th percentile 124 vs. 15 days, respectively). These findings are consistent with the idea that combination therapy with an atypical antipsychotic and another mood stabilizer may be more efficacious than conventional mood stabilizer monotherapy.

Olanzapine + fluoxetine co-therapy (OFC) in the treatment of bipolar depression has also been examined. In an 83-site, 13-country study, Tohen and colleagues (78) randomized 833 moderately-to-severely depressed bipolar I patients to 8 weeks of double-blind treatment with 5–20 mg/day of olanzapine ($n = 370$), placebo ($n = 377$), or OFC ($n = 86$). The OFC group received 6 or 12 mg/day of olanzapine, plus 25 or 50 mg/day of fluoxetine. Results showed that starting at week 1 and throughout the study, improvement in depressive symptoms in both the olanzapine and the OFC groups was greater than that shown by the placebo group, as measured by MADRS scores (olanzapine: -15.0, $p = 0.02$ and OFC: -18.5, $p = 0.001$ vs. placebo: -11.9). The improvement shown by the OFC group was significantly greater than that shown by the olanzapine group ($p = 0.014$). Additionally, the percentage of patients achieving remission (i.e., decrease in MADRS score to 12 or less) was significantly higher for the OFC group (40/71, 56.3%) than for the olanapine group (115/284, 40.5%, $p = 0.027$). The investigators concluded that OFC therapy is more effective than olanzapine monotherapy in the treatment of bipolar depression.

2. Unipolar Depression

There have been a number of uncontrolled studies of olanzapine in unipolar depression (79–82). One trial of olanzapine was conducted in psychotic patients with unipolar depression (80). Seven depressed inpatients received 10–20 mg of olanzapine daily. Primary response measures were the HAM-D, the CGI, and the Scale for the Assessment of Positive Symptoms (SAPS). Five patients completed the full 10-week trial duration; of these, four responded (by HAM-D, CGI, and SAPS scores) to treatment, where response was defined as at least a 50% reduction in symptoms from baseline to final visit. Three of the five improved at least 2 points on the CGI. Three of the five met criteria for full remission of their psychotic episodes; i.e., their HAM-D scores were no more than 7. Parker (79) reported that olanzapine augmentation in treatment of melancholia led to rapid response in 6/10 patients. Finally, Marangell et al. (82) have recently reported successful treatment of apathy in 21 individuals with unipolar depression who were maintained on SSRI treatment.

D. Quetiapine

As is the case with a number of other atypical antipsychotic compounds, there is a rapidly expanding amount of information known about the efficacy of quetiapine in patients with mood disorders. Zarate et al. (84) reported on the results of a retrospective record review that assessed the efficacy of quetiapine in the treatment of psychotic mood disorders in comparison with non-affective psychotic disorders. Patient diagnoses included bipolar disorder, major depression with psychotic features, schizophrenia, schizoaffective disorder, and delusional disorder. Similar to what has been noted with clozapine (26) and with risperidone (34), in the study by Zarate et al. (84), patients with a diagnosis of bipolar disorder and schizoaffective disorder had higher response rates compared to patients with schizophrenia. However, in the Zarate study this finding did not achieve statistical significance.

1. Bipolar Disorder

Sachs et al. (85) reported on a 3-week, double-blind placebo-controlled trial which examined the efficacy of quetiapine as adjunctive treatment with a mood stabilizer in 191 patients with acute type I bipolar mania. Primary efficacy measure was change from baseline in YMRS total score. Quetiapine produced a significantly greater improvement in YMRS total score, from baseline to last observation compared to placebo (-13.76 vs. -9.93, $p = 0.021$). Response ($\geq 50\%$ decrease in YMRS) was significantly higher in the quetiapine group than placebo (54.3% vs. 32.6%, $p = 0.005$). Mean last week dose of quetiapine was 580 mg/day in responders.

Mullen and Paulsson (86) reported on another randomized, double-blind trial of adjunct therapy with quetiapine plus mood stabilizer compared to placebo plus mood stabilizer in 402 patients with acute manic episode. Primary outcome measure was change in YMRS from baseline at day 21. Findings were similar to the report by Sachs et al. (85) with superior response in the quetiapine plus mood stabilizer group at day 21 compared to the placebo plus mood stabilizer-treated group ($p = 0.014$). More quetiapine-treated patients completed the trial, and there were fewer discontinuations due to adverse events in the quetiapine group compared to the control group. Most quetiapine responders (76.7%) at Day 21 received doses of quetiapine between 400–800 mg/day.

Paulsson and Huizar (87) recently reported on a 12-week, randomized, double-blind trial of quetiapine (up to 800 mg/day) compared to placebo in the treatment of acute mania. Patients receiving lithium (0.6–1.4 mEq/L target trough serum levels) served to control for assay sensitivity. In this study, 302 patients with type I bipolar disorder were randomized to receive either quetiapine ($n = 107$), placebo ($n = 97$), or lithium ($n = 96$). Primary efficacy endpoint in this study was change from baseline in YMRS score at day 21; a secondary endpoint was change from baseline in YMRS score at day 84. All study participants had a study entry YMRS score of 20 or greater including a score of 4 or greater on two of the core YMRS items of Irritability, Speech, Content, and Disruptive/Aggressive Behavior. More withdrawals from the study occurred in the group that received placebo (63.9%) compared to quetiapine-treated (32.7%) and lithium-treated (31.6%) groups. Mean quetiapine dose for responders was 568 mg/day at day 21 and 651 mg/day at day 84. The decrease in YMRS score from baseline was significantly greater for quetiapine-treated patients than for placebo-treated patients at both day 21 ($p < 0.001$) and at day 84

($p < 0.001$). YMRS change from baseline with lithium therapy was also significantly better ($p < 0.001$) compared to placebo, and was similar to the response on YMRS observed with quetiapine therapy. The most common side effects in quetiapine-treated patients were dry mouth, somnolence, and weight gain compared to tremor, insomnia, and headache in the lithium-treated group.

Brecher and Huizar (88) reported results of a 12-week, double-blind study of quetiapine monotherapy in acute mania in which 302 patients were randomized to quetiapine (up to 800 mg/day), placebo, or haloperidol. As with the study by Paulsson and Huizar (87), primary endpoint was change in baseline YMRS score at day 21. In the report by Brecher and Huizar (88), 53.9% of quetiapine-treated patients completed the trial compared to 41.6% of placebo-treated patients. Patients receiving quetiapine had significantly greater improvement from baseline in YMRS score compared to patients receiving placebo at both day 21 ($p = 0.01$) and at day 84 ($p < 0.001$). Haloperidol response was similar to quetiapine response with respect to change from baseline on YMRS, although tolerability was better with quetiapine, primarily due to EPS-related adverse effects with haloperidol. YMRS response and remission rates at day 84 were similar for quetiapine- and haloperidol-treated patients, and both quetiapine- and haloperidol-treated patient response and remission rates by day 84 were significantly greater compared to placebo ($p < 0.001$). Mean change in weight from baseline by day 84 was 2.1 kg for the quetiapine group and 0.1 kg for the haloperidol group. Finally, mean last week dose for quetiapine responders at day 21 was 559 mg/day.

Sajatovic et al. (89) reported an analysis of efficacy of quetiapine and risperidone against depressive symptoms in outpatients with psychotic disorders. This was part of a larger, 4-month, open-label trial comparing quetiapine to risperidone in patients with a variety of psychotic disorders including schizophrenia, schizoaffective disorder, bipolar disorder, major depression and delusional disorder. There were 316 subjects with mood disorders treated with quetiapine and 103 subjects with mood disorders treated with risperidone. Mood symptoms were evaluated with the HAM-D. Although both agents produced improvement in mean HAM-D scores quetiapine produced a slightly greater improvement compared to risperidone ($p = 0.002$). Subjects with HAM-D scores 20 or greater than had the most robust improvement with both compounds.

Sajatovic et al. (83) reported on an open-label prospective study of 10 individuals with bipolar disorder and 10 individuals with schizoaffective disorder who received 12 weeks of quetiapine therapy. Overall, subjects had significant improvement on BPRS score ($p < 0.001$), YMRS score ($p = 0.043$), and HAM-D score ($p = 0.002$). Mean quetiapine dosage was

202.9 mg/day. Ghaemi and Goodwin (90) reported results of a retrospective chart review in which two of six patients with treatment-resistant bipolar disorder exhibited moderate to marked improvement with quetiapine therapy. Ghaemi et al. (16) have also reported on the successful use of quetiapine in rapid cycling bipolar illness. As with other atypical antipsychotic compounds, possible precipitation of mania/hypomania has been reported with quetiapine (91). Adverse effects most commonly associated with quetiapine include sedation, dizziness, and orthostasis.

2. Unipolar Disorder

Use of quetiapine in major depression has been less studied compared to bipolar illness. Padia (92) recently reported on the successful treatment of depression with psychotic features in an adolescent boy. In this report quetiapine (up to 400 mg/day) was prescribed concomitantly with fluoxetine 40 mg/day. Subjects with major depression were also included in the study reported by Sajatovic et al. (89). Mean percentage change on the HAM-D for 75 subjects with major depressive disorder treated with quetiapine was 42.2% ($p < 0.05$). While mean quetiapine dose in the study by Sajatovic et al. (89) was 317 mg, under flexibly dosed, open-label conditions, there was a "spectrum" of dosing dependent on primary diagnostic status. Patients with major depressive or schizoaffective disorder were prescribed 74 mg/day or 41 mg/day respectively, less than patients with schizophrenia ($p < 0.05$).

E. Ziprasidone

Ziprasidone is an atypical antipsychotic compound approved for the treatment of schizophrenia, and its use in mood disorders has been studied to a limited extent.

1. Bipolar Disorder

Keck et al. (93) recently reported on a study of ziprasidone in the treatment of bipolar disorder. Following a screening period and discontinuation of all psychotropic medications except PRN lorazepam and temazepam, 210 manic or mixed state patients were randomized to ziprasidone 80 mg/day to 160 mg/day ($n = 140$), or placebo ($n = 70$) for 3 weeks. Patients were rated using the Schedule for Affective Disorders and Schizophrenia-Change (SADS-C), the Mania Rating Scale (MRS) from the SADS-C, the CGI-S, PANSS, and GAF. The intent-to-treat analysis showed the ziprasidone cohort with significantly greater MRS improvement than the placebo cohort from study day 2 ($p = 0.01$) and continuing throughout the duration of the study ($p = 0.001$ from study day 4 thereafter). A similar improvement was seen in the CGI-S data beginning at study day 4 ($p = 0.05$). Improvement in PANSS overall and positive symptom scores was seen from study day 7 and thereafter ($p = 0.001$). Mean endpoint GAF scores in the ziprasidone cohort were significantly greater than those of the placebo group ($p < 0.05$). Mean dose of ziprasidone was 139.1 mg/day on days 14–21, and 130.1 mg during days 15–21. An IM form of ziprasidone, which has been shown efficacious in reducing acute agitation associated with psychosis (94). This form of the medication has not been evaluated in controlled trials using a bipolar population.

2. Unipolar Disorder

There are currently no published studies of ziprasidone in unipolar disorder.

F. Aripiprazole

Aripiprazole received approval by the FDA for a schizophrenia indication in late 2002, and there have been some recent reports on the use of aripiprazole in bipolar disorder. Marcus et al. (95) reported on a 3-week, double-blind, placebo-controlled study of aripiprazole in the treatment of acute bipolar mania. In this multicenter trial patients were randomized to receive either aripiprazole 30 mg/day, with option to decrease to 15 mg ($n = 130$), or placebo ($n = 132$). Primary outcome was assessed using the YMRS and CGI, with response defined as 50% or greater improvement in YMRS. Aripiprazole produced significant improvements in YMRS total score compared to placebo ($p < 0.05$). The response rate was significantly higher in the aripiprazole group compared to the placebo group (40% vs. 19%, $p < 0.01$). Discontinuation rate and weight gain for patients treated with aripiprazole did not differ significantly from patients receiving placebo. A report by Sanchez et al. (96) was of a 12-week double-blind study of aripiprazole 15 mg/day, with option to increase to 30 mg/day ($n = 175$) compared to haloperidol ($n = 172$). The primary outcome measure was response at week 12 on the YMRS, with response defined as 50% or greater improvement on the YMRS. At week 12, significantly more patients responded to and remained on aripiprazole compared to haloperidol (50% vs. 28%, $p < 0.001$). The major reason for discontinuation in the haloperidol group was adverse events, with 36% of haloperidol-treated patients reporting EPS (c.f. 9% of the aripiprazole-treated patients). Weight gain was minimal and not different between the two treatment groups. Mean dose of aripiprazole at the end of week 3 was 22.6 mg/day and 21.6 mg/day at the end of week 12. Mean dose of haloperidol at the end of week 3 was 11.6 mg/day and 11.1 mg/day at the end of week 12.

G. Additional Compounds

There are a variety of compounds currently being investigated for efficacy as atypical antipsychotics. Reflective of the current state of knowledge regarding atypical antipsychotics as broad spectrum psychotropic agents, some of these compounds have been preliminarily studied for their effects on serious mood disorders. Further research is needed to clarify the roles of these and other investigational compounds for possible use in the treatment of individuals with serious mood disorders.

III. SPECIAL POPULATIONS

While atypical antipsychotics have become widely utilized in clinical settings for the management of mood disorders, there is still a relative scarcity of data on their use in special populations with mood disorders, such as children, older adults, and pregnant or lactating women (97).

A. Children and Adolescents

Clozapine usage in children and adolescents with mood disorders has been described in case reports (98,99), primarily in bipolar illness. In these cases clozapine was successfully combined with lithium therapy. Primary adverse effects were sedation and fatigue. Fuchs (98) noted that there may be significant adverse effects between valproic acid and clozapine in the treatment of adolescent bipolar disorder.

Preliminary data suggest that risperidone may be effective in the treatment of mania in children and adolescents. Frazier et al. (100) reported a retrospective chart review of 28 outpatient youths (mean age 10.4 years) with bipolar disorder who received risperidone therapy. Using CGI improvement scores of ≤ 2 (very much/much improved) to define robust improvement, 82% showed improvement in symptoms of mania and aggression. Mean risperidone dose was 1.7 mg/day. Schreier (101) reported on an open-label trial of risperidone therapy in 11 children/adolescents with affective symptoms and aggression. The sample was described as "mostly suggestive of bipolar disorder," and daily risperidone dosing was relatively low (0.75–2.5 mg/day). Side effects of risperidone therapy with children/adolescents primarily involve mild sedation and occasional weight gain (101). There have been rare reports of galactorrhea (102) and neuroleptic malignant syndrome (103).

Frazier et al. (104) reported on an 8-week, open-label prospective study of olanzapine monotherapy (dose range 2.5–20 mg/day) in 23 bipolar youths (age range 5–14 years). Twenty-two of the 23 completed the study. Olanzapine treatment was associated with significant improvement in mean YMRS score. Overall, olanzapine was well tolerated, and extrapyramidal symptom measures were not significantly different from baseline. Body weight increased significantly over the study (5.0 ± 2.3 kg, $p < 0.001$). Additional case reports (67,105) summarized olanzapine trials in manic adolescents. Chang and Ketter (106) reported the successful treatment of acute mania in three prepubertal children. In this report olanzapine was added to existing mood stabilizer regimens with marked improvement in manic symptoms within 3–5 days. Adverse effects included sedation and weight gain.

Quetiapine may be efficacious as adjunctive therapy to divalproex in treating manic, depressive, and psychotic symptoms in adolescents. Delbello et al. (107) reported results of a 6-week double blind, placebo-controlled, randomized clinical study comparing the efficacy and safety of adding quetiapine to a regiment of divalproex in the treatment of mania in adolescents (age 12–18 years). In this report, 22 of 30 (73%) of subjects completed this study. Mean dosage of quetiapine was 432 mg/day. Patients treated with combination therapy (quetiapine plus valproate) experienced significantly greater improvement in the manic and depressive symptoms than patients treated with valproate monotherapy. The most commonly reported adverse events for the combination therapy group vs. the monotherapy group were sedation (80% vs. 33%), nausea (27% vs. 40%), and headache (47% for both groups).

2. Older Adults

Although clozapine therapy in the elderly may be effective (108,109), its use is often limited by adverse effects including sedation, orthostasis, and cardiac effects. While the risk of agranulocytosis with clozapine is on the order of 0.3–1.0% in younger populations, there is a greater vulnerability for agranulocytosis among the elderly (110). Patients aged 55–64 may have a more robust response to clozapine therapy compared to patients aged 65 and older (109).

Risperidone therapy may be beneficial, and is generally well tolerated among older adults with bipolar disorder (111). Older adults are particularly vulnerable to tardive dyskinesia (TD). A prospective 9-month, longitudinal study compared cumulative incidence of TD with risperidone to haloperidol in older patients with a variety of conditions, including mood disorders (112). Life table analysis suggested that patients treated with haloperidol were significantly more likely to develop TD than patients treated with risperidone ($p < 0.05$). Reports of use of risperidone therapy in elderly patients with treatment-resistant depression suggest that low dose risperidone therapy may be useful when added to antidepressants, even in circumstances when psychosis is not evident (113,114).

There have been very few reports on the use of olanzapine or quetiapine in elderly individuals with primary mood disorders (115). It has been suggested that olanzapine therapy may have a role in treatment-resistant psychotic mood disorders (117). Solomons and Geiger (116) have reported that up to 60.3% of elderly individuals refractory to other antipsychotic medications may improve with olanzapine. The most common side effects of olanzapine use in the elderly include drowsiness, extrapyramidal symptoms, and delirium (116). Quetiapine may offer some advantages in the treatment of elderly patients with mood disorders with particular respect to potential for extrapyramidal symptoms (118–121). McManus et al. (121) reported a 52-week, multicenter, open-label trial of quetiapine therapy in older adults with psychosis. In this report quetiapine was associated with minimal EPS. The most common side effects were somnolence, dizziness and postural hypotension.

C. Pregnant or Lactating Women

There are a limited number of reports of clozapine therapy in pregnancy, predominantly in women with schizophrenia or related disorders (122–125). In two reports (123,126) it was speculated that gestational diabetes was exacerbated by clozapine therapy. Risks of neonatal safety may be a substantial issue with clozapine therapy during lactation (127).

Ernst and Goldberg (127) reviewed the case registry/literature reports on olanzapine therapy in pregnancy and lactation. From a total of 96 prospectively reported cases of olanzapine therapy in pregnancy, 69 (71.9%) resulted in normal births, 12 (12.5%) resulted in spontaneous abortion, 2 (2.1%) led to premature deliveries, 3 (3.1%) were stillbirths, and 1 case (1.0%) resulted in major malformations. These are all within the range of normal historical control rates (127). It is not clear if effect on birth outcome may differ between women with mood disorders and non-mood disorders who receive olanzapine therapy during pregnancy. With respect to olanzapine therapy during lactation, it has been noted that in four out of 20 cases there have been reports of adverse effects including: 1) jaundice, sedation, cardiomegaly, heart murmur, 2) lethargy, shaking, and poor sucking, 3) protruding tongue, and 4) rash, diarrhea, and sleep disorder (128).

There are no adequate human studies to evaluate safety of risperidone, quetiapine, or ziprasidone therapy in humans. In the case of risperidone, there is a single case report of agenesis of the corpus callosum

(129) with in utero exposure, and no adverse effect seen with a case report of risperidone therapy during breast feeding in a woman with puerperal psychosis (130). Tenyi et al. (131) recently reported a single case of no apparent adverse effects associated with quetiapine therapy during pregnancy in a woman with schizophrenia. There are no reports of quetiapine or ziprasidone therapy during pregnancy in women with primary mood disorders.

IV. CLINICAL IMPLICATIONS AND RECOMMENDATIONS

A core goal of treatment in bipolar disorder is the control of symptoms, thus allowing individuals with bipolar illness to maximize levels of psychosocial functioning. Rapid control of symptoms such as aggression and psychosis is critical in order to ensure patient safety and minimize negative sequelae.

Lithium, valproate, and antipsychotics are all effective treatment for acute mania (7), and the combination of an antipsychotic with either lithium or valproate may be more effective than monotherapy treatment (7). Atypical antipsychotics are generally preferred over typical agents. For less ill patients, monotherapy with lithium, valproate, or an atypical antipsychotic such as olanzapine (7) may provide sufficient symptom control. Table 1 outlines guidelines for clinicians regarding use of specific atypical antipsychotic agents in bipolar disorder. For treatment of bipolar depression, first-line treatment recommendation is usually lithium or lamotrigine (7). Antipsychotics in bipolar depression are often reserved for individuals with psychotic features. When first-line medications at therapeutic doses fail to fully control symptoms, treatment options include adding another first line agent, or alternative treatments such as adding an antipsychotic medication if it has not been already prescribed, or changing from one antipsychotic to another (7).

In the treatment of unipolar depression antidepressant agents are considered a first-line therapy (132). Patients with major depressive disorder with psychotic features require either the combined use of antidepressants plus antipsychotics or ECT (132). As noted earlier, some patients with non-psychotic depression may also benefit from the addition of an atypical antipsychotic to their antidepressant treatment regimen.

V. PATIENT EDUCATION

Treatment of bipolar illness, as with any psychiatric condition, is ideally a collaborative process in which care providers and patients have an

Table 1 Guidelines for Clinicians: Specific Antipsychotic Medications in the Management of Mood Disorders

Medication	Summary of research data results	Adverse effects and precautions	Suggested daily dose (mg/day)	Unique patient education issues	Comments
Clozapine	Reserved for use in treatment-refractory illness May be used as monotherapy in bipolar illness May be useful as an antimanic as well as a long-term mood stabilizer	Risk of agranulocytosis on the order of 0.3–1.0% Required serum blood count (WBC) monitoring Other side effects: sedation, orthostasis, weight gain, seizures	300–500	Review need for continuous serum monitoring Nutritional counseling regarding weight gain and possible effects on serum glucose, cholesterol Discuss probable need for divided daily dosing	Reports of reduced suicidality with clozapine in some psychiatric populations May be significant interaction with some SSRI antidepressants
Risperidone	FDI-approved for treatment of acute biploar mania May be useful in bipolar/unipolar depression May be used as monotherapy or adjunctive therapy	Most common adverse effects: extrapyramidal symptoms, sedation, dizziness	2–6	Review potential for EPS	Research studies include several controlled trials Dosing at or below 4 mg/day seen in most recent reports Long-acting injectable available

Drug	Indications	Most common adverse effects	Dose (mg/day)	Monitoring	Comments
Olanzapine	FDA approved for treatment of acute bipolar mania; May be used as monotherapy or adjunct; May be useful as a long-term mood stabilizer; May be useful in bipolar/unipolar depression	Most common adverse effects: weight gain, sedation	10–20	Nutritional counseling regarding weight gain and possible effects on serum glucose, cholesterol	Research studies include largest number of controlled trials; Rapid acting IM formulation under investigation
Quetiapine	FDA-approved for treatment of acute bipolar mania; May be useful in bipolar/unipolar depression; May be used as monotherapy or adjunctive therapy	Most common adverse effects: sedation and orthostasis	200–400	May need divided dosing; Review potential effects of sedation, orthostasis; May need ophthalmological monitoring	Patients with more depressive symptoms may have most robust improvement
Ziprasidone	May be useful in acute mania	Most common adverse effects: somnolence, headache, nausea	80–160	May need EKG screening/monitoring	IM formulation available, possible use in acute mania
Aripiprazole	May be useful in acute mania	Most common adverse effects: nausea, dyspepsia, somnolence	15–30	Review potential GI, sedative effects	Some patients may respond to 10 mg/day

interactive and constructive alliance with the goal of achieving optimal illness outcome. Good communication and a full awareness of treatment options and expected results are essential. In order to facilitate this, it is critical that patients and those individuals providing psychosocial support to the individual with illness, have a comprehensive understanding of pertinent psychotropic medications. While atypical antipsychotic drugs are often used to manage symptoms of bipolar illness in clinical settings, it is not surprising that patients and their families may think of these compounds as "schizophrenia medications." It is important that care providers explain the role of atypical antipsychotic medications in bipolar illness, including a discussion of possible risks, benefits, and side effects. Table 2 is an example of patient education materials that might be discussed when prescribing atypical antipsychotic medication to individuals with bipolar illness. Regular evaluation of ongoing or new adverse effects will promote treatment adherence, assist in monitoring and managing adverse effects, and facilitate achievement of optimal health outcomes.

VI. SUMMARY

There has been tremendous growth in the sophistication of psychopharmacology of mood disorders over the past decade. The proliferation of the atypical antipsychotic drugs has been accompanied by broader application of these compounds in seriously ill psychiatric populations including individuals with bipolar and unipolar illness. For bipolar illness in particular, the efficacy of atypical antipsychotic medications has substantially changed recommended treatment guidelines. Atypical antipsychotic medications are commonly utilized in clinical settings to manage acute mania, psychotic depression, and as agents to optimize long-term mood outcomes. Table 3 summarizes main points on the use of atypical antipsychotic drugs in mood disorders.

Currently, there are three atypical antipsychotic agents with an FDA-approved indication in bipolar disorder (olanzapine, risperidone and quetiapine); however, this is expected to change in the near future with the rapid growth of clinical research in this area. There is a critical need for blinded, controlled, and long-term trials of atypical antipsychotic medications in serious mood disorders to validate the findings reported in open-label and uncontrolled studies. Finally, the unique properties of the differing agents as they apply to specific subtypes of mood disorder, for example rapid cycling bipolar disorder, treatment-refractory major depression, and special populations with mood disorders need to be further explored.

Table 2 Patient Information – Antipsychotic Medications

Type of medication
Antipsychotic medication, typical group and atypical group

Medications in this group

Typical: Chlorpromazine, Chlorprothixene, Droperidol, Fluphenazine, Haloperidol, Loxapine, Mesoridazine, Molindone, Perphenazine, Pimozide, Prochlorperazine, Pimozine, Thioridazine, Thiothixene, Trifluoperazine, Triflupromazine

Atypical: Clozapine, Risperidone, Olanzapine, Quetiapine, Ziprasidone, Aripiprazole

Reasons not to take this medicine
If you have an allergy to antipsychotic medications or any other part of the medicines in this group.
Do not take mesoridazine (Serentil®), pimozide (Orap™), or thioridazine (Mellaril®) if you have a history of abnormal heartbeats.
Do not take mesoridazine (Serentil®) or thioridazine (Mellaril®) if you are taking certain heartbeat controlling medicines, such as, amiodarone (Cordarone®, Pacerone®), cisapride (Propulsid®), cyclic antidepressants, dispyramide (Norpace®, Norpace® CR), dofetilide (Tikosyn™), fluoxetine (Prozac®, Prozac® Weekly ™, Sarafem™) (should be stopped for 5 weeks before starting this medicine), fluvoxamine (Luvox®), gatifloxacin (Tequin®), moxifloxacin (ABC Pack™, Avelox®), paroxetine (Paxil®), procainamide (Procanbid®, Pronestyl®, Pronestyl-SR®), quinidine (Cardioquin®, Quinaglute® Dura-Tabs®, Quinidax® Extentabs®), sotalol (Betapace®, Betapace AF™, Sorine™), or sparfloxacin (Zagam®). Check all medicines with healthcare provider.
Do not take ziprasidone (Geodon®) if you are taking any of these medicines: Amiodarone (Cordarone ®, Pacerone®), cisapride (Propulsid®), disopyramide (Norpace®, Norpace® CR), dofetilide (Tikosyn™), mesoridazine (Serentil®), pimozide (Orap™), procainamide (Procanbid®, Pronestyl®, Pronestyl-SR®), quinidine (Cardioquin®, Quinaglute® Dura-Tabs®, Quinidex® Extentabs®), some quinolone antibiotics (moxifloxacin [ABC Pack™, Avelox®], sparfloxacin [Zagam®], gatifloxacin [Tequin®]), sotalol (Betapace®, Betapace AF™, Sorine™), or thioridazine (Mellaril®). Check all medicines with healthcare provider.
Do not use ziprasidone (Geodon®) if you have had a recent heart attack or have a severely weakened heart (congestive heart failure).

What is this medicine used for?
Treatment of psychosis which may be seen in a variety of mental disorders such as schizophrenia, manic-depressive disorder, and dementia. Other uses of antipsychotic medications include tic disorders (Tourette's disorder); severe aggressive or impulsive conditions; behavioral problems in children; Huntington's chorea; prevention of nausea and vomiting; Reye's syndrome; and spasmodic torticollis.

(continued)

Table 2 Continued

How does it work?
Antipsychotics work in various areas of the brain to help control voices, paranoia, hallucinations, aggression, agitation, delusions, and mania.

How is it best taken?
To gain the most benefit, do not miss doses.
Take all other medicines in this group with or without food. Take with food if this medicine causes an upset stomach. Be consistent, take with food every time or take on an empty stomach every time.
Do not suddenly stop using this medicine if you have been taking it for a long time. Medicine should be slowly decreased.
Take with plenty of non-caffeine-containing liquids every day unless told to drink less liquid by healthcare provider.
Use chlorpromazine (Thorazine®) and prochlorperazine (Compazine®) suppository rectally only.
A liquid (concentrate) is available for thiothixene (Navane®), trifluoperazine (Stelazine®), molindone (Moban®), loxapine (Loxitane®), fluphenazine (Permitil®, Prolixin®) (also available as an elixir), haloperidol (Haldol®), and perphenazine (Trilafon®) if you cannot swallow pills. Prochlorperazine (Compazine®) is available as a syrup. Those who have feeding tubes can also use the liquid. Flush the feeding tube before and after medicine is given. Mix 1/2 cup of water before drinking. Mesoridazine (Serentil®) is also available as a concentrate and can be mixed with distilled water, orange or grape juice before drinking. Thioridazine (Mellaril®) is available as a concentrate or suspension and can be mixed with 1/4 to 1/2 cup of water, fruit juice, carbonated drink, milk, or pudding before drinking. Chlorpromazine (Thorazine®) is available as a syrup or concentrate and can be mixed with 1/2 cup of water or soft food before drinking or eating. Do not spill liquid concentrate on skin. Can irritate your skin.
Do not mix thioridazine (Mellaril®) concentrate with carbamazepine (Carbatrol®, Epitol®, Tegretol®, Tegretol®-XR) suspension. Separate by 1–2 hours.

What do I do if I miss a dose?
Take this medicine exactly as recommended by your healthcare provider.
Do not take a double dose or extra doses.
Do not change dose or stop medicine.
Talk with healthcare provider about what you should do if you miss a dose of this medicine.

What are the precautions when taking this medicine?
Check any other medicines you may be taking with healthcare provider.
    This medicine may not mix well with other medicines.
If you are 65 or older, you may have more side effects.

(*continued*)

Table 2 Continued

May cause drowsiness. Avoid driving, doing other tasks or activities until
you see how this medicine affects you.

Avoid alcohol (includes wine, beer, and liquor), other medicines, and herbal
products that slow your actions and reactions. Talk with healthcare provider.

You can get sunburned more easily. Avoid lots of sun, sunlamps, and tanning
beds. Use sunscreen; wear protective clothing and eyewear.

Be careful in hot weather. You may be more sensitive to the heat.

Use caution with ziprasidone (Geodon®) if you have a weakened heart.
May increase the risk of effects on the heart. Talk with healthcare provider.

If you are on any heart medicines such as quinidine (Cardioquin®,
QuinagIute® DuraTabs®, Ouinidex® Extentabs®), procainamide
(Procanbid®, Pronestyl®, Pronestyl SR®), disopyramide (Norpace®,
Norpace® CR), mexiletine (Mexitil®), moriciZine (Ethmozine®), tocainide
(Tonocard ®), flecainide (Tamboocor™), propafenone™ (Rythmnol™),
arniodarone (Cordarone™, Pacerone™), or sotalol (Betapace®Betapace
AF™, Sorine™), talk with healthcare provider before taking
thioridazine (Mellaril®) mesoridazine (Serentil®), or pimozide (Orap™).

Tell healthcare provider if you are allergic to any medicine. Make sure to tell
about the allergy and how it affected you. This includes telling about
rash; hives; itching; shortness of breath; wheezing; cough; swelling of
face, lips, tongue, throat; or any other symptoms involved.

Tell healthcare provider if you are pregnant or plan on getting pregnant.

Do not use if you are breastfeeding.

What are the common side effects of this medicine?

All drugs are associated with side effects. Most side effects are mild, and
often may improve over time. Discuss side effects of this medicine
with your healthcare provider before starting therapy, including how
you should contact your healthcare provider if side effects occur. The
following side effects are more common with antipsychotic medications and
should be discussed with your healthcare provider.

Feeling sleepy or lightheaded. Avoid driving, doing other tasks or activities that
require you to be alert until you see how this medicine affects you.

Dizziness is common. Rise slowly over several minutes from sitting or lying
position.

Be careful climbing stairs.

Dry mouth. Frequent mouth care, sucking hard candy, or chewing gum
may help.

Constipation. More liquids, regular exercise, or a fiber-containing diet may
help. Talk with healthcare provider about a stool softener or laxative.

Weight gain.

Change in sexual ability or desire. This can return to normal after the
medicine is stopped.

Talk with healthcare provider about other medicines without this side effect.

(*continued*)

Table 2 Continued

What should I monitor?

Follow up with healthcare provider and report any side effects at visit.

Monitor heart rhythm as medical condition warrants if you are taking ziprasidone (Geodon®). Talk with healthcare provider.

Have an eye exam as warranted every 6 months if you are taking quetiapine (Seroquel®). Talk with healthcare provider.

Reasons to call healthcare provider immediately

Signs of a life-threatening reaction. These include wheezing; chest tightness; fever; itching; bad cough; blue skin color; fits; or swelling of face, lips, tongue, or throat.

Unable to think clearly.

Blurred vision.

Restlessness and inability to stay still or calm.

Movements not controlled by you, shakiness, difficulty moving around, or stiffness.

Change in balance, feeling shaky or unsteady.

Too tired or sleepy.

Fast heartbeats.

Passing out or fainting.

Severe dizziness.

For females, menstrual changes. These include lots of bleeding, spotting, or bleeding between cycles.

High fever.

Any rash.

If you suspect an overdose, call your local poison control center immediately or dial 911.

How should I store this medicine?

Store in a tight, light-resistant container at room temperature. Protect from heat and moisture.

General statements

Do not share your medicine with others and do not take anyone else's medicine. Know the name, spelling, and milligram dosage amount of your medicine. This may be written down on a card kept in your wallet or purse. This information is extremely important should you become suddenly ill or are involved in an emergency situation. Keep all medicine out of the reach of children and pets.

Talk with healthcare provider before starting any new medicine, including over-the-counter or natural products (herbs, vitamins).

Source: Ref. 133.

Table 3 Summary of Main Points

Atypical antipsychotic medications (APS) may be useful treatments in the
management of serious mood disorders

Largest body of literature supports APS use in bipolar disorder

Most common clinical scenario of use of APS in bipolar disorder is in acute
manic/mixed presentation

Most common clinical scenario of use of APS in unipolar disorder is in
psychotic depression

APS response may be greater in patients with bipolar and schizoaffective
disorder compared to patients with schizophrenia

Olanzapine, risperidone and quetiapine have an FDA indication for bipolar illness,
however there is a rapidly growing literature on the usefulness of other APS
as well

Patients and families should receive education regarding risks, benefits, and
expected treatment outcomes with use of APS in mood disorders

There is a critical need for controlled and long-term studies utilizing APS in
serious mood disorders to validate findings from uncontrolled/short-term
studies

REFERENCES

1. American Psychiatric Association. Practice Guideline for the Treatment of Patients with Bipolar Disorder. Washington, DC: American Psychiatric Publishing, 1994.
2. Goodwin FK, Jamison KR. Manic-Depressive Illness. New York: Oxford University Press, 1990.
3. Prien RF, Caffey EM, Klett DJ. Comparison of lithium carbonate and chlorpromazine in the treatment of mania. Report of the Veterans Administration and National Institute of Mental Health Collaborative Study Group. Arch Gen Psychiatry 1972; 26:146–153.
4. Fuller M, Sajatovic M. Drug Information for Mental Health. Cleveland, Ohio: Lexi-Comp, 2001:630–631.
5. Ghadirian AM, Annable L, Belanger MD, Chouinard G. A cross-sectional study of parkinsonism and tardive dyskinesia in lithium-treated affective disordered patients. J Clin Psychiatry 1996; 57(1):22–28.
6. Kukopoulos A, Reginaldi D, Laddamada P, Floris G, Serra G, Tondo L. Course of the manic-depressive cycle and changes caused by treatment. Pharmakopsychaitrie-Neuropsychopharmakol 1980; 13:156–167.
7. American Psychiatric Association. Practice guideline for the treatment of patients with bipolar disorder (revision). Washington, DC: American Psychiatric Press, 2002.
8. Brown ES, Thomas NR, Carmody T, Mahadi S, Nejtek, VA. Atypical antipsychotics in bipolar and schizoaffective disorders. Pharmacopyschiatry 2001; 34(2):80–81.

9. Bowden CL. Novel treatments for bipolar disorder. Expert Opin Investig Drugs 2001; 10(4):661–671.
10. Thase ME. What role do atypical antipsychotic drugs have in treatment-resistant depression? J Clin Psychiatry 2002; 63(2):95–103.
11. Buckley PF. Broad therapeutic uses of atypical antipsychotic medications. Biol Psychiatry 2001; 50(11):912–924.
12. Glick ID, Murray SR, Vasudevan P, Marder SR, Hu RJ. Treatment with atypical antipsychotics: new indications and new populations. J Psychiatr Res 2001; 35(3):187–191.
13. Buckley PF, Miller DD, Singer B, Donenwirth K. What's new with the new antipsychotics? Presented at the Annual Meeting of the American College of Neuropsychopharmacology, Acapulco, Mexico, December, 1999.
14. Tohen M, Sanger TM, McElroy SL, Tollefson GD, Chengappa KNR, Daniel DG, Petty F, Centorrino F, Wang R, Grundy SL, Greaney MG, Jacobs TG, David ST, Toma V, (Olanzapine HGEH Study Group). Olanzapine versus placebo in the treatment of acute mania. Am J Psychiatry 1999; 156:702–709.
15. Tohen M, Jacobs TG, Grundy SL, McElroy SL, Banov MC, Janicak PG, Sanger T, Risser R, Zhang F, Toma V, Francis J, Tollefson GD, Breier A, (Olanzapine HGEH Study Group). Efficacy of olanzapine in acute bipolar mania: a double-blind, placebo-controlled study. Arch Gen Psychiatry 2000; 57:841–849.
16. Ghaemi SN, Goldberg JF, Ko JY, Garno JL. Quetiapine treatment of rapid-cycling bipolar disorder: an open prospective study. Eur Neuropsychopharmacol 2001; 11(suppl 3):S251.
17. Green AI, Tohen M, Patel JK, Banov M, DuRand C, Berman I, Chang H, Zarate C, Posener J, Lee H, Dawson R, Richards C, Cole JO, Schatzberg AF. Clozapine in the treatment of refractory psychotic mania. Am J Psychiatry 2000; 157(6):982–986.
18. Miller DS, Yatham LN, Lam RW. Comparative efficacy of typical and atypical antipsychotics as add-on therapy to mood stabilizers in the treatment of acute mania. J Clin Psychiatry 2001; 62(12):975–980.
19. Siris SG. Depression in schizophrenia: perspective in the era of "Atypical" antipsychotic agents. Am J Psychiatry 2000; 157(9):1379–1389.
20. Kroeze WK, Roth BL. The molecular biology of serotonin receptors: therapeutic implications for the interface of mood and psychosis. Biol Psychiatry 1998; 1:44(11):1128–1142.
21. Palvimaki EP, Roth BL, Majasuo H, Laakso A, Kuoppamaki M, Syvalahti E, et al. Interactions of selective serotonin re-uptake inhibitors with the serotonin 5-Ht_{2C} receptor. Psychopharmacology 1996; 126:234–240.
22. Roth BL, Meltzer HY, Khan N. Binding of typical and atypical antipsychotic drugs to multiple neurotransmitter receptors. Adv Pharmacol 1998; 42:484–485.
23. Shen Y, Monsama FJ, Metcalf MA, Jose PA, Hamblin MW, Sibley DR. Molecular cloning and expression of 5-hydroxytryptamine, serotonin rector subtype. J Biol Chem 1993; 268:18200–18204.

24. Ghaemi SN, Cherry El, Katzow JA, Goodwin FK. Does olanzapine have antidepressant properties? A retrospective preliminary study. Bipolar Disord 2000; 2(3 Pt1):196–199.

25. Schmidt AW, Level LA, Howard HR, Zorn SH. Ziprasidone: a novel antipsychotic agent with a unique human receptor binding profile. Eur J Pharmacol 2001; 425:197–201.

26. Frye MA, Ketter TA, Altshuler LL, et al. Clozapine in bipolar disorder. Treatment implications for other atypical antipsychotics. J Affect Disord 1998; 48:91–104.

27. McElroy SL, Dessain ED, Pope HG, Cole JO, Keck PE, Frankenberg FR, Aizley HG, O'Brien S. Clozapine in the treatment of psychotic mood disorders, schizoaffective disorder, and schizophrenia. J Clin Psychiatry 1991; 52(10): 411–414.

28. Suppes T, Webb A, Paul B, Carmody T, Kraemer H, Rush AJ. Clinical outcome in a randomized 1-year trial of clozapine versus treatment as usual for patients with treatment-resistant illness and a history of mania. Am J Psychiatry 1999; 156:1164–1169.

29. Zarate CA, Tohen M, Baldessarini RJ. Clozapine in severe mood disorders. J Clin Psychiatry 1995; 56, 411–417.

30. Barbini G, Scherillo P, Beneditti F, Crespi G, Colombo C, Smeared E. Response to clozapine in acute mania is more rapid than that of chlor-promazine. Int Clin Psychopharmacol 1997; 109–112.

31. Banov MD, Zarate CA, Tohen M, et al. Clozapine therapy in refractory affective disorders: polarity predicts response in long-term follow-up. J Clin Psychiatry 1994; 55:295–300.

32. Ranjan R, Meltzer HY. Acute and long-term effectiveness of clozapine in treatment-resistant psychotic depression . Biol Psychiatry. 1995; 40:253–258.

33. Spina E, Avenoso A, Salemi M, Facciola G, Scordo MG, Ancione M, Madia A. Plasma concentrations of clozapine and its major metabolites during combined treatment with paroxetine or sertraline. Pharmacopsychiatry 2000; 33(6): 213–217.

34. Keck PE, Wilson DR, Strakowski SM, McElroy SL, Kizer DL, Balistreri TM, Holtman HM, DePriest M. Clinical predictors of acute risperidone response in schizophrenia, schizoaffective disorder, and psychotic mood disorder. J Clin Psychiatry 1995; 56(10):466–470.

35. Segel J, Berk M, Brook S. Risperidone compared with both lithium and haloperidol in mania: a double-blind, randomized controlled trial. Clin Neuro-pharmacol 1998; 21(3):176–180.

36. Sachs G, Risperidone Bipolar Study Group. Safety and efficacy of risperdone versus placebo as add-on therapy to mood stabilizers in the treatment of manic phase of bipolar disorder. Poster presentation at the 37th Annual Meeting of the American College of Neuropsychopharmacology, Acapulco, Mexico, December 12–16, 1999.

37. Yatham LN. Safety and efficacy of risperidone as combination therapy for the manic phase of bipolar disorder; preliminary findings of a randomized,

double-blind study (RIS-INT-46). 22nd CINP Congress Meeting, Brussels, Belgium, July 9–13, 2000.

38. Hirschfeld R, Keck PE, Karcher K, Dramer M, Grossman F. Rapid antimanic effect of risperidone monotherapy: a 3-week multicenter, double-blind, placebo-controlled trial. Bipolar Disord 2003; 1(5):84.

39. Gopal S, Steffens DC, Kramer ML, Olsen MK. Mania remission rates in a randomized controlled trial of risperidone. Bipolar Disord 2003; 1(5):51.

40. Conte G, Basi C, Pasquale L, Passino DS, Zubani D. Risperidone in the long-term treatment of bipolar patients nonresponding to mood stabilizers. 22nd Annual CINP Congress Meeting, Brussels, Belgium, July 9–13, 2000.

41. Ghaemi SN, Sachs GS, Baldassano CG, et al. Acute treatment of bipolar disorder with adjunctive risperidone in outpatients. Can J Psychiatry 1997; 42:196–199.

42. Ghaemi SN, Sachs GS. Long-term risperidone treatment in bipolar disorder: 6-month follow up. Int Clin Psychopharmacol 1997; 12:333–338.

43. Tohen M, Zarate CA, Centorrino F, et al. Risperidone in the treatment of mania. J Clin Psychiatry 1996; 57(6):249–253.

44. McIntyre R, Young LT, Hasey G, et al. Risperidone in the treatment of mania. J Clin Psychiatry 1997; 57(6):249–253.

45. Vieta E, Benabarre A, Martinez G, Fernandez A, Gasto C. Risperidone therapy in bipolar disorder: results from a 6-month long, open-label study in Spain. 113th Congress of the European College of Neuropsychopharmacology. Munich, Germany, September 9–13, 2000.

46. Shelton RC, Addington S, Augenstein E, Ball W. Risperidone and paroxetine in bipolar disorder. Poster presentation at the annual Meeting of the American Psychiatric Association, New Orleans, Louisiana, May 5–10, 2001.

47. Vieta E, Gasto C, Colom F, et al. Treatment of refractory rapid cycling bipolar disorder with risperidone. J Clin Psychopharmacol 1998; 18(2):172–174.

48. Dwight MM, Keck PE, Stanton SP, et al. Antidepressant activity and mania associated with risperidone treatment in schizoaffective disorder (letter). Lancet 1994; 344:554–555.

49. Schaffer CB, Schaffer LC. The use of risperidone in the treatment of bipolar disorder. J Clin Psychiatry 1996; 153(9):1235–1236.

50. Sajatovic M, DiGiovanni SK, Bastani B, et al. Risperidone therapy in treatment refractory acute bipolar and schizoaffective mania. Psychopharmacol Bull 1996; 32(1):55–61.

51. Ghaemi SN, Katzow JJ. The use of quetiapine for treatment-resistant bipolar disorder: a case series. Ann Clin Psychiatry 1999; 11(3):137–140.

52. Fahy S, Fahy TJ. Induction of manic symptoms by novel antipsychotic (letter). Brit J Psychiatry 2000; 176:97.

53. Ashleigh EA, Larsen PD. A syndrome of increased affect in response to risperidone among patients with schizophrenia. Psychiatric Serv 1998; 9: 526–528.

54. Aubry JM, Simon AE, Bertschy G. Possible induction of mania and hypomania by olanzapine or risperidone: a critical review of reported cases. J Clin Psychiatry 2000; 61:649–655.
55. FitzGerald MJ, Pinkofsky HB, Brannon G, et al. Olanzapine-induced mania (letter). Am J Psychiatry 1999; 156:1114.
56. Lane HY, Lin YC, Chang WH. Mania induced by risperidone: Dose related? J Clin Psychiatry 1998; 59(2):85–86.
57. Jacobsen FM. Risperidone in the treatment of affective illness and obsessive-compulsive disorder. J Clin Psychiatry 1995; 56(9):423–429.
58. Hirose S, Ashby CR. An open pilot study combining risperidone and a selective serotonin reuptake inhibitor as initial antidepressant therapy. J. Clin Psychiatry 2002; 63:733–736.
59. Ostroff RB, Nelson JC. Risperidone augmentation of selective serotonin reuptake inhibitors in major depression. J Clin Psychiatry 1999; 60:56–259.
60. Stoll AL, Haura G. Tranylcypromine plus risperidone for treatment-refractory major depression (letter). J Clin Psychopharmacol 2000; 20:495–496.
61. Zarate C, Narendran R, Tohen M, et al. Clinical predictors of acute response with olanzapine in psychotic mood disorders. J Clin Psychiatry 1998; 59:24–28.
62. McElroy S, Frye M, Denikoff K, et al. Olanzapine in treatment-resistant bipolar disorder. J Affect Disord 1998; 49:119–122.
63. Guille C, Sachs G, Ghaemi S. A naturalistic comparison of clozapine, risperidone, and olanzapine in the treatment of bipolar disorder. J Clin Psychiatry 2000; 61:638–642.
64. Ketter T, Winsberg M, DeGolia S, et al. Rapid efficacy of olanzapine augmentation in nonpsychotic bipolar mixed states. J Clin Psychiatry 1998; 59:83–85.
65. Ravindran A, Jones B, Al-Zaid K, Lapierre Y. Effective treatment of mania with olanzapine: 2 case reports. J Psychiatr Neurosci 1997; 22:345–346.
66. Sharma V, Pistor L. Treatment of bipolar mixed states with olanzapine. J Psychiatr Neurosci 1999; 24:40–44.
67. Soutullo C, Sorter M, Foster K, McElroy S, Keck P. Olanzapine in the treatment of adolescent acute mania: a report of seven cases. J Affect Disord 1999; 53:279–283.
68. Weisler R, Ahearn E, Davidson J, Wallace C. Adjunctive use of olanzapine in mood disorders: five case reports. Ann Clin Psychiatry 1997; 9:259–262.
69. Zullino D, Bauman P. Olanzapine for mixed episodes of mood disorder. J Psychopharmacol 1999; 13:198.
70. Sanger TM, Grundy SL, Gibson PJ, Namjoshi MA, Greaney MG, Tohen MF. Long-term olanzapine therapy in the treatment of bipolar I disorder: an open-label continuation phase study. J Clin Psychiatry 2001; 62(4):273–281.
71. Berk M, Ichim L, Brook S. Olanzapine compared to lithium in mania: a double-blind randomized controlled trial. Int Clin Psychopharmacology 1999; 14: 339–343.
72. Zajecka JM, Weisler R, Swann AC, Sachs G, Tracy K, Sommerville KW, Wozniak P, Martin J. Divalproex sodium vs olanzapine for the treatment of

mania in bipolar disorder. 39th American College of Neuropsychopharmacology Annual Meeting, San Juan, Puerto Rico, December 2000.

73. Tohen M, Baker RW, Altshuler LL, Zarate C, Suppes T, Milton DR, Risser R, Gilmore JA, Breier A, Tollefson G. Olanzapine versus Divalproex in the treatment of acute mania. Am J Psychiatry 2002; 159:1011–1017.

74. Tohen M, Marneros A, Bowden D, Greil W, Koukopoulis A, Belmaker H, Jacobs T, Baker RW, Williamson D, Evans AR, Dossenbach M, Cassano G. Olanzapine versus lithium in relapse prevention in bipolar disorder: a randomized double-blind controlled 12-month clinical trial. Bipolar Disord 2003; 1(5):89(P200).

75. Tohen M, Bowden C, Calabrese J, Chou JC, Jacobs T, Baker RW, Williamson D, Evans AR. Olanzapine's efficacy for relapse prevention in bipolar disorder: a randomized double-blind placebo-controlled 12-month clinical trial. Bipolar Disord 2003; 1(5):89(P201).

76. Meehan K, Zhang F, David S, et al. A double-blind, randomized comparison of the efficacy and safety of intramuscular injections of olanzapine, lorazepam, or placebo in treating acutely agitated patients diagnosed with bipolar mania. J Clin Neuropsychopharmacol 2001; 21:389–397.

77. Tohen M, Chengappa KNR, Suppes T, et al. Olanzapine combined with lithium or valproate in prevention of recurrence in bipolar disorder: an 18-month study. Poster presented at the 155th Annual Meeting of the American Psychiatric Association, Philadelphia, 2002.

78. Tohen M, Vieta E, Ketter T, et al. Olanzapine and olanzapine-fluoxetine combination (OFC) in the treatment of bipolar depression. Poster presented at the 155th Annual Meeting of the American Psychiatric Association, Philadelphia, 2002.

79. Parker G. Olanzapine augmentation in the treatment of melancholia: the trajectory of improvement in rapid responders. Int Clin Psychopharmacol 2002; 17(2):7–89.

80. Nelson E, Rielage E, Welge J, Keck P. An open trial of olanzapine in the treatment of patients with psychotic depression. Ann Clin Psychiatry 2001; 13:147–151.

81. Schmitt A, Baus DF. Effective treatment of depressive disorder with psychotic symptoms by olanzapine combination therapy. Dtsch Med Wochenschr 2000; 125(50):526–529.

82. Marangall LB, Johnson CR, Kertz B, Zboyan HA, Martinez JM. Olanzapine in the treatment of apathy in previously depressed participants maintained with selective serotonin reuptake inhibitors: an open-label, flexible-dose study. J Clin Psychiatry 2002; 63(5):91–395.

83. Sajatovic M, Brescan DW, Perez DE, DiGiovanni SK, Hattab H, Belton JR, Bingham CR. Quetiapine alone and added to a mood stabilizer for serious mood disorder. J Clin Psychiatry 2001; 62:728–732.

84. Zarate CA, Rothschild A, Fletch KE, Madrid A, Zapatel J. Clinical predictors of acute response with quetiapine in psychotic mood disorder. J Clin Psychiatry 2000; 61(3):85–189.

85. Sachs G, Mullen JA, Sweitzer DE. Quetiapine versus placebo as adjunct to mood stabilizer for the treatment of acute bipolar mania. Presented at the 3rd European Stanley Foundation Conference on Bipolar Disorder, Freiburg, Germany, September 12–14, 2002.

86. Mullen J, Paulsson B. Quetiapine in combination with mood stabilizer for the treatment of acute mania associated with bipolar disorder. Bipolar Disord 2003; 1(5):70(P140).

87. Paulsson B, Huizar K. Quetiapine monotherapy for the treatment of bipolar mania. Bipolar Disord 2003; 1(5):74(P153).

88. Brecher M, Huizar K. Quetiapine monotherapy for acute mania associated with bipolar disorder. Bipolar Disord 2003; 1(5):35(P27).

89. Sajatovic J, Mullen J, Sweitzer D. Efficacy of quetiapine and risperidone against depressive symptoms in outpatients with psychotic disorder. J Clin Psychiatry 2002; 63(12):1156–1163.

90. Ghaemi SN, Goodwin FK. Use of atypical antipsychotic agents in bipolar and schizoaffective disorders: review of the empirical literature. J Clin Psychopharmacol 1999; 19(4):354–361.

91. Benazzi F. Quetiapine-associated hypomania in a woman with schizoaffective disorder. Can J Psychiatry 2001; 46(2):182–183.

92. Padia D. Quetiapine resolves psychotic depression in an adolescent boy. J Child Adolesc Psychopharmacol 2001; 11(2):207–208.

93. Keck PE, Versiani M, Potkin S, West SA, Giller E, Ice K. Ziprasidone in the treatment of acute bipolar mania: a three week, placebo-controlled, double-blind, randomized trial. Am J Psychiatry 2003; 160:741–748.

94. Daniel D, Potkin S, Reeves K, et al. Intramuscular (IM) ziprasidone 20 mg is effective in reducing state agitation associated with psychosis: a double-blind, randomized trial. Psychopharmacology 2001; 155:128–134.

95. Marcus R, Keck PE, Saha AR, Iwamoto T, Jody DN, Tourkodimitris S, Archibald DG, Sanchez R. Aripiprazole vs placebo in acute mania. Bipolar Disord 2003; 1(5):66.

96. Sanchez R, Bourin M, Auby P, Swanik R, Marcus R, McQuade RD, Iwamoto T, Stock G. Aripiprazole vs haloperidol for maintained treatment effect in acute mania. Bipolar Disord 2003; 1(5):80.

97. Collaborative Working Group on Clinical Trial Evaluations. Treatment of special populations with the atypical antipsychotics. J Clin Psychiatry 1998; 509(suppl 12):6–52.

98. Fuchs DC. Clozapine treatment of bipolar disorder in a young adolescent. J Am Acad Child Adolesc Psychiatry 1994; 33(9):1299–1302.

99. Masi G, Milone A. Clozapine treatment in an adolescent with bipolar disorder. Panminerva Med 1998; 40(3):254–257.

100. Frazier JA, Meyer MD, Biederman J, Wozniak J, Wilens TE, Spencer TJ, Kim GS, Shapiro S. Risperidone treatment for juvenile bipolar disorder: a retrospective chart review. J Am Acad Child Adolesc Psychiatry 1999; 38(8):960–965.

101. Schreier HA. Risperidone for young children with mood disorders and aggressive behavior. J Child Adolesc Psychopharmacol 1998; 8(1):49–59.

102. Gupta S, Frank B, Madhusoodanan S. Risperidone-associated galactorrhea in a male teenager. J Am Acad Child Adolesc Psychiatry 2001; 40(5):504–505.
103. Robb AS, Chang W, Lee HK, Cook MS. Case study: risperidone-induced neuroleptic malignant syndrome in an adolescent. J Child Adolesc Psychopharmacol 2000; 10(4):227–330.
104. Frazier JA, Biederman J, Tohen M, Feldman PD, Jacobs TG, Toma V, Rater MA, Tarazi RA, Kim GS, Garfield SB, Sohma M, Gonzalex-Heydrich J, Risser RC, Nowlin ZM. A prospective trial of open-label treatment of olanzapine monotherapy in children and adolescents with bipolar disorder. J Child Adolesc Psychopharmacol 2001; 11(3):239–250.
105. Khouzam H, El-Gablawi F. Treatment of bipolar I disorder in an adolescent with olanzapine. J Child Adolesc Psychopharmacol 2000; 10:147–151.
106. Chang K, Ketter T. Mood stabilizer augmentation with olanzapine in acutely manic children. J Child Adolesc Psychopharmacol 2000; 10:45–49.
107. Delbello MP, Schwiers ML, Rosenberg HL, Strakowski SM. A double-blind, randomized, placebo-controlled study of quetiapine as adjunctive treatment for adolescent mania. J Am Acad Child Adolesc Psychiatry 2002; 41:1216–1223.
108. Sajatovic M, Madhusoodanan S, Buckley P. Schizophrenia in the elderly: guidelines for its recognition and treatment. CNS Drugs 2000; 13(2):103–115.
109. Sajatovic M, Ramirez LF, Garver D, Thompson P, Ripper G, Lehmann LS. Clozapine therapy for older veterans. Psychiatric Serv 1998; 49:340–344.
110. Alvir JM, Lieberman JA, Safferman AZ, Schwimmer JL, Schaaf JA. Clozapine-induced agranulocytosis: incidence and risk factor in the United States. N Engl J Med 1993; 329:162–167.
111. Williams R. Optimal dosing with risperidone: updated recommendations. J Clin Psychiatry 2001; 62(4):282–289.
112. Jeste DV, Lacro JP, Bailey A, Rockwell E, Harris MJ, Caligiuri MP. Lower incidence of tardive dyskinesia with risperdone compared with haloperidol in older patients. J Am Geriatr Soc 1999; 47(6):716–719.
113. Rubin NJ, Arcenaux JM. Intractable depression or psychosis. Acta Psychiatr Scand 2001; 104(5):402–405.
114. Knopf U, Hubrich-Ungureanu P, Thome J. Paroxetine augmentation with risperidone in therapy-resistant depression. Psychiatr Prax 2001; 28(8):405–406.
115. Sajatovic M. Treatment of bipolar disorder in older adults. Int J Geriatric Psychiatry 2002; 17:865–873.
116. Solomons K, Geiger O. Olanzapine use in the elderly: a retrospective analysis. Can J Psychiatry 2000; 5(2):151–155.
117. Narendran R, Young CM, Valenti AM, Pristach CA, Pato MT, Grace JJ. Olanzapine therapy in treatment-resistant psychotic mood disorder: a long-term follow-up study. J Clin Psychiatry 2001; 62(7):509–516.
118. Yeung PR, Mintzer JE, Mullen JA, Sweitzer DE. Extrapyramidal symptoms in elderly outpatients treated with either quetiapine or risperidone. Presented at the Annual Meeting of the American College of Neuropsychopharmacology, Acapulco, Mexico, December 12–16, 1999.

119. Jeste DV, Glazer WM, Morgenstern H, Pultz JA, Yeung PR. Rarity of persistent tardive dyskinesia with quetiapine treatment of psychotic disorders in the elderly. Presented at the Annual Meeting of the American College of Neuropsychopharmacology, Acapulco, Mexico, December 12–16, 1999.

120. Tariot P, Salzman C, Yeung P, Pultz J, Raniwalla J. Clinical improvement and tolerability is maintained long-term in elderly patients with psychotic disorders treated with quetiapine. Presented at the Annual Meeting of the American College of Neuropsychopharmacology, Acapulco, Mexico, December 12–16, 1999.

121. McManus DQ, Arvanitis LA, Kowalcyk GG, for the Seroquel Trial 48 Study Group. Quetiapine: a novel antipsychotic: experience in elderly patients with psychotic disorders. J Clin Psychiatry 1999; 60(5):292–298.

122. Olbrich HM, Marin P. Drug treatment of schizophrenic psychoses in puerperium Nervenarzt 1994; 65(7):482–485.

123. Dickson RA, Hogg L. Pregnancy of a patient treated with clozapine. Psychiatr Serv 1998; 49(8):1081–1083.

124. Stoner SC, Sommi RW, Marken PA, Anya I, Vaughn J. Clozapine use in two full-term pregnancies. J Clin Psychiatry 1998; 59(5):57.

125. Currier GW, Simpson GM. Pregnancy and clozapine. Psychiatr Serv 1998; 49(8):97.

126. Waldman MD, Safferman AZ. Pregnancy and clozapine. Am J Psychiatry 1993; 150:68–169.

127. Ernst CL, Goldberg JF. The reproductive safety profile of mood stabilizers, atypical antipsychotics, and broad-spectrum psychotropics. J Clin Psychiatry 2002; 63(suppl 4):42–55.

128. Goldstein DJ, Corbin LA, Fung MC. Olanzapine-exposed pregnancies and lactation: early experience. J Clin Psychopharmacol 2000; 20:399–403.

129. Physician's Desk Reference. Montvale, NJ: Medical Economics, 2001.

130. Hill RC, McEvor RJ, Wojnar-Horton RE, et al. Risperidone distribution and excretion into human milk: case report and estimated infant exposure during breast-feeding. J Clin Psychopharmacol 2000; 20:285–286.

131. Tenyi T, Trixler M, Kereszetes A. Quetiapine and pregnancy. Am J Psychiatry 2002; 159(4):674.

132. American Psychiatric Association. Practice Guideline for the Treatment of Patients with Major Depressive Disorder (revision). Washington, DC: American Psychiatric Press, 2000.

133. Drug Information Handbook for Psychiatry. 3rd edn. Cleveland, OH: Lexi-Comp.

12

New Targets for Antipsychotic Drugs

Donald C. Goff and Oliver Freudenreich

*Massachusetts General Hospital and
Harvard Medical School,
Boston, Massachusetts, U.S.A.*

I. INTRODUCTION

New targets for antipsychotic drug development may follow from several lines of inquiry. These include efforts to understand mechanisms of action of currently available drugs with the aim of capitalizing upon potentially beneficial characteristics – in particular using clozapine as a model. A second approach augments current treatments based upon theoretical or empirical leads. In another approach, animal models of schizophrenia are developed and drugs identified which ameliorate aberrant behaviors. Finally, it is hoped that genetic studies will link schizophrenia to polymorphic alleles that regulate proteins amenable to pharmacological intervention, although this goal has not yet been realized.

Current drug targets are generally focused on extracelluar receptors. As a result, pharmacological approaches remain limited to influencing neuronal systems through manipulating the initiation phase rather than the adaptation phase (1). Very likely, future understanding of pathophysiology will shift the focus from receptors to downstream (postreceptor) signal transduction pathways located inside the cell and more specifically influencing gene expression. A case in point is the phosphoprotein DARPP-32 which integrates dopaminergic and other signaling pathways (2). Its central position in dopamine signaling makes it an attractive target for disorders of dopamine regulation. Other potential approaches which do not follow traditional receptor binding strategies are recent attempts to alter neuronal membrane properties with polyunsaturated fatty acids (3), and the more speculative goal of producing drugs that influence brain development (4,5), perhaps by enhancing myelination-stimulating neurotrophic factors, or protecting the brain against putative neurotoxic factors such as free radicals from impaired or overwhelmed oxidative stress defenses (6) (Table 1).

Table 1 Potential Targets for Drug Development in Schizophrenia

Pharmacological target	Clinical target
Dopamine (stimulants,[c] L-dopa,[c] COMT,[d] or MAO inhibitors[c])	Cognition, negative sxs
D_1 agonist[c]	Working memory
D_2 partial antagonist[a]	Psychosis, reduced EPS
D_3 antagonist[d]	Psychosis, negative sxs
D_4 antagonist[b]	Psychosis
Serotonin (SSRIs)[c]	Negative sxs
5-HT_{2A} antagonist[a]	Negative sxs, reduced EPS
5-HT_{1A} agonist[c]	Anxiety, tension
5-HT_3 agonist[d]	Cognition
Noradrenergic (stimulants)[c]	Cognition
Alpha 1 antagonist[a]	Cognition, reduce relapse
Alpha 2 agonist[a]	Attention, cognition
Glutamate (inhibitors – lamotrigine[c])	Psychosis
NMDA agonists (glycine reuptake blockers[d], D-serine[a])	Negative sxs, positive sxs, cognition
AMPA agonists[a]	Attention, cognition
Nicotine	
Alpha 7 partial agonist[d]	Attention, cognition
Membrane stabilization (omega-3 fatty acids[c])	Psychosis
Neurotrophic factors[d] (BDNF – "ampakines")	Cognition, negative sxs
Myelination promoters[d]	Cognition
Neuroprotective agents[d] (antioxidants, memantadine)	Halt progression of illness

Data from published trials in schizophrenia patients have been:
[a]Positive/encouraging
[b]Negative/discouraging
[c]Inconsistent/difficult to interpret
[d]Inadequate human data available.

Progress in the pharmacotherapy of schizophrenia has advanced during a period in which a far more complex model of the illness has replaced an earlier, nearly exclusive focus upon psychotic symptoms and dopamine neurotransmission. Schizophrenia is now recognized as a heterogeneous disorder linked to multiple genes which individually exert relatively small effects and which are believed to interact with numerous environmental factors (7). Not surprisingly, the phenotype is similarly heterogeneous, composed of at least four or five distinct symptom clusters, including psychotic symptoms, disorganization, negative symptoms, cognitive deficits, and affective symptoms (8). The pattern of symptom expression is diverse within patient samples; medications also differ in patterns of symptom response. Future advances in drug development may first require identification of subgroups of patients that share biological defects in common and may also take into account different pathogenic mechanisms associated with different stages of the disease (9). In addition, pharmacological interventions that target specific symptoms may be necessary rather than continued attempts to treat the full syndrome with a single agent.

Two types of models for schizophrenia have particular relevance to pharmacology: models based on structural lesioning experiments and models based on pharmacological challenges. Lesioning models are best illustrated by a series of experiments performed by Lipska and colleagues (10,11) in which excitotoxic ventral hippocampal ablations in neonatal rats resulted in abnormal prepulse inhibition (PPI) and behavioral hypersensitivity to dopamine and stress first exhibited in young adulthood. Although aberrant behaviors exhibited by lesioned rats often improve in response to antipsychotic medication, a model based on structural defects consigns pharmacotherapy to the rather limited role of producing compensatory changes without much hope for reversing etiological impairments. Unless pharmacological interventions can be directed at pathological processes involved in early brain development, expectations for full syndromal response must be low.

In contrast, pharmacological challenge models are more encouraging for drug development. The classic pharmacological model, stimulant intoxication, produces delusions and hallucinations that closely resemble psychotic symptoms of schizophrenia and generally can be fully attenuated by dopamine antagonists (12). Stimulant intoxication is less informative for other symptoms of schizophrenia, however. Currently, the most compelling evidence of catecholaminergic dysregulation in schizophrenia comes from studies of amphetamine-induced dopamine release in striatum. Although considerable overlap is found between normal and schizophrenia samples, a subgroup of schizophrenia patients exhibit increased dopamine release which positively correlates with response to conventional antipsychotic medication (13).

An additional pharmacological challenge of interest to schizophrenia drug development involves infusion of noncompetitive antagonists that block the glutamatergic-NMDA gated ion channel (14). Drugs such as phencyclidine (PCP) and the lower-affinity dissociative anesthetic, ketamine, produce a broad spectrum of schizophrenia-like symptoms in normal subjects, including psychosis, negative symptoms and memory deficits (15). Ketamine also exacerbates symptoms in schizophrenia patients who have been stabilized on haloperidol – an effect that is blocked by clozapine (16,17). Furthermore, the abnormality in amphetamine-induced striatal dopamine release characteristic of some patients with schizophrenia can be reproduced in normal subjects with ketamine (18). NMDA antagonists disrupt prepulse inhibition (PPI) in rats, which mimics the attentional deficit characteristic of patients with schizophrenia and produce several behavioral effects in rodents, including social isolation and hyperactivity – all of which demonstrate preferential response to atypical antipsychotics compared to conventional agents (19).

Several genes with biologically relevant functions recently have been linked preliminarily to schizophrenia. For example, a gene on chromosome 8p, associated with expression of neureglin, has been linked to schizophrenia (20). Neureglin plays a role in brain development, particularly the expression of NMDA receptors. Transgenic mice heterozygous for the neureglin allele express 16% fewer NMDA receptors compared to normal mice, and exhibit hyperactivity and abnormal PPI; the abnormal behaviors respond to clozapine. In a related finding, Mohn and colleagues (21) produced transgenic mice with an approximately 95% reduction in functional NMDA receptors (by deletion of the NMDAR1 subunit) and found that mice exhibited hyperactivity, sterotypies, and social isolation. Hyperactivity and stereotypy improved with haloperidol, whereas only clozapine improved social withdrawal.

In addition, two genes involved in expression and activation of D-amino acid oxidase (DAAO) have also been linked to schizophrenia (22). DAAO metabolizes D-serine, a neurotransmitter believed to play an important role in activating the glycine co-agonist site of the NMDA receptor. It is hypothesized that a polymorphism that results in heightened activity of DAAO might lower brain concentrations of D-serine, decrease activation of NMDA receptors, and hence place individuals at risk for schizophrenia. An additional gene is involved in expression of catecholamine-O-methyl transferase (COMT), an enzyme that metabolizes intrasynaptic dopamine (23). While the presence of a polymorphism that would increase COMT activity and decrease dopamine concentrations has only a modest impact upon risk (1.5 odds ratio), COMT status does predict phenotypic expression (24).

II. DOPAMINE SYSTEMS

To identify potential dopaminergic targets for new antipsychotic agents, it is necessary to briefly review certain aspects of dopamine neurotransmission and pharmacology (25). Dysregulation of nigrostriatal pathways, originating from the A9 dopamine neurons in the substantia nigra, is thought to underlie extrapyramidal side effects of antipsychotic drugs and tardive dyskinesia. Dopaminergic projections from the A10 ventral tegmental midbrain dopamine neurons to frontal and temporal cortex (mesocortical) and nucleus accumbens (mesolimbic) have been linked to negative and positive symptoms of schizophrenia, respectively (26). Firing of ventral tegmental dopamine neurons is modulated by D_2 and NMDA autoreceptors (27). Dopamine released in the prefrontal cortex acts on excitatory glutamatergic pyramidal neurons via D_1 receptors and on GABAergic inhibitory neurons via D_4 receptors. Activation of D_1 receptors is crucial to working memory and attention (28). The primary target of the mesolimbic DA system projections to the ventral striatum is the D_3 receptor. The ventral striatum projects via the ventral pallidum to the mediodorsal and anteroventral thalamic nuclei and, ultimately, the anterior prefrontal cortex. Medication-free schizophrenia patients were found to have elevated levels of D_3 receptors in ventral striatum which were down-regulated by antipsychotic drugs (29). Within the hippocampus, dopamine acts on D_1 and D_2 receptors to influence the process of novelty detection and may in part determine whether sensory information is processed as a new memory or is recognized as redundant with previously encoded experience. Excessive dopaminergic activity in the hippocampus has been conjectured to cause inappropriate blocking of new stimuli and misinterpretation of previously coded memories (30).

Although debated, conventional antipsychotics are generally believed to produce depolarization blockade in A9 and A10 dopamine neurons via antagonism of D_2 autoreceptors (31,32). After approximately 4 weeks of exposure to D_2 antagonists, a substantial portion of dopamine neurons become electrically silent and remain in an inactive, depolarized state – dramatically reducing dopamine release and disrupting normal patterns of neuronal firing. Conventional neuroleptics may cause acute EPS by blockade of striatal postsynaptic D_2 receptors and delayed EPS by depolarization blockade of A9 dopamine neurons. EPS occur when occupancy of striatal D_2 receptors is in excess of approximately 78%, making dose titration necessary to avoid neurological side effects (33,34).

Atypical antipsychotics incorporate three approaches to minimize EPS compared to conventional neuroleptics. Firing of A9 dopamine neurons is believed to be preserved by serotonergic 5-HT_{2A} and alpha 2 adrenergic antagonism, producing relative protection against EPS (35). Risperidone is an example of a drug with a relatively high 5-HT_{2A}-to-D_2 receptor affinity ratio and a high affinity for alpha 2 adrenergic receptors (36). In comparison with high-dose haloperidol, risperidone produced significantly fewer EPS, although this advantage was less marked as the dose of risperidone increased and the relative ratio of 5-HT_{2A} receptor-to-D2 receptor occupancy decreased (37). Second, clozapine and quetiapine have large dissociation constants for binding to the D_2 receptor, indicating that these drugs may be rapidly displaced by endogenous dopamine (38). As a result, neither drug approaches the EPS threshold of roughly 78% striatal D_2 occupancy. Finally, aripiprazole is the first antipsychotic with D_2 partial agonist activity (39). It binds to D_2 receptors with relatively high affinity, but reduces intrinsic activity by only 70% compared to dopamine. The partial, 30% activation of striatal D_2 receptors by aripiprazole (combined with 5-HT_{2A} antagonism) appears sufficient to prevent EPS and elevation of prolactin (40).

Both conventional and atypical antipsychotics cause depolarization blockade of A10 ventral tegmental neurons and increase C-fos production in nucleus accumbens (41). These actions are believed to underlie antipsychotic efficacy. It is important to note that full occupancy of D_2 receptors can be achieved within hours of drug administration, whereas antipsychotic efficacy is usually not achieved for several weeks. This finding suggests that D_2 occupancy is only a proximal cause of antipsychotic effect; delayed depolarization blockade with loss of dopamine release acting on limbic or hippocampal dopamine receptors is one possible explanation for antipsychotic efficacy. The antipsychotic efficacy of agents such as quetiapine and clozapine that produce very low levels of D_2 blockade further challenges the relationship of D_2 occupancy and antipsychotic effect.

A. Dopamine: Future Directions

Preservation of nigrostriatal dopaminergic function remains an important goal for novel antipsychotics – one that can be partially realized by addition of 5-HT_{2A} antagonism combined with careful clinical titration of dose, or more successfully by a high dissociation constant for binding to the D_2 receptor, or by partial agonist activity at the D_2 receptor. It is also possible that atypical agents preferentially bind to D_2 and D_3 receptors in thalamis and temporal cortex compared to striatum (42,43). While atypical agents appear to preserve nigrostriatal function, depolarization blockade of A10 dopamine neurons by atypical agents, which probably is necessary for antipsychotic efficacy, may disrupt cognitive functions associated with the phasic release of dopamine in the prefrontal cortex. Efforts to enhance dopaminergic release in prefrontal cortex have included augmentation with psychostimulants. Preliminary evidence suggests that stimulants (amphetamine) may improve prefrontal cortical activation and negative symptoms when administered as a single dose (44,45), but repeated dose trials of stimulant augmentation have generally been negative (46,47). Alternative strategies could include antagonism of dopamine metabolism (COMT or MAOI inhibitors) and augmentation with selective D_1 agonists. Clozapine, risperidone and olanzapine have been shown to increase dopamine release in prefrontal cortex, an effect possibly mediated by 5-HT_{2A} and adrenergic antagonism (29,48).

Unfortunately, since the mechanism by which D_2 blockade produces antipsychotic effects remains unclear, it is difficult to design strategies that will preserve or enhance antipsychotic efficacy while minimizing side effects. Targeting D_3 receptors is an interesting approach, since a selective D_3 antagonist might modulate limbic dopamine activity without affecting ventral tegmental or nigrostriatal neuronal firing (29). Amisulpiride has been reported to preferentially block D_3 receptors, to which has been attributed its very favorable clinical profile of efficacy for positive and negative symptoms with minimal EPS (49). Other, more selective D_3 antagonists are currently in development. Whether the combination of relatively weak D_2 antagonism with relatively strong D_1 antagonism, as typified by clozapine, is a model worth replicating in new agents also requires further work. Despite considerable interest in D_4 antagonists following the discovery of clozapine's high affinity for this receptor, trials of selective D_4 antagonists have been disappointing (50,51).

III. SEROTONIN

Blockade of serotonin 5-HT_{2A} receptors is a characteristic of all atypical antipsychotic agents except amisulpiride (52). Early studies by Paul Janssen's group demonstrated that 5-HT_{2A} antagonism reverses EPS in haloperidol treated animals and in schizophrenia subjects and may improve negative symptoms of schizophrenia (36,53). More recently, selective 5-HT_{2A} antagonists have demonstrated the ability to reverse some behavioral effects of NMDA antagonism, possibly by increasing release of glutamate (54,55). However, M100907, a selective 5-HT_{2A} antagonist, was not adequately effective compared with haloperidol in early clinical trials to merit development as an antipsychotic agent (56). Antagonism of 5-HT_{2A} continues to be a desirable characteristic of antipsychotic agents when combined with D_2

antagonist effects. The relative value of activity at other serotonergic receptors remains unclear. Serotonin5-HT$_{1A}$ partial agonists also appear to reverse neurological side effects of D$_2$ antagonists. In an open augmentation study, the 5-HT$_{1A}$ partial agonist, buspirone, improved ratings of EPS and tension when added to haloperidol (57). Both ziprasidone and aripiprazole exhibit agonist activity at the5-HT$_{1A}$ receptor – the potential contribution of this activity to clinical response requires study. Serotonin-reuptake blockers have also demonstrated efficacy for negative symptoms when added to conventional neuroleptics (58). This finding has been relatively consistent with fluoxetine and fluvoxamine, but less consistent with other selective serotonin reuptake inhibitors (SSRIs) – the reason for this inconsistency is unclear.

IV. NOREPINEPHRINE

Dysregulation of norepinephrine release or of adrenergic receptors has not been well established in schizophrenia, although adrenergic effects may contribute to clinical benefits of certain atypical antipsychotics (59). Clozapine's marked elevation of plasma norepinephrine concentrations is possibly the most striking of all measurable effects (60). Risperidone, which recently has demonstrated superior efficacy for prevention of relapse compared to haloperidol (61), also possesses relatively high affinity for alpha 1 and alpha 2 adrenergic receptors and elevates plasma norepinephrine (62). Litman and colleagues (63) previously demonstrated that augmentation of fluphenazine with the alpha 2 antagonist idazoxan significantly improved psychosis and negative symptoms. Antagonism of postsynaptic alpha 2 adrenoreceptors appears to enhance release of dopamine in prefrontal cortex (64,65) and may have cognitive benefits (66). The selective alpha 1 receptor antagonist, prazosin is also reported to prevent depolarization blockade of A9 dopamine neurons following administration of conventional neuroleptics (67). While less well studied than D$_2$ and 5-HT$_{2A}$ receptors, adrenergic antagonism is shared by most atypical antipsychotics and may contribute to clinical benefit. It is an intriguing hypothesis that extraordinarily high concentrations of norepinephrine produced by clozapine via unclear mechanisms may reduce sensitivity to environmental stress and hence protect against relapse – an effect possibly also achieved by adrenergic receptor blockade.

V. GLUTAMATERGIC STRATEGIES

Glutamatergic approaches have received considerable attention in light of reported abnormalities of glutamatergic receptor density and subunit composition in schizophrenia brain, the production of a broad range of symptoms characteristic of schizophrenia by infusion of NMDA antagonists in normal subjects, and preliminary success with agonists at the glycine site of the NMDA receptor (19). Several placebo-controlled trials have demonstrated improvement of negative symptoms with the addition of the full agonists, glycine and D-serine, or the partial agonist, D-cycloserine, to antipsychotics other than clozapine (68–70). Because glycine poorly penetrates the blood–brain barrier, large doses (30–60 g/d) are required to achieve clinical effects (69,71). Glycine reuptake inhibitors are currently under development and represent a promising alternative approach (72). D-Cycloserine, a partial agonist, has produced improvement of negative symptoms over a narrow therapeutic dose range; psychotic exacerbation has been reported at higher doses and in approximately 10% of patients receiving a typical therapeutic dose of 50 mg/d (68). Glycine and D-serine have demonstrated a broader range of efficacy in preliminary studies; negative symptoms, psychosis, and relatively rudimentary measures of cognitive function have all improved in augmentation studies. Clinical trials with D-serine have been delayed in the United States pending safety studies. If found safe, D-serine is particularly attractive since it crosses the blood–brain barrier more readily than glycine, is not removed from the synapse as rapidly by active transport, and has been implicated by recent genetic linkage studies between schizophrenia and genes regulating activity of D-amino acid oxidase.

Trials of glycine site agonists added to clozapine have tended to find no clinical improvement (73,74) and the partial agonist, D-cycloserine, worsened negative symptoms when added to clozapine in two studies (75,76). The relative efficacy of glycine site agonists when added to other atypicals is less well studied, although a large clinical trial (the CONSIST study) is currently underway to examine this question. These findings suggest that targeting the glycine site may enhance efficacy of most antipsychotic drugs, but probably will not improve upon clozapine's efficacy. This further raises the question of whether clozapine's superior efficacy may in part reflect activity at the glycine site, mediated by as yet unclear indirect mechanisms.

Metabotropic (mGlu) receptor agonists have recently gained attention as a promising new target for antipsychotic development. mGlu receptor ligands have been shown to modulate dopamine neuronal activity in striatum and nucleus accumbens (77,78). The group II mGlu receptor agonists have been demonstrated to selectively regulate glutamate release in cortex and hippocampus (79). In rat models, group II mGlu receptor agonists attenuated phencyclidine behavioral effects (80) but did not prevent disruption of prepulse inhibition (81).

A final glutamatergic receptor class which may hold promise as an area of drug development in schizophrenia is the AMPA receptor. AMPA receptor positive modulators, or "ampakines," are currently under development. Ampakines augment opening of voltage-dependent NMDA receptors by facilitating early depolarization (82). In animal studies, ampakines have produced improvements in learning and memory and have acted synergistically when combined with low doses of antipsychotics to attenuate rearing behaviors in response to methamphetamine (83–85). In one very preliminary placebo-controlled dose-finding trial, addition of an ampakine to clozapine in 19 schizophrenia subjects was well tolerated and produced some evidence of improvement in memory and attention (86).

VI. NICOTINE

Nicotinic acetylcholine receptors have also received considerable attention for their possible role in cognitive deficits of schizophrenia. Nicotine normalizes a sensory gating abnormality measured by the inhibition of P50 evoked response to paired stimuli; this deficit in information processing is found in about 85% of schizophrenia patients and in about half of first degree relatives and has been linked to the alpha 7 nicotinic receptor (87). The gene that expresses the alpha 7 nicotinic receptor, CHRNA7, is decreased by approximately 50% in post-mortem hippocampus from schizophrenia patients compared to normal controls (88). A polymorphism in the promoter region of the CHRNA7 gene has also been linked to schizophrenia (89). Pharmacological targeting of the alpha 7 nicotinic receptor is complicated because it is highly sensitive to down-regulation in response to agonists. Nicotine transiently normalizes P50 gating deficits, but this effect is lost with repeated dosing. Clozapine uniquely appears capable of improving P50 deficits, apparently via alpha 7 receptors, although the mechanism remains uncertain (90). It has been suggested that alpha 7 activation by clozapine might be mediated by serotonin $5-HT_3$ agonist effects which enhance release of acetylcholine (90). A selective alpha 7 agonist, DMXB-A appears to produce sustained improvement of P50 sensory gating with repeated dosing in animal models (91). Trials in schizophrenia patients will be of great interest to determine whether this compound enhances attention, even in subjects prone to maintain high levels of nicotine from heavy smoking.

VII. MEMBRANE THEORIES OF SCHIZOPHRENIA

One of the few approaches to schizophrenia treatment that do not focus upon receptor ligands is based on the conceptualization of schizophrenia as a brain lipid disorder. In this model, first proposed by Horrobin as a prostaglandin deficiency (92), the focus is on alterations of the physicochemical properties of the biomembrane of the cell. In its simplest form, the theory posits an aberrant composition of constituents of the cell membrane leading to a multitude of biological changes. The focus has been on phospholipids and polyunsaturated fatty acids (PUFAs), especially deficiency of omega-3 fatty acids (3). Clinical evidence for the usefulness of supplementation with omega-3 fatty acids has been mixed, several small studies showing excellent improvement, one double-blind trial being negative (93–95).

VIII. TROPHIC FACTORS

The prototypical course of schizophrenia can be characterized as a *time-limited* progression of illness to a defect state (9,96). Whatever the mechanism, its deleterious effect seems to be turned on and shut off again, not operational beyond the period of decline. Efforts to understand the neurobiological conditions and mechanisms that are responsible for this deterioration might lead to secondary prevention. It is likely that targets beyond classic receptors must be targeted, possibly within a critical phase of brain development. Possible targets include neurotrophic factors that regulate processes putatively disturbed in schizophrenia: neuronal and glial differentiation, migration, and proliferation (97). If some aspect of schizophrenia can be understood as a fault in synaptic pruning as first formulated by Feinberg (98), timely intervention seems key. A clearer understanding of the cellular pathways that maintain synaptic connectivity and control apoptosis (such as the role of bcl-2 (99)) and their role in schizophrenia is necessary. These pathways might provide important targets for disease-modifying treatments or at a minimum lead to drugs that do not add additional neurotoxicity.

White matter abnormalities can be seen with diffusion MRI (100) and recently abnormal expression of genes involved in myelination has been found in schizophrenia brain (101). It is of interest that clozapine significantly affects lipid metabolism (102); whether such an effect might influence myelin or neuronal membrane composition remains unclear. It is hoped, however, that progress in our understanding of myelination might lead to another set of drug targets (5).

IX. CONCLUSION

The absence of a fundamental understanding of the pathophysiology of schizophrenia makes the prediction of potential drug targets a highly unreliable exercise. Because a single gene or dysregulation of a single neuroreceptor is unlikely to emerge as a primary cause of the illness in most patients, treatment advances will probably require identification of biologically homogeneous subgroups and targeting of specific symptoms with multiple agents. The mechanisms responsible for the remarkable therapeutic advance represented by clozapine remain largely a mystery but have prompted advances involving combinations of D_2/D_3 blockade with 5-HT$_{2A}$ antagonists. The contributions of glutamatergic and noradrenergic effects of clozapine remain to be systematically investigated. On a more speculative front, enhancement or protection of neuronal function is of great interest and currently includes studies of fatty acid augmentation but in the future may target myelin, putative neurotoxic factors, and neurotrophic factors.

REFERENCES

1. Hyman SE, Nestler EJ. Initiation and adaptation: a paradigm for understanding psychotropic drug action. Am J Psychiatry 1996; 153(2):151–162.
2. Fienberg AA, Hiroi N, Mermelstein PG, Song W, Snyder GL, Nishi A, Cheramy A, O'Callaghan JP, Miller DB, Cole DG, Corbett R, Haile CN, Cooper DC, Onn SP, Grace AA, Ouimet CC, White FJ, Hyman SE, Surmeier DJ, Girault J, Nestler EJ, Greengard P. DARPP-32: regulator of the efficacy of dopaminergic neurotransmission. Science 1998; 281(5378):838–842.
3. Peet M. Essential fatty acids: theoretical aspects and treatment implications for schizophrenia and depression. Adv Psychiatr Treat 2002; 8:223–229.
4. DeLisi LE. Is schizophrenia a lifetime disorder of brain plasticity, growth and aging? Schizophr Res 1997; 23:119–129.
5. Bartzokis G. Schizophrenia: breakdown in the well-regulated lifelong process of brain development and maturation. Neuropsychopharmacology 2002; 27(4): 672–683.
6. Mahadik SP, Mukherjee S. Free radical pathology and antioxidant defense in schizophrenia: a review. Schizophr Res 1996; 19(1):1–17.
7. Tsuang M. Schizophrenia: genes and environment. Biol Psychiatry 2000; 47:210–220.
8. Peralta V, Cuesta MJ, de Leon J. An empirical analysis of latent structures underlying schizophrenic symptoms: a four-syndrome model. Biol Psychiatry 1994; 36:726–736.
9. Lieberman JA. Schizophrenia: comments on genes, development, risk factors, phenotype, and course. Biol Psychiatry 1999; 46(7):869–870.
10. Lipska BK, Swerdlow NR, Geyer MA, Jaskiw GE, Braff DL, Weinberger DR. Neonatal excitotoxic hippocampal damage in rats causes post-pubertal changes in prepulse inhibition of startle and its disruption by apomorphine. Psychopharmacology 1995; 122:35–43.

11. Lipska B, al-Amin H, Weinberger D. Excitotoxic lesions of the rat medial prefrontal cortex. Effects on abnormal behaviors associated with neonatal hippocampal damage. Neuropsychopharmacology 1998; 19:451–464.

12. Goff DC, Ciraulo DA. Stimulants. In: Shader RI, ed. Clinical Manual of Chemical Dependence. Washington, DC: American Psychiatric Press, 1991: 133–258.

13. Laruelle M, Abi-Dargham A, van Dyck CH. Single photon emission computerized tomography imaging of amphetamine-induced dopamine release in drug-free schizophrenic subjects. Proc Natl Acad Sci USA 1996; 93: 9235–9240.

14. Javitt D, Zukin S. Recent advances in the phencyclidine model of schizophrenia. Am J Psychiatry 1991; 148:1301–1308.

15. Krystal JH, Karper LP, Seibyl JP, Freeman GK, Delaney R, Bremner JD, Heninger GR, Bowers MBJ, Charney DS. Subanesthetic effects of the noncompetitive NMDA antagonist, ketamine, in humans: psychotomimetic, perceptual, cognitive, and neuroendocrine responses. Arch Gen Psychiatry 1994; 51:199–214.

16. Lahti AC, Holcomb HH, Medoff DR, Tamminga CA. Ketamine activates psychosis and alters limbic blood flow in schizophrenia. Neuroreport 1995; 6:869–872.

17. Malhotra A, Adler C, Kennison S, Elman I, Pickar D, Breier A. Clozapine blunts N-methyl-D-aspartate antagonist-induced psychosis: a study with ketamine. Biol Psychiatry 1997; 42:664–668.

18. Breier A, Adler CM, Weisenfeld N, Su TP, Elman I, Picken L, Malhotra AK, Pickar D. Effects of NMDA antagonism on striatal dopamine release in healthy subjects: application of a novel PET approach. Synapse 1998; 29:142–147.

19. Goff DC, Coyle JT. The emerging role of glutamate in the pathophysiology and treatment of schizophrenia. Am J Psychiatry 2001; 158:1367–1377.

20. Stefansson H, Sigurdsson E, Steinthorsdottir V, Bjornsdottir S, Sigmundsson T, Ghosh S, Brynjolfsson J, Gunnarsdottir S, Ivarsson O, Chou TT, Hjaltason O, Birgisdottir B, Jonsson H, Gudnadottir VG, Gudmundsdottir E, Bjornsson A, Ingvarsson B, Ingason A, Sigfusson S, Hardardottir H, Harvey RP, Lai D, Zhou M, Brunner D, Mutel V, Gonzalo A, Lemke G, Sainz J, Johannesson G, Andresson T, Gudbjartsson D, Manolescu A, Frigge ML, Gurney ME, Kong A, Gulcher JR, Petursson H, Stefansson K. Neuregulin 1 and susceptibility to schizophrenia. Am J Hum Genet 2002; 71(4):877–892.

21. Mohn A, Gainetdinov P, Caron M, Koller B. Mice with reduced NMDA receptor expression display behaviors related to schizophrenia. Cell 1999; 98:427–436.

22. Chumakov I, Blumenfeld M, Guerassimenko O, Cavarec L, Palicio M, Abderrahim H, Bougueleret L, Barry C, Tanaka H, La Rosa P, Puech A, Tahri N, Cohen-Akenine A, Delabrosse S, Lissarrague S, Picard FP, Maurice K, Essioux L, Millasseau P, Grel P, Debailleul V, Simon AM, Caterina D, Dufaure I, Malekzadeh K, Belova M, Luan JJ, Bouillot M, Sambucy JL, Primas G, Saumier M, Boubkiri N, Martin-Saumier S, Nasroune M, Peixoto H,

Delaye A, Pinchot V, Bastucci M, Guillou S, Chevillon M, Sainz-Fuertes R, Meguenni S, Aurich-Costa J, Cherif D, Gimalac A, Van Duijn C, Gauvreau D, Ouellette G, Fortier I, Raelson J, Sherbatich T, Riazanskaia N, Rogaev E, Raeymaekers P, Aerssens J, Konings F, Luyten W, Macciardi F, Sham PC, Straub RE, Weinberger DR, Cohen N, Cohen D, Ouelette G, Realson J. Genetic and physiological data implicating the new human gene G72 and the gene for D-amino acid oxidase in schizophrenia. Proc Natl Acad Sci USA 2002; 99(21):13675–13680.

23. Shifman S, Bronstein M, Sternfeld M, Pisante-Shalom A, Lev-Lehman E, Weizman A, Reznik I, Spivak B, Grisaru N, Karp L, Schiffer R, Kotler M, Strous RD, Swartz-Vanetik M, Knobler HY, Shinar E, Beckmann JS, Yakir B, Risch N, Zak NB, Darvasi A. A highly significant association between a COMT haplotype and schizophrenia. Am J Hum Genet 2002; 71(6):1296–1302.

24. Weinberger DR, Egan MF, Bertolino A, Callicott JH, Mattay VS, Lipska BK, Berman KF, Goldberg TE. Prefrontal neurons and the genetics of schizophrenia. Biol Psychiatry 2001; 50:825–844.

25. Heckers S, Goff DC. Neural circuitry and signaling in schizophrenia, In: Hammer RP Jr, ed. Brain Circuitry and Signaling in Psychiatry. Washington, DC: American Psychiatric Press, 2002:67–98.

26. Davis K, Kahn R, Ko G, Davidson M. Dopamine in schizophrenia: a review and reconceptualization. Am J Psychiatry 1991; 148:1474–1486.

27. Grace AA. Phasic versus tonic dopamine release and the modulation of dopamine system responsivity: a hypothesis for the etiology of schizophrenia. Neuroscience 1991; 41:1–24.

28. Sawaguchi T, Goldman-Rakic PS. D1 dopamine receptors in prefrontal cortex: involvement in working memory. Science 1991; 251(4996):947–950.

29. Gurevich EV, Bordelon Y, Shapiro RM, Arnold SE, Gur RE, Joyce JN. Mesolimbic dopamine D3 receptors and use of antipsychotics in patients with schizophrenia. Arch Gen Psychiatry 1997; 54:225–232.

30. Lisman JE, Otmakhova NA. Storage, recall, and novelty detection of sequences by the hippocampus: elaborating on the SOCRATIC model to account for normal and aberrant effects of dopamine. Hippocampus 2001; 11:551–568.

31. Grace AA, Bunney BS. Induction of depolarization block in midbrain dopamine neurons by repeated administration of haloperidol: analysis using in vivo intracellular recording. J Pharmacol Exp Ther 1986; 283:1092–1100.

32. Hollerman JR, Abercrombie ED, Grace AA. Electrophysiological, biochemical, and behavioral studies of acute haloperidol-induced depolarization block of nigral dopamine neurons. Neuroscience 1992; 47:589–601.

33. Farde L, Nordstrom AL, Wiesel FA, Pauli S, Halldin C, Sedvall G. Positron emission tomographic analysis of central D1 and D2 dopamine receptor occupancy in patients treated with classical neuroleptics and clozapine: relation to extrapyramidal side effects. Arch Gen Psychiatry 1992; 49:538–544.

34. Kapur S, Zipursky R, Jones C, Remington G, Houle S. Relationship between dopamine D2 occupancy, clinical response, and side effects: a double-blind PET study of first-episode schizophrenia. Am J Psychiatry 2000; 157:514–520.

35. Svensson TH, Mathe JM, Andersson JL, Nomikos GG, Hildebrand BE, Marcus M. Mode of action of atypical neuroleptics in relation to the phencyclidine model of schizophrenia: role of 5-HT2 receptor and alpha$_1$-adrenoreceptor antagonism. J Clin Psychopharmacol 1995; 15:11s–18s.

36. Janssen PAJ, Niemegeers CJE, Awouters F, Schellekens KHL, Megens AAHP, Meert TF. Pharmacology of risperidone (R 64 766), a new antipsychotic with serotonin-S2 and dopamine D2 antagonist properties. J Pharmacol Exp Ther 1988; 244:685–693.

37. Marder SR, Meibach RC. Risperidone in the treatment of schizophrenia. Am J Psychiatry 1994; 151(6):825–835.

38. Kapur S, Seeman P. Does fast dissociation from the dopamine D2 receptor explain the action of atypical antipsychotics?: a new hypothesis. Am J Psychiatry 2001; 158:360–369.

39. Burris KD, Molski TF, Xu C, Ryan E, Tottori K, Kikuchi T, Yocca FD, Molinoff PB: Aripiprazole, a novel antipsychotic, is a high-affinity partial agonist at human dopamine D2 receptors. J Pharmacol Exp Ther 2002; 302(1):381–389.

40. Kane JM, Carson WH, Saha AR, McQuade RD, Ingenito GG, Zimbroff DL, Ali MW. Efficacy and safety of aripiprazole and haloperidol versus placebo in patients with schizophrenia and schizoaffective disorder. J Clin Psychiatry 2002; 63(9):763–771.

41. Deutch AY. Identification of the neural systems subserving the actions of clozapine: clues from the immediate-early gene expression. J Clin Psychiatry 1994; 55 (9 suppl B):37–42.

42. Pilowsky LS, Mulligan RS, Acton PD, Ell PJ, Costa DC, Kerwin RW. Limbic selectivity of clozapine. Lancet 1997; 350(9076):490–491.

43. Bressan RA, Erlandsson K, Jones HM, Mulligan RS, Ell PJ, Pilowsky LS. Optimizing limbic selective D2/D3 receptor occupancy by risperidone: a [123I]-Epidepride SPET study. J Clin Psychopharmacol 2003; 23(1):5–14.

44. Angrist B, Peselow E, Rubinstein M, Rotrosen J. Partial improvement in negative schizophrenic symptoms after amphetamine. Psychopharmacology 1983; 78:128–130.

45. Daniel DG, Weinberger DR, Jones DW, Zigun JR, Coppola R, Handel S, Bigelow LB, Goldberg TE, Berman KF, Kleinman JE. The effect of amphetamine on regional cerebral blood flow during cognitive activation in schizophrenia. J Neuroscience 1991; 11(7):1907–1917.

46. Casey JF, Hollister LE, Klett CJ, Lasky JJ, Caffey EM. Combined drug therapy of chronic schizophrenics: controlled evaluation of placebo, dexto-amphetamine, imipramine, isocarboxazid and trifluoperazine added to main-tenance doses of chlorpromazine. Am J Psychiatry 1961; 117:997–1003.

47. Goff D, Evins A. Negative symptoms in schizophrenia: neurobiological models and treatment response. Harvard Rev Psychiatry 1998; 6(2):59–77.

48. Yamamoto BK, Pehek EA, Meltzer HY. Brain region effects of clozapine on amino acid and monoamine transmission. J Clin Psychiatry 1994; 55(9(suppl B)):8–14.

49. Kerwin R. From pharmacological profiles to clinical outcomes. Int Clin Psychopharmacol 2000; 15(Suppl 4):S1–S4.
50. Kramer MS, Last B, Getson A, Reines SA. The effects of a selective D4 dopamine receptor antagonist (L-745,870) in acutely psychotic inpatients with schizophrenia. D4 Dopamine Antagonist Group. Arch Gen Psychiatry 1997; 54(6):567–572.
51. Truffinet P, Tamminga CA, Fabre LF, Meltzer HY, Rivicre ME, Papillon-Downey C. Placebo-controlled study of the D4/5-HT2A antagonist fananserin in the treatment of schizophrenia. Am J Psychiatry 1999; 156(3): 419–425.
52. Meltzer HY. The mechanism of action of novel antipsychotic drugs. Schizophr Bull 1992; 17:263–287.
53. Leysen JE, Janssen PMF, Schotte A, Luyten WHML, Megens AAHP. Interaction of antipsychotic drugs with neurotransmitter receptor sites in vitro and in vivo in relation to pharmacological and clinical effects: role of 5HT2 receptors. Psychopharmacology 1993; 112:S40–S54.
54. Wang RY, Liang X. M100907 and clozapine, but not haloperidol or raclopride, prevent phencyclidine-induced blockade of NMDA responses in pyramidal neurons of the rat medial prefrontal cortical slice. Neuropsychopharmacology 1998; 19:74–85.
55. Varty GB, Bakshi VP, Geyer MA. M100907, a serotonin 5HT2A receptor antagonist and putative antipsychotic, blocks dizocilpine-induced prepulse inhibition deficits in Sprague-Dawley and Wistar rats. Neuropsychopharmacology 1999; 20:311–321.
56. Rowley M, Bristow LJ, Hutson PH. Current and novel approaches to the drug treatment of schizophrenia. J Med Chem 2001; 44(4):477–501.
57. Goff D, Midha K, Brotman A, McCormick S, Waites M, Amico E. An open trial of buspirone added to neuroleptics in schizophrenic patients. J Clin Psychopharmacol 1991; 11:193.
58. Evins A, Goff D. Adjunctive antidepressant drug therapies in the treatment of negative symptoms of schizophrenia. CNS Drugs 1996; 6: 130–147.
59. Baldessarini R, Huston-Lyons D, Campbell A, Marsh E, Cohen B. Do central antiadrenergic actions contribute to the atypical properties of clozapine? Brit J Psychiatry 1992; 160 (suppl. 17):12–16.
60. Breier A, Buchanan RW, Waltrip RWn, Listwak S, Holmes C, Goldstein DS. The effect of clozapine on plasma norepinephrine: relationship to clinical efficacy. Neuropsychopharmacology 1994; 1:1–7.
61. Csernansky JG, Mahmoud R, Brenner R. A comparison of risperidone and haloperidol for the prevention of relapse in patients with schizophrenia. N Engl J Med 2002; 346:16–22.
62. Elman I, Goldstein DS, Green AI, Eisenhofer G, Folio CJ, Holmes CS, Pickar D, Breier A. Effects of risperidone on the peripheral noradrenegic system in patients with schizophrenia: a comparison with clozapine and placebo. Neuropsychopharmacology 2002; 27(2):293–300.

63. Litman RE, Su T-P, Potter WZ, Hong WW, Pickar D. Idazozan and response to typical neuroleptics in treatment-resistant schizophrenia. Brit J Psychiatry 1996; 168:571–579.

64. Hertel P, Fagerquist MV, Svensson TH: Enhanced cortical dopamine output and antipsychotic-like effects of raclopride by alpha2 adrenoceptor blockade. Science 1999; 286(5437):105–107.

65. Hertel P, Nomikos GG, Svensson TH. Idazoxan preferentially increases dopamine output in the rat medial prefrontal cortex at the nerve terminal level. Eur J Pharmacol 1999; 371(2–3):153–158.

66. Coull JT. Pharmacological manipulations of the alpha 2-noradrenergic system. Effects on cognition. Drugs Aging 1994; 5(2):116–126.

67. Grenhoff J, Svensson TH. Prazosin modulates the firing pattern of dopamine neurons in rat ventral tegmental area. Eur J Pharmacol 1993; 233:79–84.

68. Goff D, Tsai G, Levitt J, Amico E, Manoach D, Schoenfeld D, Hayden D, McCarley R, Coyle J. A placebo-controlled trial of D-cycloserine added to conventional neuroleptics in patients with schizophrenia. Arch Gen Psychiatry 1999; 56:21–27.

69. Heresco-Levy U, Javitt D, Ermilov M, Mordel C, Silipo G, Lichenstein M. Efficacy of high-dose glycine in the treatment of enduring negative symptoms of schizophrenia. Arch Gen Psychiatry 1999; 56:29–36.

70. Tsai G, Yang P, Chung L-C, Lange N, Coyle J. D-Serine added to antipsychotics for the treatment of schizophrenia. Biol Psychiatry 1998; 44:1081–1089.

71. Javitt DC, Zylberman I, Zukin SR, Heresco LU, Lindenmayer JP. Amelioration of negative symptoms in schizophrenia by glycine. Am J Psychiatry 1994; 151(8):1234–1236.

72. Javitt DC, Balla A, Sershen H, Lajtha A. Reversal of the behavioral and neurochemical effects of phencylidine by glycine and glycine transport inhibitors. Biol Psychiatry 1999; 45:668–679.

73. Evins A, Fitzgerald S, Wine L, Roselli R, Goff D: A placebo controlled trial of glycine added to clozapine in schizophrenia. Am J Psychiatry 2000; 157:826–828.

74. Tsai G, Yang P, Chung L-C, Tsai I-C, Tsai C-W, Coyle J. D-Serine added to clozapine for the treatment of schizophrenia. Am J Psychiatry 1999; 156:1822–1825.

75. Goff DC, Tsai G, Manoach DS, Flood J, Darby DG, Coyle JT. D-cycloserine added to clozapine for patients with schizophrenia. Am J Psychiatry 1996; 153:1628–1630.

76. Goff D, Henderson D, Evins A, Amico E. A placebo-controlled crossover trial of D-cycloserine added to clozapine in patients with schizophrenia. Biol Psychiatry 1999; 45:512–514.

77. Attarian S, Amalric M. Microinfusion of the metabotropic glutamate receptor agonist 1S,3R-1-aminocyclopentane-1,3-dicarboxylic acid into the nucleus accumbens induces dopamine-dependent locomotor activation in the rat. Eur J Neurosci 1997; 9(4):809–816.

78. Ohno M, Watanabe S. Persistent increase in dopamine release following activation of metabotropic glutamate receptors in the rat nucleus accumbens. Neurosci Lett 1995; 200(2):113–116.
79. Petralia RS, Wang YX, Niedzielski AS, Wenthold RJ. The metabotropic glutamate receptors, mGluR2 and mGluR3, show unique postsynaptic, presynaptic and glial localizations. Neuroscience 1996; 71(4):949–976.
80. Moghaddam B, Adams B. Reversal of phencyclidine effects by a group II metabotropic glutamate receptor agonist. Science 1998; 281:1349–1352.
81. Schreiber R, Lowe D, Voerste A, De Vry J. LY354740 affects startle responding but not sensorimotor gating or discriminative effects of phencyclidine. Eur J Pharmacol 2000; 388(2):R3–R4.
82. Staubli U, Perez Y, Xu F, Rogers G, Ingvar M, Stone-Elander S, Lynch G. Centrally active modulators of glutamate receptors facilitate the induction of long-term potentiation in vivo. Proc Natl Acad Sci USA 1994; 91:11158–11162.
83. Granger R, Deadwyler S, Davis M, Moskovitz B, Kessler M, Rogers G, Lynch G. Facilitation of glutamate receptors reverses an age-associated memory impairment in rats. Synapse 1996; 22:332–337.
84. Larson J, Quach CN, LeDuc BQ, Nguyen A, Rogers GA, Lynch G. Effects of an AMPA receptor modulator on methamphetamine-induced hyperactivity in rats. Brain Res 1996; 738:353–356.
85. Johnson S, Luu N, Herbst T, Knapp R, Lutz D, Arai A, Rogers G, Lynch G. Synergistic interactions between ampakines and antipsychotic drugs. J Pharmacol Exp Ther 1999; 289:392–397.
86. Goff D, Leahy L, Berman I, Posever T, Herz L, Leon A, Johnson S. A placebo-controlled pilot study of the ampakine, CX516, added to clozapine in schizophrenia. J Clin Psychopharmacol 2001; 21:484–487.
87. Freedman R, Adler LE, Bickford P, Byerley W, Coon H, Cullum CM, Griffith JM, Harris JG, Leonard S, Miller C, Myles-Worsley M, Nagamoto HT, Rose G, Waldo M. Schizophrenia and nicotinic receptors. Harvard Rev Psychiatry 1994; 2:179–192.
88. Freedman R, Hall M, Adler LE, Leonard S. Evidence in postmortem brain tissue for decreased numbers of hippocampal nicotinic receptors in schizophrenia. Biol Psychiatry 1995; 38:22–33.
89. Leonard S, Gault J, Hopkins J, Logel J, Vianzon R, Short M, Drebing C, Berger R, Venn D, Sirota P, Zerbe G, Olincy A, Ross RG, Adler LE, Freedman R. Association of promoter variants in the alpha7 nicotinic acetylcholine receptor subunit gene with an inhibitory deficit found in schizophrenia. Arch Gen Psychiatry 2002; 59:1085–1096.
90. Simosky JK, Stevens KE, Adler LE, Freedman R. Clozapine improves deficient inhibitory auditory processing in DBA/2 mice, via a nicotinic cholinergic mechanism. Psychopharmacology 2003; 165:386–396.
91. Simosky JK, Stevens KE, Freedman R. Nicotinic agonists and psychosis. Curr Drug Target CNS Neurol Disord 2002; 1:149–162.
92. Horrobin DF. Schizophrenia as a prostaglandin deficiency disease. Lancet 1977; i(8018):936–937.

93. Peet M, Brind J, Ramchand CN, Shah S, Vankar GK. Two double-blind placebo-controlled pilot studies of eicosapentaenoic acid in the treatment of schizophrenia. Schizophr Res 2001; 49(3):243–251.

94. Peet M, Horrobin DF. A dose-ranging exploratory study of the effects of ethyl-eicosapentaenoate in patients with persistent schizophrenic symptoms. J Psychiatr Res 2002; 36(1):7–18.

95. Fenton WS, Dickerson F, Boronow J, Hibbeln JR, Knable M. A placebo-controlled trial of omega-3 fatty acid (ethyl eicosapentaenoic acid) supplementation for residual symptoms and cognitive impairment in schizophrenia. Am J Psychiatry 2001; 158(12):2071–2074.

96. Bleuler E. Dementia Praecox and the Group of Schizophrenias. New York: International Universities Press, 1950.

97. McGlashan TH, Hoffman RE. Schizophrenia as a disorder of developmentally reduced synaptic connectivity. Arch Gen Psychiatry 2000; 57:637–648.

98. Feinberg I. Schizophrenia: caused by a fault in programmed synaptic elimination during adolescence? J Psychiatr Res 1982; 17(4):319–334.

99. Jarskog LF, Gilmore JH, Selinger ES, Lieberman JA. Cortical bcl-2 protein expression and apoptotic regulation in schizophrenia. Biol Psychiatry 2000; 48(7):641–650.

100. Buchsbaum MS, Tang CY, Peled S, Gudbjartsson H, Lu D, Hazlett EA, Downhill J, Haznedar M, Fallon JH, Atlas SW. MRI white matter diffusion anisotropy and PET metabolic rate in schizophrenia. Neuroreport 1998; 9(3):425–430.

101. Hakak Y, Walker JR, Li C, Wong WH, Davis KL, Buxbaum JD, Haroutunian V, Fienberg AA. Genome-wide expression analysis reveals dysregulation of myelination-related genes in chronic schizophrenia. Proc Natl Acad Sci USA 2001; 98:4746–4751.

102. Henderson D, Cagliero E, Gray C, Nasrallah R, Hayden D, Schoenfeld D, Goff D. Clozapine, diabetes mellitus, weight gain, and lipid abnormalities: a five year naturalistic study. Am J Psychiatry 2000; 157:975–981.

Index

About the Editors

John G. Csernansky is the Gregory B. Couch Professor of Psychiatry at the Washington University School of Medicine, St. Louis, Missouri. The author or coauthor of numerous journal articles, book chapters, and books, including *Schizophrenia* (Marcel Dekker, Inc.), he is an associate editor for the *Schizophrenia Bulletin*. A Fellow of the American Psychiatric Association and the American College of Neuropsychopharmacology, he is a member of the Society of Biological Psychiatry and the Society for Neuroscience. The recipient of the Donovan-Shear Award (2000) from the Mental Illness Coalition of St. Louis, Dr. Csernansky received the B.A. degree (1975) from Northwestern University, Evanston, Illinois, and the M.D. degree (1979) from the New York University School of Medicine, New York.

John Lauriello is Associate Professor and Vice Chairman of the Department of Psychiatry; Executive Medical Director of the UNM Psychiatric Center; Psychiatry Chief of Clinical Operations; and Director of the Schizophrenia Research Group, University of New Mexico, Albuquerque. Dr. Lauriello serves as a reviewer for the *Journal of Clinical Psychiatry*, the *American Journal of Psychiatry*, and the *International Journal of Neuropsychopharmacology*, among others, and has written over 30 journal articles and six book chapters. Named an Exemplary Psychiatrist by the National Alliance for the Mentally Ill, Dr. Lauriello completed his psychiatry residency at the New York Hospital–Payne Whitney Clinic, which he followed with fellowships in clinical psychopharmacology at the University of California at San Diego and the Stanford University/Palo Alto VAMC. He received the M.D. degree from Temple University Medical School, Philadelphia, Pennsylvania.

ISBN 0-8247-5412-3

90000